Essential
Neonatal
Medicine

ʻore

Companion website

This book has a companion website at:
www.essentialneonatalmed.com
with:
- Figures from the book in PowerPoint format
- Interactive self-assessment questions and answers
- Further reading list

Essential Neonatal Medicine

Sunil Sinha
Professor of Paediatrics & Neonatal Medicine
University of Durham & James Cook University Hospital
Middlesbrough, UK

Lawrence Miall
Consultant in Neonatal Medicine, Neonatal Intensive Care Unit
Leeds General Infirmary
Leeds, UK

Luke Jardine
Neonatologist, Mater Mothers' Hospital
South Brisbane and Senior Lecturer
University of Queensland
Australia

Fifth edition

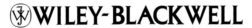

WILEY-BLACKWELL

A John Wiley & Sons, Ltd., Publication

This edition first published 2012 © 2012 by John Wiley & Sons, Ltd

First published 1987
Second edition 1993
Third edition 2000
Fourth edition 2008
Fifth edition 2012

Wiley-Blackwell is an imprint of John Wiley & Sons, formed by the merger of Wiley's global Scientific, Technical and Medical business with Blackwell Publishing.

Registered office: John Wiley & Sons, Ltd, The Atrium, Southern Gate, Chichester, West Sussex, PO19 8SQ, UK
Editorial offices: 9600 Garsington Road, Oxford, OX4 2DQ, UK
　　　　　　　　The Atrium, Southern Gate, Chichester, West Sussex, PO19 8SQ, UK
　　　　　　　　111 River Street, Hoboken, NJ 07030-5774, USA

For details of our global editorial offices, for customer services and for information about how to apply for permission to reuse the copyright material in this book please see our website at www.wiley.com/wiley-blackwell.

Library of Congress Cataloging-in-Publication Data
Sinha, Sunil K., M.D., Ph.D.
　Essential neonatal medicine / Sunil Sinha, Lawrence Miall, Luke Jardine. –
5th ed.
　　　　p. ; cm. – (Essentials)
　Rev. ed. of: Essential neonatal medicine / Malcolm I. Levene, David I.
Tudehope, Sunil K. Sinha. 4th ed. c2008.
　Includes bibliographical references and index.
　ISBN 978-0-470-67040-8 (pbk. : alk. paper)
　I. Miall, Lawrence.　II. Jardine, Luke.　III. Levene, Malcolm I. Essential
neonatal medicine.　IV. Title.　V. Series: Essentials (Wiley-Blackwell)
　[DNLM: 1. Infant, Newborn, Diseases.　2. Neonatology.　WS 421]
　618.92'01–dc23
　　　　　　　　　　　　　　　2011049098

A catalogue record for this book is available from the British Library.

Wiley also publishes its books in a variety of electronic formats. Some content that appears in print may not be available in electronic books.

Cover image © Michael Blackburn/istockphoto 1279386
Cover design by Fortiori Design

Set in 10/12 pt Adobe Garamond Pro by Toppan Best-set Premedia Limited
Printed and bound in Malaysia by Vivar Printing Sdn Bhd

1　2012

Contents

Companion website
This book has a companion website at:
www.essentialneonatalmed.com
with:
- Figures from the book in PowerPoint format
- Interactive self-assessment questions and answers
- Further reading list

Preface to the fifth edition

Modern neonatology is still a relatively new specialty: the first positive pressure ventilation for respiratory distress syndrome was practiced in the 1960s. In the 1970s and 1980s the focus was on survival of increasingly preterm infants and exogenous surfactant therapy began. The first edition of this book was published 25 years ago, at a time of great excitement about the new therapeutic options available. In the 1990s survival began to be the norm and increasingly neonatologists started to consider the evidence for therapies: antenatal steroids became a standard of care and the first concerns were expressed about the effect of post natal steroids on the developing brain.

The fifth edition of this book is published in a new era where survival of even the most preterm infants has come to be expected, and the focus now is on the quality of care and achieving the best long term outcomes with the least invasive therapy. The importance of family-centred developmental care and supporting breastfeeding and attachment are now regarded as equally important standards of care.

This book is also developing and maturing: we have tried to present complex information in a visually appealing format and we now have full colour diagrams and photographs. The authors offer the benefit of their clinical expertise with a series of "clinical tips" throughout the text and there are links to our sister title, *Nursing the Neonate*. Self-assessment questions for each chapter are available online. We have tried to present the latest evidence and therapies and addressed modern controversies and changes in practice. The result is a comprehensive text that provides an international insight into the current practice of neonatal care in a user-friendly format.

We believe this book offers an excellent introduction to state-of-the-art neonatal medicine for trainee doctors, nurses, midwives and allied health professionals. We would also like to pay tribute to two of the original authors of the first edition, Malcolm Levene and David Tudehope who have recently retired and handed over the baton of *Essential Neonatal Medicine* to a new generation of neonatologists.

Sunil Sinha
Lawrence Miall
Luke Jardine

Acknowledgements

We would like to thank Dr Michael Griksaitis for help with revising and updating the chapter on practical procedures, Dr Fiona Wood, Dr Shalabh Garg, Dr Sam Richmond and Dr Jonathan Wyllie for various images, Dr Tracey Glanville for reviewing the obstetric chapter, and Dr Jayne Shillito, Dr Mike Weston and Dr Liz McKechnie for providing clinical images.

This edition of the book would also not have been possible without the efforts of many "behind the scenes" individuals, including – Madeleine Hurd (Associate Editor, Medical Education, Wiley) and Elizabeth Norton (Production Editor, Medical Education, Wiley) and the editors are grateful to them for their patience and guidance.

We would especially like to thank our families for their patience and understanding during the many evenings we spent writing this book.

And finally we are indebted to the babies and their families that it has been our privilege to treat, who have taught us so much over the years.

Preface to the first edition

There has been an explosion of knowledge over the last decade in fetal physiology, antenatal management and neonatal intensive care. This has brought with it confusion concerning novel methods of treatment and procedures as well as the application of new techniques for investigating and monitoring high-risk neonates. The original idea for this book was conceived in Brisbane, and a *Primer of Neonatal Medicine* was produced with Australian conditions in mind. We have now entirely rewritten the book, and it is the result of cooperation between Australian and British neonatologists with, we hope, an international perspective.

We are aware of the need for a short book on neonatal medicine which gives more background discussion and is less dogmatic than other works currently available. We have written this book to give more basic information concerning physiology, development and a perspective to treatment which will be of value equally to neonatal nurses, paediatricians in training, medical students and midwives. Whilst collaborating on a project such as this we are constantly aware of the variety of ways for managing the same condition. This is inevitable in any rapidly growing acute speciality, and we make no apologies for describing alternative methods of treatment where appropriate. Too rigid an approach will be to the detriment of our patients!

A detailed account of all neonatal disorders is not possible but common problems and their management are outlined giving an overall perspective of neonatology. Attention has been given to rare medical and surgical conditions where early diagnosis and treatment may be lifesaving. It is easy to be carried away with the excitement of neonatal intensive care and forget the parents sitting at the cotside. Our approach is to care for the parents as well as their baby, and we have included two chapters on parent–infant attachment as well as death and dying. The final chapter deals with practical procedures and gives an outline of the commonly performed techniques used in the care of the high-risk newborn. We have also provided an up-to-date neonatal Pharmacopoeia as well as useful tables and charts for normal age-related ranges.

Malcolm I. Levene
David I. Tudehope
M. John Thearle

Abbreviations

ABR	auditory brainstem response
ADHD	attention deficit hyperactivity disorder
ALTE	acute life-threatening events
ART	assisted reproductive technology
ASD	atrial septal defect
BE	base excess
BPD	bronchopulmonary dysplasia
CAH	congenital adrenal hyperplasia
CCAM	congenital cystic adenomatous malformation
CDH	congenital diaphragmatic hernia
CFM	cerebral function monitoring
CHARGE	coloboma, heart defects, choanal atresia, retardation, genital and/or urinary abnormalities, ear abnormalities
CHD	congenital heart disease
CLD	chronic lung disease
CPAP	continuous positive airway pressure
CVP	central venous pressure
DDH	developmental dysplasia of the hip
DIC	disseminated intravascular coagulation
EBM	expressed breast milk
ELBW	extremely low birthweight
FASD	fetal alcohol spectrum disorder
FES	fractional excretion of sodium
FHR	fetal heart rate
FRC	functional residual capacity
GFR	glomerular filtration rate
GIFT	gamete intrafallopian transfer
GORD	gastro-oesophageal reflux disease
HCV	hepatitis C virus
HIE	hypoxic–ischaemic encephalopathy
HMF	human milk fortifiers
ICH	intracerebral haemorrhage
IDM	infants of diabetic mothers
IPPV	intermittent positive pressure ventilation
ITP	idiopathic thrombocytopenic purpura
IUGR	intrauterine growth restriction
IVF	*in vitro* fertilization
IVH	intraventricular haemorrhage
LBW	low birthweight
LMP	last menstrual period
LVH	left ventricular hypertrophy
MAS	meconium aspiration syndrome
NAS	neonatal abstinence syndrome
NCPAP	nasal continuous positive airway pressure
NICU	neonatal intensive care unit
NIPPV	non-invasive positive pressure ventilation
NTD	neural tube defects
PCV	pneumococcal conjugate vaccine
PDA	patent ductus arteriosus
PEEP	positive end-expiratory pressure
PET	pre-eclampsia
PICC	peripherally inserted central catheter
PIE	pulmonary interstitial emphysema
PIP	peak inspiratory pressure
PMR	perinatal mortality rate
PPHN	persistent pulmonary hypertension of the newborn
PROM	premature rupture of membranes
RDS	respiratory distress syndrome
ROP	retinopathy of prematurity
RVH	right ventricular hypertrophy
SGA	small for gestational age
SIDS	sudden infant death syndrome
SLE	systemic lupus erythematosus
TAR	thrombocytopenia with absent radii
TGA	transposition of the great arteries
ToF	tetralogy of Fallot
TORCH	toxoplasmosis, other infections, rubella, cytomegalovirus, herpes simplex virus
TPN	total parenteral nutrition
TSH	thyroid-stimulating hormone
TTN	tachypnoea of the newborn
TTTS	twin-to-twin transfusion syndrome
UAC	umbilical arterial catheter
UVC	umbilical venous catheter
VACTERL	vertebral anomalies, anal atresia, cardiovascular anomalies,

	tracheoesophageal fistula,	VILI	ventilator-induced lung injury
	oesophageal atresia, renal and/or	VLBW	very low birthweight
	radial anomalies, limb defects	VSD	ventricular septal defect
VAPS	volume-assured pressure support	VUR	vesico-ureteric reflux
VCV	volume-controlled ventilation	WHO	World Health Organization

How to get the best out of your textbook

Welcome to the new edition of *Essential Neonatal Medicine*. Over the next few pages you will be shown how to make the most of the learning features included in the textbook.

The Anytime, Anywhere Textbook ▶

For the first time, your textbook comes with free access to a **Wiley Desktop Edition** – a digital, interactive version of this textbook which you own as soon as you download it.

Your Wiley Desktop Edition allows you to:
Search: Save time by finding terms and topics instantly in your book, your notes, even your whole library (once you've downloaded more textbooks)
Note and Highlight: Colour code, highlight and make digital notes right in the text so you can find them quickly and easily
Organize: Keep books, notes and class materials organized in folders inside the application
Share: Exchange notes and highlights with friends, classmates and study groups
Upgrade: Your textbook can be transferred when you need to change or upgrade computers
Link: Link directly from the page of your interactive textbook to all of the material contained on the companion website

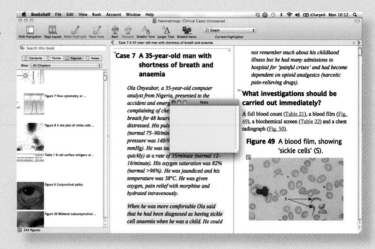

Wiley DESKTOP EDITION

To access your Wiley Desktop Edition:

- Find the redemption code on the inside front cover of this book and carefully scratch away the top coating of the label.
- Visit **www.vitalsource.com/software/bookshelf/downloads** to download the Bookshelf application.
- If you have purchased this title as an e-book, access to your Wiley Desktop Edition is available with proof of purchase within 90 days. Visit **http://support.wiley.com** to request a redemption code via the 'Live Chat' or 'Ask A Question' tabs.
- Open the Bookshelf application on your computer and register for an account.
- Follow the registration process and enter your redemption code to download your digital book.
- For full access instructions, visit:
  www.essentialneonatalmed.com.

CourseSmart gives you instant access (via computer or mobile device) to this Wiley-Blackwell eTextbook and its extra electronic functionality, at 40% off the recommended retail print price. See all the benefits at **www.coursesmart.com/students**.

Instructors . . . receive your own digital desk copies! ▶
It also offers instructors an immediate, efficient, and environmentally-friendly way to review this textbook for your course.

For more information visit **www.coursesmart.com/instructors**.
With CourseSmart, you can create lecture notes quickly with copy and paste, and share pages and notes with your students. Access your Wiley CourseSmart digital textbook from your computer or mobile device instantly for evaluation, class preparation, and as a teaching tool in the classroom.

Simply sign in at **http://instructors. coursesmart.com/bookshelf** to download your Bookshelf and get started. To request your desk copy, hit 'Request Online Copy' on your search results or book product page.

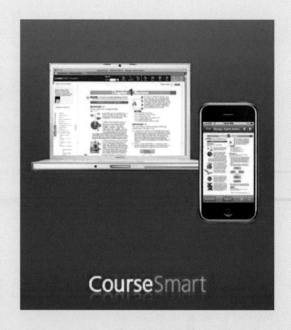

A companion website

Your textbook is also accompanied by a FREE companion website that contains:
- Figures from the book in PowerPoint format
- Interactive self-assessment questions and answers
- Further reading list

Log on to www.essentialneonatalmed.com to find out more.

Features contained within your textbook

Every chapter begins with a list of key topics contained within the chapter and an introduction to the topic.

Clinical tips give further insight into topics. ▼

CLINICAL TIP: It is important to remember that screening tests give a *risk* for Down's syndrome (higher or lower than the age-related risk) but they do not give a definitive diagnosis. Some parents find it very difficult to understand that even if the risk is only 1 in 100, they may still be the couple that go on to have an affected child. Parents need to be counselled carefully before undertaking screening.

Link to *Nursing the Neonate*: Obstetric issues relating to neonatal care. Chapter 2, pp.14–19.

◄ There are also helpful cross-references to the Wiley title *Nursing the Neonate*.

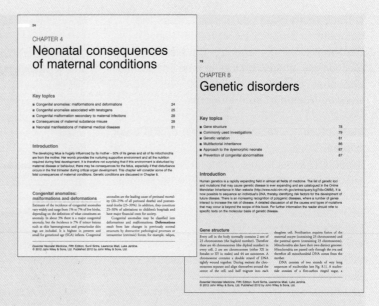

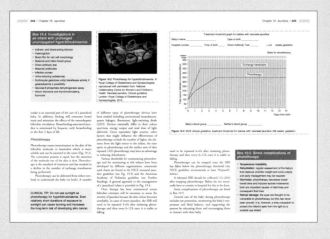

▶ Your textbook is full of useful photographs, illustrations and tables. The Desktop Edition version of your textbook will allow you to copy and paste any photograph or illustration into assignments, presentations and your own notes.

Every chapter ends with a summary which ▶ can be used for both study and revision purposes, as well as MCQs to test your learning and understanding.

There have been huge advances in the understanding of fetal development and conditions such as severe anaemia and pleural effusion are now amenable to treatment *in utero*. Screening for congenital abnormality has become more reliable.

Ultrasound monitoring of fetal well-being, including Doppler measurements, allows intervention but the risk of continued fetal compromise must be balanced against those of preterm delivery. Good communication between the perinatal team is essential.

SUMMARY

We hope you enjoy using your new textbook. Good luck with your studies!

CHAPTER 1
Fetal well-being and adaptation at birth

Key topics

Introduction

The discipline of 'perinatal medicine' spans the specialties of fetal medicine and neonatology. The obstetrician must have a thorough knowledge of pregnancy and its effects on the mother and fetus, as well as fetal development and physiology. The neonatologist specializes in the medical care of the infant immediately after birth but must also have a thorough understanding of fetal development and physiology. This chapter reviews fetal assessment and physiology to provide the paediatrician and neonatal nurse with a better understanding of normal perinatal adaptation and the adverse consequences arising from maladaptation.

Placental function

The placenta is a fetal organ that has three major functions: transport, immunity and metabolism.

The uterus is supplied with blood from the uterine arteries, which dilate throughout pregnancy, increasing blood supply 10-fold by term. Maternal blood bathes the intervillous space and is separated from fetal blood by the chorionic plate. Transport of nutrients and toxins occurs at this level. Oxygenated fetal blood in the capillaries of the chorionic plate leaves the placenta via the umbilical vein to the fetus (Fig. 1.1).

Essential Neonatal Medicine, Fifth Edition. Sunil Sinha, Lawrence Miall, Luke Jardine.
© 2012 John Wiley & Sons, Ltd. Published 2012 by John Wiley & Sons, Ltd.

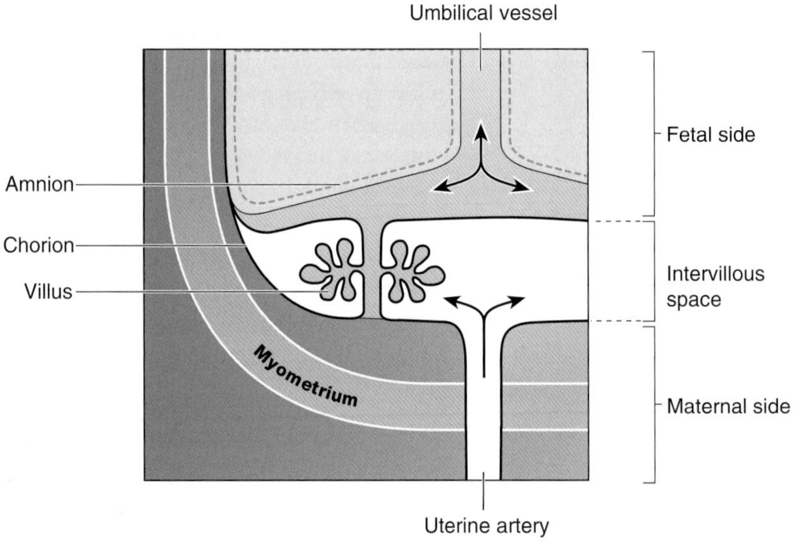

Figure 1.1 Diagram of placental structures showing blood perfusion.

Transport

The placenta transports nutrients from the mother to the fetus, and waste products in the other direction. This occurs in a number of ways, including simple diffusion (for small molecules) and active transport, which is used for larger molecules. The placenta is crucially also responsible for gaseous exchange of oxygen and carbon dioxide. Oxygen diffuses from the mother (PO_2 = 10–14 kPa, 75–105 mmHg) to the fetus (PO_2 = 2–4 kPa, 15–30 mmHg) where it binds to fetal haemoglobin. This has a higher affinity for oxygen than maternal haemoglobin for a given PO_2. This off-loading of maternal haemoglobin is also facilitated by a change in maternal blood pH.

Immunity

The placenta trophoblast prevents the maternal immune system from reacting against 'foreign' fetal antigens. Rejection does not occur because the trophoblastic cells appear to be non-antigenic, although it is known that fetal cells can cross into the maternal circulation where they can trigger an immune reaction (e.g. rhesus haemolytic disease). Maternal IgG antibody, the smallest of the immunoglobulins, can cross the placenta where it provides the newborn with innate immunity to infectious diseases. These IgG antibodies can also cause perinatal disease such as transient hyperthyroidism (see Chapter 21).

> CLINICAL TIP: Because IgG antibody crosses the placenta, the presence of IgG antibody in the newborn's blood does not mean it has been exposed to the disease. This is of particular relevance when testing newborns for HIV infection or syphilis, where a positive IgG may just reflect maternal exposure. Instead, direct tests (e.g. viral RNA by PCR) are required (see Chapter 10).

Metabolism

The placenta is metabolically active and produces hormones, including human chorionic gonadotropin (hCG) and human chorionic thyrotropin (hCT). It also detoxifies drugs and metabolites. Oestriol cannot be produced by the placenta alone. This is done by the fetal liver and adrenal glands. The metabolites are then sulphated by the placenta to form oestrogens, one of which is oestriol.

Because of its metabolic activity, the placenta has very high energy demands and consumes over 50% of the total oxygen and glucose transported across it.

Fetal homeostasis

The placenta is an essential organ for maintaining fetal homeostasis but the fetus is capable of performing a variety of physiological functions:

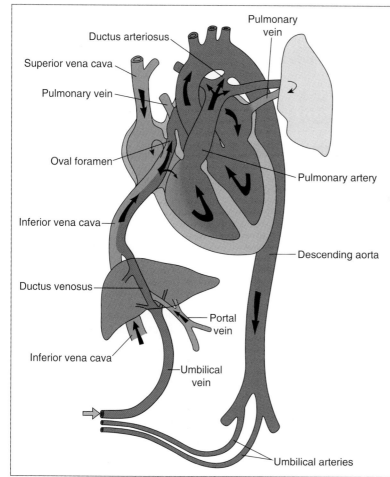

Figure 1.2 Diagram of the fetal circulation through the heart and lungs, showing the direction of flow through the foramen ovale and ductus arteriosus (DA).

- The liver produces albumin, coagulation factors and red blood cells.
- The kidney excretes large volumes of dilute urine from 10–11 weeks' gestation, which contributes to amniotic fluid.
- Fetal endocrine organs produce thyroid hormones, corticosteroids, mineralocorticoids, parathormone and insulin from 12 weeks' gestation.
- Some immunoglobulins are produced by the fetus from the end of the first trimester.

Fetal circulation

The fetal circulation is quite different from the newborn or adult circulation. The umbilical arteries are branches of the internal iliac arteries. These carry deoxygenated blood from the fetus to the placenta where it is oxygenated as it comes into close apposition with maternal blood in the intervillous spaces. Oxygenated fetal blood is carried in the single umbilical vein which bypasses the liver via the ductus venosus to reach the inferior vena cava. It then passes into the inferior vena cava and enters the right atrium as a 'jet', which is shunted to the left atrium across the foramen ovale (Fig. 1.2). From here it passes into the left ventricle and is pumped to the coronary arteries and cerebral vessels. In this way the fetal brain receives the most oxygenated blood. Some deoxygenated blood is pumped by the right ventricle into the pulmonary artery, but the majority bypasses the lungs via the ductus arteriosus to flow into the aorta where it is carried back to the placenta. Only 7% of the combined ventricular output of blood passes into the lungs. The right ventricle is the dominant ventricle, ejecting 66% of the combined ventricular output.

In summary, there are three shunts:

1 The **ductus venosus** bypasses blood away from the liver to the IVC.

2 The **foramen ovale** shunts blood from the right atrium to the left atrium.

3 The **ductus arteriosus** shunts blood from the pulmonary artery to the aorta.

The last two shunts only occur because of the very high fetal pulmonary vascular resistance and the high pulmonary artery pressure that is characteristic of fetal circulation.

Umbilical vessels

There are two umbilical arteries and one umbilical vein, surrounded by protective 'Wharton's jelly'. In 1% of babies there is only one umbilical artery, and this may be associated with growth retardation and congenital malformations, especially of the renal tract. Chromosomal anomalies are also slightly more common.

Assessment of fetal well-being

Assessment of fetal well-being is an integral part of antenatal care. It includes diagnosis of fetal abnormality, assessment of the fetoplacental unit and fetal maturity, monitoring of growth and well-being monitoring in the third trimester and during labour (Fig. 1.3).

Assessment of maturity

Clinical assessment

Assessment of gestational age depends on the date of the last menstrual period (LMP) and clinical measurement of fundal height: fundal height (cm) = gestational age (weeks). This is most accurate in early pregnancy. Fetal 'quickening' can help in dating the duration of pregnancy: in primiparas movements are first felt at about 20–21 weeks, and in multiparas at 18 weeks.

Ultrasound

Early measurement of fetal size is the most reliable way to estimate gestation and is considered to be even more reliable than calculation from the date of the LMP. Ultrasound measurements that correlate well with gestational age include crown–rump length (until 14 weeks), biparietal diameter (BPD) and femur length. The BPD measurement at 14–18 weeks appears to be the best method for assessing the duration of pregnancy.

Assessment of fetal growth and well-being

Clinical assessment

Monitoring fundal height is a time-honoured method of assessing fetal growth. Unfortunately, up to 50% of growth-restricted infants are not detected clinically.

Ultrasound

Serial estimates of BPD, head circumference, abdominal circumference and femur length are widely used to monitor growth, often on customized fetal growth charts. In fetuses suffering IUGR, head growth is usually the last to slow down. Estimating fetal weight by ultrasound has become very accurate and provides critical information for perinatal decision-making about the timing of delivery.

Link to *Nursing the Neonate*: Obstetric issues relating to neonatal care. Chapter 2, pp.14–19.

Ultrasound imaging and Doppler blood flow

The location of the placenta can be confidently established by ultrasound. Doppler flow velocity waveforms of the umbilical artery are now used as a major determinant of fetal well-being. In IUGR fetuses, abnormal Doppler waveforms are a reliable prognostic feature. As fetal blood flow become compromised there is reduced, then absent or reversed flow during diastole. Reversed diastolic flow is an ominous sign and is associated with a high risk of imminent fetal demise (see Fig. 1.4). If end-diastolic flow (EDF) is absent, detailed Doppler studies of the middle cerebral artery (MCA) and ductus venosus are indicated. Evidence of cerebral

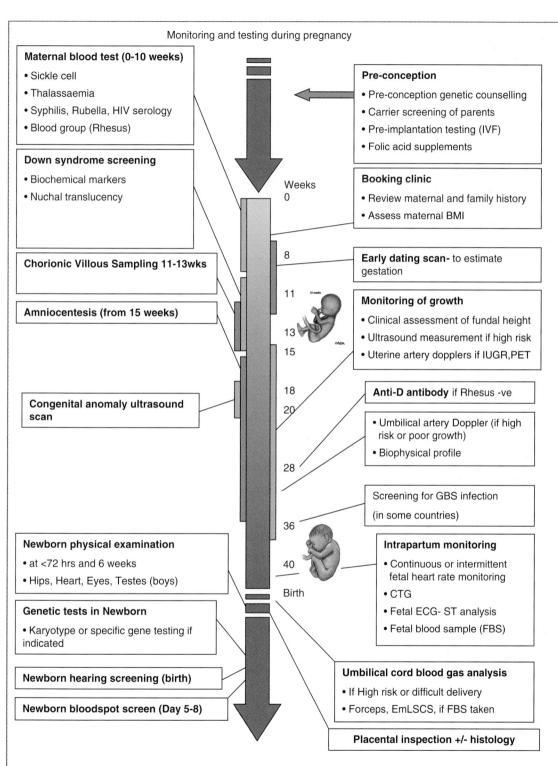

Figure 1.3 A timeline for fetal assessment and monitoring during pregnancy.

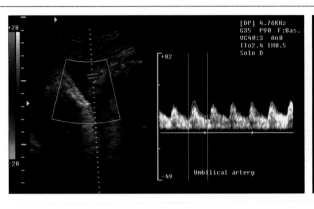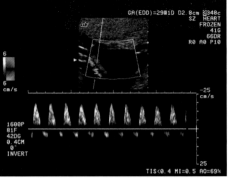

Figure 1.4 Doppler measurement of blood flow in the fetal umbilical artery. Left hand panel shows normal forward flow throughout the cardiac cycle. Right hand panel shows pathological reversed flow during diastole.

redistribution should trigger intensive regular monitoring. Timing of delivery will be based on Dopplers, gestation and estimated fetal weight. Recently, Doppler measurement of peak systolic blood flow velocity in the MCA has become a part of the assessment of fetal anaemia and isoimmunization. As anaemia becomes severe the velocity increases (see Chapter 20).

Amniotic fluid volume

Amniotic fluid is easily seen on ultrasound and the maximum pool size in four quadrants is measured (amniotic fluid index). This is often combined with non-stress testing (NST), counting movement and breathing. Both excess (polyhydramnios) and reduced (oligohydramnios) amniotic fluid volumes can be associated with adverse fetal outcome. See Table 1.1.

Fetal breathing movements

The breathing movements of the fetus show marked variability. The fetus breathes from about 11 weeks' gestation, but this is irregular until 20 weeks. Fetal breathing promotes a tracheal flux of fetal lung fluid into the amniotic fluid. An absence of amniotic fluid (oligohydramnios) can lead to pulmonary hypoplasia. Abnormal gasping respiration, extreme irregularity of breathing in a term fetus and complete cessation of breathing are visible by ultrasound.

Table 1.1 Fetal problems associated with abnormal amniotic fluid volumes

Polyhydramnios	Oligohydramnios
Maternal diabetes	Preterm rupture of membranes (PPROM)
Twin-to-twin transfusion syndrome (recipient)	Twin-to-twin transfusion (donor)
Obstruction to swallowing	Severe fetal growth restriction (IUGR)
Oesophageal atresia	Renal anomalies
Duodenal atresia	Renal agenesis (Potter's syndrome)
Abnormal swallowing	ARPCKD
Abnormal swallowing	Posterior urethral valves (in males)
Congenital myotonic dystrophy	Chromosomal anomalies
Trisomy 18	Increased risk of pulmonary hypoplasia
Increased risk of preterm labour and PPROM	If severe, risk of fetal deformation

Fetal heart rate monitoring, non-stress test and biophysical profile

The response of the fetal heart to naturally occurring Braxton Hicks contractions or fetal movements provides information on fetal health during the third trimester. A normal fetal heart trace is reactive (≥2 accelerations) in response to fetal movements. If it is not reactive, further assessment with ultrasound is indicated.

In late pregnancy the biophysical profile combines the NST and ultrasound assessment of fetal movements. A score (2) is given for each of heart rate accelerations, fetal breathing movements, fetal limb movements, movement of the trunk and adequate amniotic fluid depth. A normal well fetus will score 10/10 and a score of less than 8 is abnormal.

Screening during pregnancy

Maternal blood screening

Screening programmes vary from country to country. In the UK all pregnant women are routinely screened for syphilis, hepatitis B, immunity to rubella and haemoglobinopathies (sickle cell disease, thalassaemia), and HIV screening is strongly encouraged.

Fetal imaging

Ultrasound examination of the fetus for congenital abnormalities is now offered as a routine procedure. Major malformations of the central nervous system, bowel, heart, genitourinary system and limbs should be detected. Some disorders, such as twin-to-twin transfusion, pleural effusion and posterior urethral valves are amenable to fetal 'surgery'. Advanced '4D' (3D seen in real time) ultrasonography allows visualization of the external features of the fetus, such as the presence of cleft lip (see Fig. 1.5).

Fetal MRI is now feasible and appears safe in pregnancy. The large field of view, excellent soft tissue contrast and multiple planes of construction make MRI an appealing imaging modality to overcome the problems with ultrasound in cases such as maternal obesity and oligohydramnios, but MRI cannot be used for routine screening. It is useful in

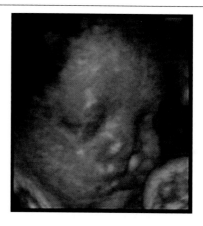

Figure 1.5 Cleft lip. Courtesy of Dr Jason Ong.

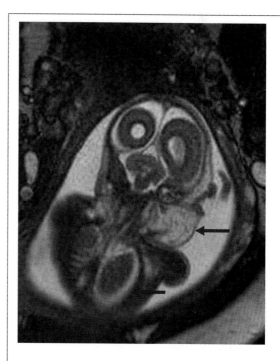

Figure 1.6 Fetal MRI scan (coronal view) showing large cystic hygroma on the left side of the neck (arrow) and an associated pleural effusion (arrow). Courtesy of Dr Mike Weston.

the assessment of complex anomalies such as urogenital and spinal anomalies, complex brain malformation and congenital diaphragmatic hernia as well as for some fetal cardiac disorders (Fig 1.6).

Link to *Nursing the Neonate*:
Obstetric issues relating to neonatal
care. Chapter 2, pp. 14–19.

Down's syndrome screening

Trisomy 21 affects 1 in 600 fetuses and 1 in 1000
live births. Incidence rises with maternal age (1 in
880 at 30 years to 1 in 100 at 40 years) but as more
younger women are pregnant, in the UK screening
is offered to all pregnant women regardless of age.
The screening tests vary and are summarized in
Table 1.2. If the risks after screening are high then
a diagnostic test (amniocentesis or chorionic villus
sampling, CVS) is offered.

CLINICAL TIP: It is important to remember
that screening tests give a *risk* for Down's
syndrome (higher or lower than the age-
related risk) but they do not give a definitive
diagnosis. Some parents find it very difficult
to understand that even if the risk is only 1
in 100, they may still be the couple that go
on to have an affected child. Parents need
to be counselled carefully before
undertaking screening.

Amniocentesis

Amniocentesis is valuable for the diagnosis of a
variety of fetal abnormalities. Trisomy 13, 18 and
21 can be detected by PCR within 48 h and the
cells cultured for chromosome analysis (14 days)
or to study enzyme activity. Ultrasound-guided
amniocentesis is undertaken by passing a needle
through the anterior abdominal wall into the
uterine cavity. The risk of miscarriage is less than
1%. Larger volumes of amniotic fluid may be
removed (amnioreduction) as a treatment for polyhydramnios, although this treatment normally
needs to be repeated weekly.

Chorionic villus sampling

CVS involves the transcervical or transabdominal
passage of a needle into the chorionic surface of the

Table 1.2 Screening tests for Down's syndrome in UK

Screening test	Timing (weeks of gestation)	Comments
Nuchal fold thickness	11–13	Measures translucency at nape of neck, which is increased in trisomy 18 and some cardiac defects. Gives age-related risk
Triple test AFP hCG Oestriol	10–14	Gives age-related risk. AFP very high with neural tube defects
Combined test Nuchal fold hCG h-PAPP	11–13	Biochemical screening with nuchal fold measurement to give age-related risk
Quadruple test hCG AFP Oestriol Inhibin A	15–20	Suitable for late booking when nuchal fold measurement no longer reliable. Gives age-related risk

AFP, alpha-fetoprotein; hCG, human chorionic gonadotropin; PAPP, pregnancy-associated plasma protein A.

placenta after 11 weeks' gestation to withdraw a
small sample of tissue. Because of the 1% risk of
miscarriage, the test is reserved for detection of
genetic or chromosomal abnormalities in at-risk
pregnancies, rather than as a mere screening test.
Preliminary chromosomal results can be obtained
within 24–48 hours by fluorescent *in situ* hybridiza-

tion (FISH) or PCR. Direct analysis requires cell culture (14 days)

Fetal blood sampling (cordocentesis)

Fetal blood sampling is an ultrasound-guided technique for sampling blood from the umbilical cord to assist in the diagnosis of chromosome abnormality, intrauterine infection, coagulation disturbance, haemolytic disease or severe anaemia. It can also be used for treatment, with *in utero* transfusion of packed red blood cells during the same procedure. There is a 1% risk of fetal death.

Fetal monitoring during labour

Intrapartum monitoring

In low-risk pregnancies intermittent auscultation of the fetal heart rate (FHR) is all that is required. Continuous electronic monitoring of the FHR can be performed non-invasively with a cardiotocograph (CTG) strapped to the abdominal wall, or invasively with a fetal scalp electrode.

The CTG trace allows observation of four features:
- Baseline heart rate
- Beat to beat variability
- Decelerations:
  - *Early:* slowing of the FHR early in the contraction with return to baseline by the end of the contraction
  - *Late:* repetitive, periodic slowing of FHR with onset at middle to end of the contraction
  - *Variable:* *v*ariable, intermittent slowing of FHR with rapid onset and recovery
  - *Prolonged:* abrupt fall in FHR to below baseline lasting at least 60–90 s; pathological if last >3 min
- *Accelerations:* transient increases in FHR >15 bpm lasting 15 s or more. These are normal and are reassuring. The significance of absent accelerations as a single feature is not known.

The interpretation of the CTG must then be classified as normal, suspicious or pathological (Box 1.1; see also Table 1.3 and Fig. 1.7).

Box 1.1 Interpretations of the cardiotocograph

- *Normal:* all four features fall into a reassuring category.
- *Suspicious:* one non-reassuring feature, but all three others are reassuring. Assess for uterine hypercontractility, infection and hypotension and optimize treatment. Consider fetal scalp electrode.
- *Pathological:* two or more non-reassuring features. Put mother in the left lateral position and check fetal blood sample or expedite delivery.

Although FHR monitoring has been in widespread use of for over 30 years it has not been shown to reduce morbidity in term infants. It has, however, increased the rate of instrumental and caesarean section delivery. There is no evidence that routine FHR monitoring in the low-risk fetus improves outcome. Intermittent auscultation seems to be acceptable in these cases.

Fetal scalp pH

Used in conjunction with CTG monitoring. In the presence of abnormal FHR, fetal scalp pH measurement may be helpful. Clinical decisions are made on the severity of the blood acidosis (Table 1.4).

Fetal electrocardiogram

Direct measurement of fetal ECG via a fetal scalp electrode, in conjunction with a CTG allows S-T waveform analysis (STAN). This has been shown to reduce fetal blood sampling and operative delivery and improve fetal condition at birth compared with CTG alone.

Fetal compromise

'Fetal distress' is a commonly used but emotive clinical term which usually refers to a stressed fetus showing signs of compromise due to lack of oxygen. 'Fetal compromise' may be used to describe

Table 1.3 Features of a CTG

Parameter	'Reassuring'	'Non-reassuring'	'Abnormal'
Baseline heart rate	110–160 bpm	100–109 or 161–180 bpm	<100 or >180 bpm Sinusoidal for >10 min
Beat to beat variability	>5 bpm variation	<5 bpm variation for 40–90 min	<5 bpm for >90 min
Decelerations	No decelerations	Typical variable decelerations >50% of contractions over 90 min Single prolonged deceleration <3 min	Atypical variable decelerations >50% of contractions over 30 min Late decelerations over 30 min Single prolonged deceleration >3 min
Accelerations	Present	Not present	Not present

Table 1.4 Clinical decisions based on blood acidosis

pH	Action
≥7.25	No action, continue to monitor fetus electronically
7.21–7.24	Repeat pH within 30 min
≤7.20	Deliver urgently

Table 1.5 Causes of fetal compromise

Maternal	Hypotension Hypertension, including pre-eclampsia Diabetes mellitus Cardiovascular disease Anaemia Malnutrition Dehydration
Uterine	Hypercontractability, usually due to excessive use of oxytocin (Syntocinon)
Placental	Abnormal placentation Abruption Vascular degeneration
Umbilical	Cord prolapse True knot in cord Strangulation; either in monoamniotic twin pregnancy or if cord tightly around the neck (normally cord around the neck does not cause harm)

the 'at-risk' fetus, e.g. evidence of severe IUGR or abnormal Doppler flow. Factors causing fetal compromise are listed in Table 1.5.

Fetal compromise may lead to
• reduction in fetal movements
• passage of thick meconium into the amniotic fluid (this can be normal at term)
• FHR abnormality on CTG or fetal scalp electrode as described above
• metabolic acidosis (pH <7.20) on fetal scalp sample or arterial umbilical cord blood gas sample.

Physiological changes at birth

At birth the baby changes from being in a fluid environment, with oxygen provided via the umbilical vein, to an air environment, with oxygenation dependent on breathing. This remarkable adaptation requires considerable changes to the respiratory and cardiovascular systems within the first minutes after delivery. Other adaptations required include

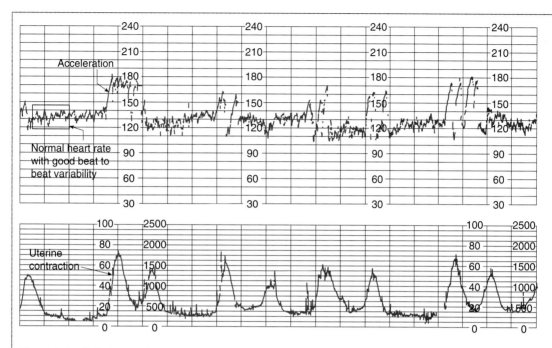

Figure 1.7a CTG showing fetal heart rate accelerations.

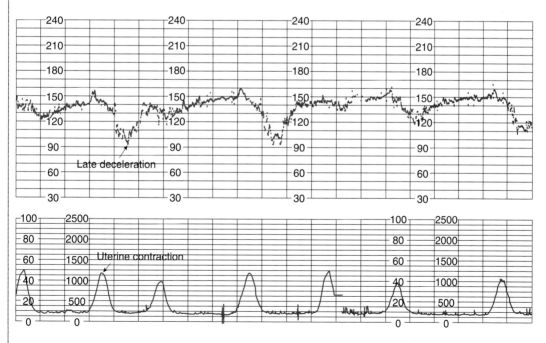

Figure 1.7b CTG showing late decelerations.

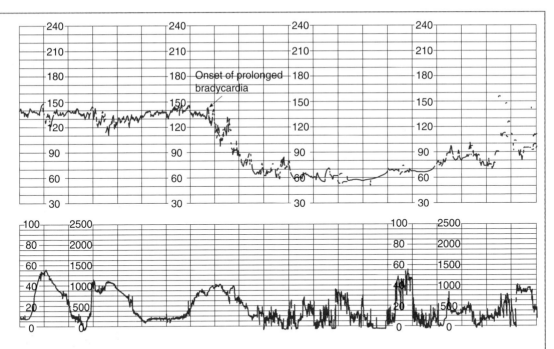

Figure 1.7c CTG showing normal heart rate followed by severe prolonged fetal bradycardia.

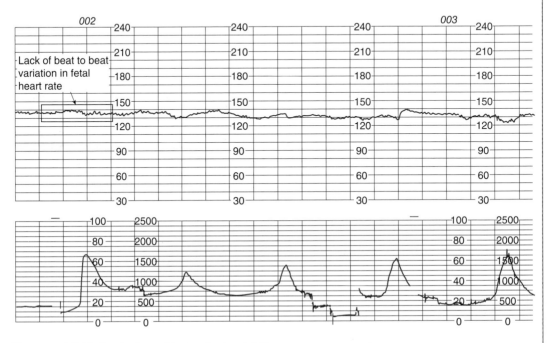

Figure 1.7d CTG showing loss of beat to beat variability.

maintenance of glucose homeostasis (see Chapter 21) and thermoregulation (see Chapter 24).

While the fetus is *in utero* the lungs are filled with lung fluid, which is produced at up to 5 mL/ kg per hour in response to secretion of chloride ions in pulmonary epithelium. During labour rising adrenaline levels 'switch off' lung fluid secretion and reabsorption begins. At birth the baby generates enormous negative pressures (−60 cmH$_2$O) which fill the lungs with air. With the first two or three breaths much of the fetal lung fluid is expelled. The remainder is absorbed into pulmonary lymphatics and capillaries over the first 6–12 h. Sometimes these clearance mechanisms fail and the lungs remain 'wet'. This is known as transient tachypnoea of the newborn (see Chapter 13). The stimulus for the first breath is a combination of cold, physical touch, rising carbon dioxide levels and cessation of placental adenosine. It is also in part a reflex reaction to the emptying of the lungs of fluid (Hering–Breuer deflation reflex).

With the first few breaths the arterial oxygen tension (P_aO_2) increases from 2–3.5 kPa (15–25 mmHg) to 9–13 kPa (68–98 mmHg). This rise in oxygen tension results in constriction of the ductus arteriosus: this is functionally closed by 10–15 h, but not anatomically closed until 4–7 days. There is also marked fall in pulmonary vascular resistance, so that pulmonary blood flow increases, right ventricular pressure falls, and blood stops shunting from the right to left atrium across the foramen ovale.

The foramen ovale takes some time to close, and in 10% it remains patent through life. With cord occlusion there is a marked decrease in blood flow in the IVC, and the ductus venosus closes.

Many factors may interfere with these physiological changes at birth. If there is severe birth asphyxia or respiratory distress then blood may continue to be shunted through fetal channels, leading to persistent pulmonary hypertension of the newborn (PPHN) (see Chapter 16).

> **CLINICAL TIP:** If a fetus is born to a mother who has not been through labour, then the molecular lung fluid reabsorption mechanisms are not fully activated and the baby may remain breathless for several hours after birth (TTN). This is more common after elective caesarean section.

SUMMARY

There have been huge advances in the understanding of fetal development and conditions such as severe anaemia and pleural effusion are now amenable to treatment *in utero*. Screening for congenital abnormality has become more reliable.

Ultrasound monitoring of fetal well-being, including Doppler measurements, allows intervention but the risk of continued fetal compromise must be balanced against those of preterm delivery. Good communication between the perinatal team is essential.

 Now visit **www.essentialneonatalmed.com** to test yourself on this chapter.

CHAPTER 2
Perinatal epidemiology and audit

Key topics

Introduction

Conception, embryonic and fetal development, parturition and subsequent neonatal growth and development form a continuum. Obstetricians and neonatologists have, however, arbitrarily divided this into rigid categories, which are used to audit standards of care during the perinatal and subsequent periods. Unfortunately, international agreement regarding some of the terminology is lacking, and definitions within this developmental continuum given here are those used in the UK and Australia.

Definitions of terms commonly used in perinatal medicine

- *Gestational age*: this is calculated from the first day of the last normal menstrual period to the date of birth, and is expressed in completed weeks.
- *Term delivery* occurs when the infant is born at or after 37 and before 42 weeks' gestation.
- *Preterm delivery* occurs if the infant is born less than 37 weeks' gestation. In the UK and Australia, 6–9% of infants are born preterm.
- *Post-term delivery* occurs if the infant is born at or after 42 completed weeks of gestation. Approximately 1% of infants are born post-term.
- A *live birth* is one in which there are signs of life (breathing, heartbeat or spontaneous movement) after complete expulsion from the mother, irrespective of the gestational age or birthweight.
- A *stillbirth*, or fetal death, is defined as an infant expelled from the birth canal at or after 24 weeks

Essential Neonatal Medicine, Fifth Edition. Sunil Sinha, Lawrence Miall, Luke Jardine.

of pregnancy who shows no signs of life and has no heartbeat. In Australia, stillbirth is defined as an infant born at or after 20 weeks' gestation and/or weighing 400 g with no signs of life. As the definition varies from country to country, comparison of figures may be misleading.

The stillbirth rate is expressed as the number of infants born dead at or after 24 weeks per 1000 live births and stillbirths.

• *Low birthweight* (LBW) refers to any infant who weighs less than 2500 g at birth (WHO). In the UK and Australia, approximately 6% of live births are LBW. These infants are either born too early (preterm), or have grown inadequately in the uterus and are classed as 'small for gestational age'. Some low birthweight infants may be both preterm and small for gestational age.

• *Very low birthweight* (VLBW) infants are those who weigh less than 1500 g at birth. Approximately 1–1.5% of liveborn infants are VLBW.

• *Extremely low birthweight* (ELBW) infants are those who weigh less than 1000 g at birth. This category accounts for approximately 0.7% of all births.

• *Small for gestational age* (SGA). This term is generally synonymous with the fetus who has suffered intrauterine growth restriction (IUGR). Diagnosis depends on accurate assessment of gestational age (see p. 4) and plotting of weight on an appropriate growth chart. There is no international consensus on the definition of SGA, which varies from less than the 10th, 5th or 3rd percentiles or more than two standard deviations below the mean birthweight. Accordingly, incidence figures will vary. In the UK, SGA is defined as a baby weighing below the 10th centile for gestational age. Asymmetrical SGA refers to a baby whose weight is below the 10th centile, but whose head is above the 10th centile. This usually indicates late-onset IUGR (p. 139).

• *Perinatal mortality rate* (PMR):

$$PMR = \frac{\text{Number of still births and neonatal deaths}}{\text{Number of stillbirths and live births}} \times 1000$$

Different definitions are used depending upon location (see Table 2.1).

• *Neonatal death* is death occurring within 28 days of birth in an infant whose birthweight was at least 500 g or, if the weight was not known, an infant born after at least 22 weeks' gestation.

• *Neonatal death rate in the* UK and Australia refers to the number of deaths within 28 days of birth of any child who had evidence of life after birth. Birthweight and/or gestational age criteria apply as for PMR.

Table 2.1 Classification of perinatal deaths according to institution

Institution	Perinatal deaths		
	Fetal deaths		**Neonatal deaths**
	Birthweight (g)	**Gestational age (weeks)**	
WHO	1000	28 (only if birth weight unavailable)	<7 days
Australian National reporting	500	22 (only if birth weight is unavailable)	<7 days
Australian States	400	20 (only if birth weight is unavailable)	<28 days
NHDD and NPSU	400	20	<28 days

NHDD, National Health Data Dictionary (Australia); NPSU, National Perinatal Statistics Unit (Australia); WHO, World Health Organization.

• *Postneonatal death rate* (or late infant deaths) refers to the number of deaths of liveborn infants dying after 28 days but before 1 year of age per 1000 live births.

• *Infant death* is death occurring within 1 year of birth in a liveborn infant whose birthweight was at least 500 g, or at least 22 weeks' gestation if the birthweight was not known. This category includes neonatal deaths as defined above.

The role of perinatal and neonatal audit

By collecting epidemiological data and monitoring clinical indicators, it is hoped to improve care and clinical practice. Audit may identify variations in morbidity or mortality which warrants further investigation. The process can also facilitate collaboration and research.

Outcomes for preterm infants are discussed in Chapter 11. In Australia and New Zealand, the Australia and New Zealand Neonatal Network (ANZNN) audits information on all babies born at less than 32 weeks' gestation or with a birth weight of less than 1500 g and babies who received assisted ventilation or major surgery. Other large networks that collect data include the National Institute of Child Health and Human Development (NICHD) and the Vermont Oxford Network in the USA, and The Canadian Neonatal Intensive Care Unit Network.

Classification of perinatal deaths

It is often difficult for clinicians to agree on the cause of death in a diverse group of patients. In Australia, the Perinatal Society of Australia and New Zealand (PSANZ) have developed a hierarchical classification, the PSANZ Perinatal Death Classification (PSANZ-PDC), to aid in the identification of the single most important factor which led to the chain of events which resulted in the perinatal death, and the PSANZ-Neonatal Death Classification (PSANZ-NDC) to identify the single most important factor in the neonatal period which caused the death (Chan 2004).

All perinatal deaths should be reviewed by a Perinatal Mortality Committee (or a Death Review Committee), including deaths of infants born within the service who may have died elsewhere. Membership of the committee should be multidisciplinary. The committee serves a number of functions which may include:

• consistent classification of all deaths according to local requirements
• evaluation of factors surrounding and contributing to death
• development of recommendations for improving processes of care
• feedback to clinicians and parents based on above recommendations
• implementation of action required based on above recommendations
• data collection and documentation of perinatal deaths.

Perinatal loss can have significant social and psychological impacts on the family and staff. Following a perinatal death, parents should be allowed to spend private time with their baby, they should be offered the opportunity to create mementos (e.g. footprints, lock of hair). Pastoral care services should be available if requested. Mothers may require advice with regards to lactation and ongoing support services may be necessary.

The role of autopsy

The most reliable cause of death is obtained by an experienced perinatal pathologist conducting an autopsy examination, but even following such examination the precise cause of death may remain undetermined, particularly when the infant dies before birth. Even if the cause of death is known, autopsy can still have a valuable role in confirming this and may sometimes identify previously unrecognized abnormalities. Unfortunately, autopsy rates appear to be declining. If still possible, the placenta should also be examined by a perinatal pathologist and in some cases this alone may elicit the aetiology of a perinatal death.

The role of the coroner

Most jurisdictions have a Coroners Act (or equivalent) which requires all reportable deaths, including those where cause of death cannot be explained with certainty or those dying in an unusual circumstances, to be reported to the coroner or other responsible official. Usually a stillborn child is not reportable.

Factors affecting perinatal death rates

Perinatal deaths have a wide range of causes. They can result from maternal conditions, problems in the placenta, conditions affecting the fetus or newborn or a combination of the above. Sometimes the cause of perinatal death is not identifiable. In Australia in 2008 the PMR was 10.2 per 1000 live births, comprised of 72.5% fetal deaths and 27.5% neonatal deaths (Laws 2008). The main causes of perinatal death were congenital abnormalities (24.9%), spontaneous preterm birth (15.4%) and maternal conditions (14.5%).

Maternal factors which may be associated with perinatal mortality include age, infection, parity, social class, coexisting medical condition, nutrition and underutilization of antenatal services. For mothers under the age of 20 years, or aged 40 or over, the PMRs are 19.6 and 13.8 per 1000 births respectively. Social class is also an important factor. In the UK, there is almost a 100% difference in PMR between women in socioeconomic class I (professional groups) and those in class V (unskilled occupations). In Australia, babies born to indigenous mothers have almost one and half times the PMR of non-indigenous mothers. The perinatal death rate is almost 50% higher for women giving birth after receiving assisted reproductive technology (ART) compared to non-ART women.

Maturity is of course an important factor in the PMR: about half of all deaths occurred in babies who weighed less than 2000 g at birth, and of this group more than half weighed less than 1000 g. The extreme preterm infant is discussed in Chapter 11. Multiple births have a much higher PMR and this is discussed in Chapter 3. In Australia, the PMR for twins was 3.9 times higher than for singletons and for higher-order multiples the PMR was almost 10 times greater. The sex of the fetus or infant is also important. In Australia, the male perinatal death rate was 8.6 per 1000 in 1993–1995, compared to 7.4 per 1000 for females.

Prevention of perinatal mortality and low birthweight

Implementation of preventative measures, particularly in developing countries, could substantially improve perinatal outcomes. Factors which may reduce perinatal mortality and low birthweight include improvement in maternal health and education, reduction in unplanned pregnancy, and providing prenatal care in a comprehensive and coordinated manner.

Changing trends

In developed countries such as the UK and Australia, the PMR has decreased by almost two thirds in the last 30 years.

Reasons for decreasing death rates include improved survival in low birthweight and preterm infants, improved antenatal care and increased use of antenatal steroids.

Despite the inconsistency in classification, collection of epidemiological data has an important role in improving the outcomes for mothers and babies. The main causes of perinatal death are congenital abnormalities, preterm birth and maternal conditions. All perinatal deaths should be reviewed and classified by a Perinatal Mortality Committee. Implementation of a number of preventive measures could help to reduce the PMR, particularly in developing countries.

SUMMARY

 Now visit **www.essentialneonatalmed.com** to test yourself on this chapter.

CHAPTER 3
Multiple births

Key topics

Introduction

Multiple pregnancies are a common problem in the neonatal nursery. Rates have increased since the introduction of assisted reproductive technology (ART). This chapter briefly discusses the physiology of fertilization and placenta formation and their relevance in multiple gestations. Specific complications of multiple gestations are discussed in detail.

Physiology of fertilization, implantation and placenta formation

Fertilization

Normal fertilization occurs in the fallopian tube. Once a sperm enters the ovum, the process of rapid mitotic cell division begins. At about 3 days a ball of 12–16 blastomeres enters the uterine cavity and is called a **morula**. Cell division continues and spaces begin to appear between the cells within the morula forming the blastocyst cavity. The outer surface of this cavity (called the trophoblast) has two layers, an inner cytotrophoblast and outer syncytiotrophoblast. At this point the embryo is referred to as a **blastocyst**.

Implantation

At about 6 days after fertilization, the syncytiotrophoblast comes into contact with the uterine epithelium. If conditions are favourable, there is rapid proliferation and erosion into the endometrium. The process of eroding into the endometrium is referred to as implantation. As cell division of the cytotrophoblast continues a small space appears between the inner cell mass and the outer layers; this is the beginning of the amniotic cavity. The inner cell mass will ultimately go on to form the embryo and amnion. The outer layers will go on to form the chorion and placenta. The cells in between the outer cytotrophoblast and inner cell mass are the extraembryonic mesoderm. Spaces (the chorionic cavity) then also develop in the extraembryonic mesoderm forming the extraembryonic somatic mesoderm which lines the trophoblast and covers the amnion, and the extraembryonic splanchnic mesoderm which surrounds the yolk sac.

Placenta

After implantation the syncytiotrophoblast erodes the endometrial blood vessels allowing maternal blood to form networks of lacunae. These networks are the beginning of the decidual (or maternal) layer of the placenta. The fetal layer of the placenta is due to proliferation of the synctiotrophoblasts and formation of the primary chorionic villi at approximately 2 weeks after fertilization. The external layers of the trophoblast and the extraembryonic somatic mesoderm constitute the **chorion**.

Amniotic cavity

The chorion forms the chorionic sac and within lies the embryo, in its amniotic sac. The amniotic sac continues to enlarge much faster than the chorionic sac. This causes their walls to fuse, obliterating the chorionic cavity and forming the amniochorionic membrane which in turn comes in contact with the decidual layer of the placenta. The developing embryo is now suspended from the placenta by the umbilical cord and is contained within the amniotic cavity.

Classification of multiple pregnancy

Multiple pregnancies are normally classified by the number of placentas and the number of amniotic sacs. A multiple pregnancy may arise from the spontaneous splitting of a single zygote (monozygotic) or through the fertilization of more than one oocyte (dizygotic). If they are dizygotic or if division occurs before implantation they will have separate placentas and separate amniotic cavities. If the division occurs after implantation then they will share the placenta (monochorionic) and either share the

amniotic cavity (monoamniotic) or have their own (diamniotic). Higher-order multiples are usually multizygotic (from multiple ovum) but can arise from zygotic splitting and then resplitting again. They are also classified by the number of placentas and amniotic sacs. For example, triplets may each have their own placenta (trichorionic) and their own amnion (triamniotic) or may be combinations of the above.

> **CLINICAL TIP: Twins of different sexes must be dizygotic. Dizygotic twins must have separate placentas and amnions. The placentas may be fused along a ridge. Monochorionic (MC) twins must be identical irrespective of whether or not they are monoamniotic (MA) or diamniotic (DA). About one in four like-sexed twins who are dichorionic (DC) are identical, but determination of zygosity is not possible without DNA testing.**

Assisted reproductive technology

Assisted reproductive technologies essentially involve manipulation of the egg or sperm to facilitate pregnancy. Technically, ART does not include therapies that simply stimulate the ovaries to produce more eggs (e.g. clomiphene). Techniques include *in vitro* fertilization (IVF), intracytoplasmic sperm injection (ICSI), gamete intrafallopian transfer (GIFT) and zygote intrafallopian transfer (ZIFT).

With the advent of ART there was an increased incidence of multiple-fetus pregnancies. This now appears to be falling again in the UK and Australia since the introduction of legislation and professional guidelines to limit the number of embryos transferred. This is not the case in other countries where no such legislation exists.

Incidence of multiple pregnancies

The incidence of multiple births was first studied by Hellin in 1895. Following this work the Hellinic law was described, which stated that the incidence of twins was 1/89 pregnancies and of triplets $1/89^2$

(1/7921) and quadruplets $1/89^3$ (1/704 969). The actual incidence of multiple births varies greatly between countries due to differing rates of dizygotic twins. Factors influencing the increased rate of dizygotic twinning other than ART are maternal age 35–39 years, high parity, tall stature, periconceptual folate and familial factors (increased risk ×4 if mother, or ×2 if sister is a dizygotic twin). As opposed to dizygotic twins, the incidence of monozygotic twins is relatively stable occurring in approximately 3.5 per 1000 births. Reasons for the development of monozygotic twins are poorly understood. There is fivefold increased risk of monozygotic twinning of an IVF embryo.

Of all naturally conceived twins, 40% are monozygotic, and of all monozygotic twins, 63% are monochorionic diamniotic (MCDA), 33% are dichorionic diamniotic (DCDA) with either separate or fused placentas, and 4% are monochorionic monoamniotic (MCMA).

In developed countries with routine antenatal care and ultrasound assessment the birth of undiagnosed twins is a rare event. Antenatal diagnosis enables assessment of chorionicity, and detection of malpresentation and complications of multiple gestation.

Parental counselling

The perinatal mortality rate is much higher for multiple pregnancies than for singletons, with a fivefold increase for twin pregnancies and 14-fold increase for triplet pregnancies for birth, stillbirth and neonatal death. Similarly, multiple pregnancy is markedly overrepresented in neonatal morbidity (see below). Knowing the increased risks, selective reduction is an option for some parents.

Parents of multiple gestations need a great deal of support and advice with the care of their children. The mother particularly needs encouragement to breastfeed her infants. Voluntary community groups, such as the Twins Club and Twins and Multiple Birth Association, may be helpful in providing support and counselling.

Parents often wish to know if their twins are identical or not. This may be of benefit in terms of rearing practices, the known concordance of medical conditions in 70–90% of twins, and if solid organ transplant is required. The medical profession is notorious for imprecise counselling, and multiple birth support groups have requested that zygosity testing is provided as a routine service in cases of multiple births regardless of the high cost of DNA testing.

Complications of multiple pregnancy

Discordant growth rates

Normally both twins will continue to grow at the rate of a singleton fetus until 30 weeks' gestation, after which growth restriction may occur. As the number of fetuses increases from twins to triplets to quadruplets, the gestational age at which birthweight first falls below that of a singleton fetus also decreases. Twins have birthweights similar to singletons up to 30 weeks, but thereafter are below singleton levels; similarly, birthweights in triplets deviate from the singleton curve at 27–28 weeks, and in quadruplets at approximately 26 weeks. In addition, as the fetal number increases the rate of individual fetal growth in the third trimester decreases. Thus, the further the multiple gestation advances and the higher the fetal number, the more individual birthweights will differ from singleton values.

Twins usually grow at nearly identical rates, the mean intertwin birthweight difference being 11%. Small for gestational age (SGA) infants have been reported in 24–40% of twin gestations. In one study, 13% of twin gestations resulted in one SGA fetus and 9.4% of gestations resulted in two SGA fetuses. Monozygotic twins grow less well than dizygotic twins, and major discrepancies in weight are commoner in monozygotic twins. Causes of discrepancy are poor insertion of the cord into the placenta in one twin and, in dichorionic twins, poor placentation of one twin. The commonest cause is fetofetal transfusion (see below).

Disappearing twin phenomenon

Ultrasound studies have shown that up to 50% of pregnancies initially found containing twins in the first 8 weeks of gestation absorb one conceptus and continue as singleton pregnancies. This has been referred to as the 'disappearing twin' or 'vanishing twin' phenomenon. Rarely, the dead twin is not reabsorbed and fetus papyraceus ensues. It is suggested that the disruption to the surviving twin as a result of the early fetal loss of the co-twin predisposes the baby to cerebral palsy, but there is currently little direct evidence for this.

> CLINICAL TIP: Fetus papyraceous occurs if one twin dies early in the first trimester and becomes mummified. The other twin continues to grow normally. There is a strong association with the occurrence of embolic phenomena (from the dead fetus) affecting the surviving twin. Multicystic encephaloleukomalacia and multiple cutis aplasia have been reported in the surviving twin.

Conjoined twins

Conjoined twins are rare, occurring in 1–2 per 100 000 pregnancies. The fetuses can be connected via the head (craniopagus), chest (thoracopagus), or abdomen and will often share organs as well (e.g. heart, liver). The site of connection and nature of organ sharing will ultimately determine the prognosis. The condition is often incompatible with life (Fig. 3.1).

Prematurity

The incidence of premature delivery in twin pregnancies is 20–30%, and the incidence is greater in higher-order multiple pregnancies. Fifty per cent of twins weigh less than 2500 g at birth. Premature birth relates to increased intrauterine volume, premature rupture of the membranes, complications of multiple pregnancy (e.g. disconcordant growth, twin-to-twin transfusion syndrome) and third-trimester bleeding.

Malpresentation

Multiple gestations may present in the uterus in many ways, some of which predispose them to trauma. Locked twins may occur as a result of unstable lies and cause obstruction to delivery. The types and frequency of presentation in twin pregnancies are listed in Table 3.1.

Congenital malformations

In multiple gestations, the incidence of major malformation is 2%, and of minor malformation 4%. It is often stated that monozygotic twinning results

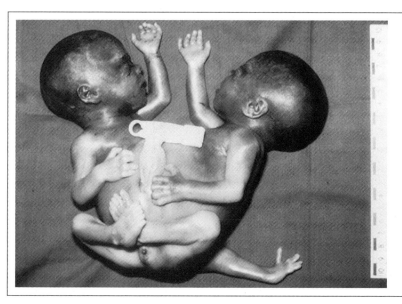

Figure 3.1 Conjoined twins attached from chest to buttocks.

Table 3.1 Types and frequency of presentation in twin pregnancies	
Type of presentation	**Percentage of pregnancies**
Vertex and vertex	45%
Vertex and breech	40%
Breech and breech	10%
Vertex and transverse	3%
Breech and transverse	1.5%
Transverse and transverse	0.5%

from a chance teratogenic event. Malformations due to the event of twinning itself are conjoined twins, amorphous twins, sirenomelia, holoprosencephaly, neural tube defects and anencephaly. Other malformations result from vascular interchange between monozygotic twins, and include acardia in one twin, disseminated intravascular coagulation (DIC) from embolization, with defects such as microcephaly, hydranencephaly, intestinal atresia, cutis aplasia and limb amputation. There is an increased incidence of major birth defects in infants conceived via ICSI and IVF.

Postural deformities

Deformations such as talipes and hip dysplasia result from intrauterine crowding occur in multiple gestations and are independent of zygosity.

Twin-to-twin transfusion

In monochorionic twins, there are connections on the placenta that join the twins' circulations. The majority of these connections are balanced but in up to 15% of cases they are unbalanced. When the connection is unbalanced, one twin (the donor twin) will donate some blood volume to the other twin (the recipient twin). The donor twin will have decreased urine output, causing oligohydramnios, and the recipient twin will have increased urine output, causing polyhydramnios. In its most severe form the donor twin with very severe oligohydramnios becomes 'stuck' and immobile. Twin-to-twin

transfusion syndrome (TTTS) is normally diagnosed on ultrasound when the amniotic fluid around the donor twin is 2 cm or less and the amniotic fluid around the recipient is 8 cm or more. There may also be changes in the umbilical cord blood flow and in severe cases hydrops fetalis may develop in the recipient. It is recognized in the neonatal unit by either discordant growth (>20% birthweight difference), which is referred to as chronic TTTS, or a haemoglobin difference or more than 5 g/dL (acute TTTS).

If one of the twins dies *in utero*, this may result in acute transfusion from the surviving twin. This can cause subsequent death of the other fetus, or if it survives can result in significant long-term disability. Overall, untreated TTTS will result in a fetal loss of up to 90% and is associated with significant morbidity in survivors. Fetoscopic laser ablation of the communicating vessels can be used to successfully stop the process of TTTS and allows recovery in the twins. It is normally performed between 16 and 28 weeks' gestation. It has been shown to decrease the risk of cerebral palsy and neurodevelopmental disability in survivors. The risks of fetal laser ablation include preterm labour, preterm premature rupture of membranes and fetal loss. Fetal medicine specialists now recommend scanning all monochorionic twins every 2 weeks to detect discordant amniotic fluid volume.

In the neonate rapid treatment of the anaemic twin may be necessary (see p. 254), and the plethoric twin may require a dilutional exchange transfusion. Because of the high risk of long-term neurodevelopmental disability, all TTTS survivors should receive long-term follow-up.

Cord entanglement

If the twins share the same amniotic cavity there is a chance that their umbilical cords can become intertwined, resulting in potential obstruction of blood supply from the placenta to one (or both) of the fetuses. The umbilical cords of monoamniotic twins can start to become entwined within the first trimester of pregnancy. As the pregnancy progresses there is increased risk of cord compression. Cord entanglement can be monitored by Doppler ultrasound. As the pregnancy progresses, there is an increased risk of fetal loss particularly after 32 weeks' gestation.

> **CLINICAL TIP:** Elective delivery at 32 weeks gestation is recommended for monoamniotic twins. Appropriate antenatal steroids should be administered prior to elective delivery.

Infection

This occurs much more commonly in the first twin and probably relates to premature rupture of the membranes of the first amniotic sac.

Hypoxic ischaemic encephalopathy

The second twin is more vulnerable to hypoxic ischaemic encephalopathy (HIE) than the first twin. This is related to delayed delivery, cord prolapse, placental separation and malpresentation.

> **CLINICAL TIP:** Not only are second twins at higher risk of HIE, they also have higher rates of respiratory distress syndrome and hypoglycaemia.

Respiratory distress syndrome

Overall, there is an 8.5% incidence of respiratory distress syndrome (RDS) in twins, with 29% of preterm twins being diagnosed as having RDS.

Neurodevelopmental outcomes

Children born from multiple pregnancies have much higher rates of cerebral palsy, learning difficulties and behavioural problems. Probable antecedents are premature birth, growth restriction, birth trauma, infection, hypoxia and intrauterine demise of one twin. However, there still appears to be an increased risk even when the above confounders are accounted for.

Twins are over-represented in populations with cerebral palsy (5–10% in most studies), particularly spastic diplegia. The risk of a twin developing cerebral palsy is 5–6 times higher than in a singleton pregnancy, and the risk in a triplet is 17–20 times higher than in a singleton. Typical rates of cerebral palsy per 1000 births are singleton 2.3, twin 12.6 and triplet 44.8. This risk is particularly increased where a monozygotic co-twin has died *in utero*. In all such cases the brain of the surviving twin must be carefully examined with ultrasound or MRI to detect evidence of cerebral infarction (most probably periventricular leukomalacia). It is estimated that the risk of cerebral palsy in a surviving monozygotic twin whose co-twin dies is 12 times greater than when both twins survive.

SUMMARY

Multiple gestations may arise spontaneously or be due to ART. The introduction of ART significantly increased the incidence of multiple gestations, but careful implementation of legislation and guidelines can reduce their occurrence. Multiple gestations require a significant burden of surveillance and treatment, both antenatally and postnatally. Multiple gestations carry increased risk of mortality and morbidity. Parents need to be counselled extensively about risks prior to undergoing ART and early in multiple pregnancy.

 Now visit **www.essentialneonatalmed.com** to test yourself on this chapter.

CHAPTER 4
Neonatal consequences of maternal conditions

Key topics

Introduction

The developing fetus is hugely influenced by its mother – 50% of its genes and all of its mitochondria are from the mother. Her womb provides the nurturing supportive environment and all the nutrition required during fetal development. It is therefore not surprising that if this environment is disturbed by maternal disease or behaviour, there may be consequences for the fetus, especially if that disturbance occurs in the first trimester during critical organ development. This chapter will consider some of the fetal consequences of maternal conditions. Genetic conditions are discussed in Chapter 8.

Congenital anomalies: malformations and deformations

Estimates of the incidence of congenital anomalies vary widely and range from 1% to 7% of live births, depending on the definition of what constitutes an anomaly. In about 3% there is a major congenital anomaly, but the incidence is 7% if minor lesions such as skin haemangiomas and preauricular skin tags are included. It is highest in preterm and small for gestational age (SGA) infants. Congenital anomalies are the leading cause of perinatal mortality (20–25% of all perinatal deaths) and postneonatal deaths (25–30%). In addition, they constitute 25–30% of admissions to children's hospitals and have major financial costs for society.

Congenital anomalies may be classified into deformations and malformations. **Deformations** result from late changes in previously normal structures by destructive pathological processes or intrauterine (extrinsic) forces; for example, talipes, hydrocephalus and bowel atresia. **Malformations** result from a disturbance of growth during embryogenesis; for example, congenital heart disease. Some defects may arise by both mechanisms.

Deformations

Deformations may be single or multiple. They have many common aetiological factors, which are listed in Box 4.1.

Extrinsic forces may cause a single localized deformation, such as talipes equinovarus or a **deformation sequence**. Examples of the latter are the oligohydramnios sequence, with contractures, facial dysmorphism and pulmonary hypoplasia, or the breech deformation sequence. Intrauterine contractures that give rise to joint fixation are known as arthrogryposis. The types of problems that lead to prenatal joint contractures are shown in Fig. 4.1.

Malformations

Incidence

Major congenital anomalies are either lethal or significantly affect the individual's function or appear-

Box 4.1 Risk factors for deformation

- Oligohydramnios
- Uterine abnormalities, e.g. fibroids, bicornuate or septate uterus
- Multiple pregnancy
- Abnormal presentation, e.g. breech position
- Intrauterine growth restriction

ance. Minor anomalies have no functional or major cosmetic importance.

National registers of congenital malformations are available, but it is difficult to compare overall rates because of reporting differences. Most registers only include abnormalities present at birth. Due to miscarriage, stillbirth or termination of pregnancy the overall incidence may be much higher. There may also be large regional variations within a single country. Registers are increasingly including metabolic disorders and genetic disorders (e.g. cystic fibrosis) even if they have no physical characteristics present at birth.

The incidence of congenital malformations reported for South Australia from 1986 to 2003 was 5.7%, with annual variations from 4.5% to 6.0%. The UK figures are similar. The commonest major congenital anomalies involve the central nervous and cardiovascular systems. Table 4.1 lists the incidence of some congenital malformations.

Causes of congenital malformations

Congenital anomalies result from a wide variety of mechanisms ranging from genetic (monogenic and polygenic) to environmental factors (teratogenesis), maternal metabolic disease, drugs and chemicals, infectious agents and irradiation (Table 4.2).

Genetic malformations

These are discussed in Chapters 6 and 8.

Congenital anomalies associated with teratogens

A **teratogen** is an agent (chemical, drug, virus or radiation) that affects the well-being of the fetus. A

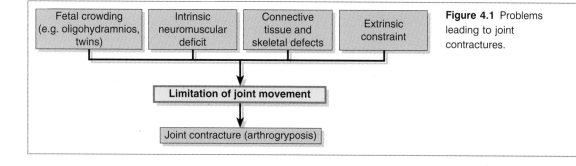

Figure 4.1 Problems leading to joint contractures.

Table 4.1 Major congenital anomalies by major anatomical systems (Australia 2002–2003)

Congenital anomaly	Rate (per 1000 total births, including fetal deaths)	Rate (per 1000 total births and ToP before 20 weeks)
Central nervous system		
Spina bifida	0.27	0.47
Anencephaly	0.12	0.41
Encephalocoele	0.05	0.1
Congenital hydrocephalus	0.54	0.68
Cardiovascular system		
Transposition of great vessels	0.40	0.47
Hypoplastic left heart	0.16	0.21
Coarctation of aorta	0.38	0.41
Respiratory system		
Congenital diaphragmatic hernia	0.25	0.28
Gastrointestinal system		
Cleft lip ± cleft palate	0.91	0.97
Oesophageal atresia	0.2	0.22
Gastroschisis	0.22	0.25
Urogenital system		
Hypospadias	0.47	0.47
Cystic kidney	0.47	0.53
Renal agenesis/dysgenesis	0.48	0.56
Limb		
Polydactyly	0.92	0.97
Chromosomal		
Trisomy 21	1.1	2.6
Trisomy 13	0.07	0.26
Trisomy 18	0.2	0.7

ToP, termination of pregnancy.

fetotoxin is an agent causing damage of any kind to the fetus, and a **mutagen** is an agent that causes a permanent transmissible change in the genetic material. The commonest potential teratogens are medications and so in general drugs should be avoided during pregnancy and, if essential, their safety profile must be checked before prescribing. Unfortunately with some newer agents, human safety data is lacking and animal data must be used to make a careful risk-benefit assessment. This is why congenital anomaly registers are important, to identify unexpected clusters of congenital anomalies.

Table 4.2 Causes of congenital malformations

Cause	Estimated contribution (%)
Genetic (mendelian inheritance)	20
Chromosomal	10
Polygenic	25–30
Teratogenic effect:	6–9
Congenital infection	2–3
Drugs and environmental pollutants/insecticides	2–3
Maternal metabolic disease	1–2
Radiation exposure	<1
Unknown/idiopathic	35–40

Table 4.3 Major organ system risk periods

Organ	Risk period (days after conception)
Brain	15–25
Eye	25–40
Heart	20–40
Limbs	24–36
Ear	40–60

Table 4.4 Drugs as teratogens

Hormones	Progestogens, diethyl stilboestrol, male sex hormones
Antipsychotics, hypnotics, anticonvulsants	Lithium, haloperidol, thalidomide
Anticonvulsants	Hydantoins, sodium valproate, carbamazepine, primidone, phenobarbitone
Antimicrobials	Tetracycline, chloramphenicol, streptomycin, flucytosine, amphotericin B
Antineoplastics	Alkylating agents, folic acid antagonists
Anticoagulants	Warfarin
Antithyroids	Iodine, carbimazole, propylthiouracil
Antivirals	Ribavirin
Hypoglycaemics	Biguanides, sulphonylureas
Vitamin A analogues	Isotretinoin, etretinate
Others	Toluene, alcohol, marijuana, narcotics

The critical periods in embryogenic development have been extrapolated from the effects of rubella exposure and are expressed in days from time of conception (not last menstrual period) in Table 4.3.

During the first 2 weeks of development from conception to the first missed period the embryo is resistant to any teratogenic effects of medicines. The critical period begins when organ development starts at 17 days after conception, and extends until this is complete at 60–70 days. In general, exposure to medicines beyond 70 days after conception is not associated with major birth defects. However, drugs can interfere with functional development of organ systems in the second and third trimesters.

Pharmaceutical agents

Drugs may act by interfering with embryogenesis or by exerting their pharmacological actions on developing fetal organs. The timing and dose of agent, the efficiency with which the mother metabolizes the agent, placental transfer and the individual susceptibility of the fetus are important. Table 4.4 lists some of the more common teratogenic drugs.

Irradiation

Exposure to radiation in pregnancy is now rare, but previous experience with X-rays and atomic bomb irradiation confirmed major teratogenic effects including microcephaly. Carcinogenic effects and mutagenic effects (changes to DNA which can be passed to future generations) are also described.

Chemicals

Pesticides and waste products have not been subjected to rigorous teratogenic studies in humans. However, recent experience with the dioxin contaminant in the insecticide 2,4,5-T and its possible association with spina bifida and Potter's syndrome suggest that a much more rigorous surveillance of chemicals is necessary in the future. Long-term prenatal exposure to organic mercury causes disturbed brain development. Methyl isocyanate gas released in the Bhopal disaster led to an increase in congenital anomalies in the offspring of those exposed (mutagenic effect).

Congenital malformation secondary to maternal infections

Prenatal infections cause inflammation which interferes with cell division. This can lead to congenital deafness, cataracts and limb defects. Examples are outlined in Table 4.5. Infections are described in Chapter 10.

Fever

Studies suggest that it may be the high fever associated with viral infection (e.g. influenza) that causes malformation. Sauna baths and faulty electric blankets producing very high body temperatures at a critical period of embryogenesis may be teratogenic.

Consequences of maternal substance misuse

All drug ingestion during pregnancy carries risk to the developing fetus, and maternal substance misuse can cause fetal malformation and sometimes neonatal withdrawal. Cigarettes, alcohol, opiates, amphetamines and cocaine are all known to cause harm.

Table 4.5 Teratogenic effects of maternal infection

Infection	Effect
Rubella	Heart defects CNS defects Eye defects (cataract) Deafness
Toxoplasmosis	Cerebral calcification Epilepsy, Hydrocephalus Chorioretinitis
Syphilis	Skin lesions, saddle nose, osteochondritis
Varicella (herpes zoster)	Brain, skeletal and eye defects Dermatomal scarring
Parvovirus B19	Severe fetal anaemia, hydrops
Cytomegalovirus (CMV)	Microcephaly, retinitis, deafness
Herpes simplex	Microcephaly or hydranencephaly
Influenza	Teratogenic effects from fever. Increased risk of schizophrenia

Fetal alcohol spectrum disorder

Fetal alcohol spectrum disorder (FASD) is the generic term covering fetal alcohol syndrome, fetal alcohol effects and alcohol-related neurodevelopmental disorders.

Excessive alcohol intake during fetal organogenesis can result in a specific syndrome of facial abnormalities, growth failure, microcephaly and skeletal and visceral abnormalities. This syndrome was identified in 1973 as the fetal alcohol syndrome. The facial features include hypoplasia of the mid-face, with beaking of the forehead; sunken nasal bridge; small upturned nose; micrognathia, a prominent philtrum and ear deformities (Fig. 4.2). Intrauterine growth retardation (IUGR) is usual, with poor postnatal growth. Major abnormalities include cleft lip and palate, and limb, ocular, cardiac and renal

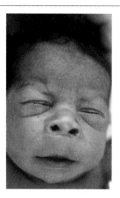

Figure 4.2 Infant with typical features of fetal alcohol syndrome. From Lissauer, T. and Fanaroff, A. A. Neonatology at a Glance, 2nd edition. © 2011 Blackwell Publishing Ltd.

Box 4.2 The four-digit diagnostic code

Diagnosis is made using four key diagnostic features:

- Growth restriction (weight or length <10th centile)
- Fetal alcohol syndrome facial phenotype (small eye openings, smooth philtrum, thin upper lip)
- CNS damage/dysfunction
- Prenatal alcohol exposure

malformations. There is usually delayed psycho-motor development. Approximately one-third of infants born to chronic alcoholic women develop the fetal alcohol syndrome, whereas others may be growth restricted or demonstrate only minor features. Neonatal withdrawal symptoms, including convulsions, may occur.

It is not known whether social drinking of alcohol in pregnancy is associated with IUGR, but it is unlikely that very occasional consumption of small quantities of alcohol during later pregnancy will seriously adversely affect the fetus. However, current recommendation is to avoid all alcohol consumption during pregnancy.

There is no laboratory test for FASD. Diagnosis relies on a pattern of abnormalities that makes up the disorder, along with a history of alcohol misuse during pregnancy. Sometimes the phenotype becomes more obvious in childhood. Various scoring systems are in use, such as the four-digit diagnostic code (see Box 4.2).

Smoking in pregnancy

Although there is overwhelming evidence of harm to the fetus and mother from smoking, up to 25% of pregnant women still smoke. Smoking has a dose-dependent effect on growth due to impaired uterine perfusion, with placental changes, increased carboxyhaemoglobin levels and increased fetal erythropoiesis. The risks of pre-eclampsia are slightly reduced. Passive exposure to paternal smoking has nearly as great an effect. Complications in smokers include subfertility, spontaneous abortion, impaired fetal growth, placenta praevia, placental abruption, amniotic fluid infection and premature rupture of the membranes. Children of smokers demonstrate increased hyperactivity at 4 years, reduced stature and mental function, and increased risk of sudden infant death syndrome (SIDS) and malignancy. Smoking is not associated with any specific congenital abnormalities.

Infants of substance-misusing mothers

Neonatal withdrawal symptoms have been reported with alcohol, amphetamines, barbiturates, codeine, ethchlorvynol, heroin, pethidine, methadone, morphine and pentazocine. Methamphetamine ('ice') and 'crack' cocaine are currently of major concern, but drug-using practices vary according to availability, geography and price.

Link to *Nursing the Neonate*: Neonatal neurology. Chapter 14, pp. 252–254.

Opiate use in pregnancy

Heroin and methadone are the narcotic drugs most frequently abused during pregnancy. Their illicit use has been associated with increased fetal and neonatal deaths. Increased IUGR and prematurity means that the average birthweight of infants born to

Table 4.6 Withdrawal symptoms seen in neonates born to opiate-abusing mothers

Central nervous system	Irritability and high-pitched cry Hyperactivity with reduced periods of sleep Tremors Increased tone Convulsions (rare)
Gastrointestinal	Poor feeding Vomiting Diarrhoea
Other autonomic symptoms	Sweating Fever Frequent yawning Snuffles and sneezing Tachycardia

heroin addicts is 2500 g. The fetal brain becomes acclimatized to the chronic stimulation of opiate receptors in the brainstem. After birth the baby experiences sudden cessation of this stimulation and increased adrenergic activity of the locus caeruleus causes 'withdrawal' symptoms. Women should be encouraged to attend an addiction unit that can manage their antenatal care and switch them to a safer alternative, e.g. prescribed methadone.

About 70% of exposed infants exhibit withdrawal symptoms, usually within 48 h of birth. They can be delayed for up to a week. Signs include extreme jitteriness, tachycardia, vomiting, diarrhoea and fever (see Table 4.6). Convulsions occur rarely. Infants born to drug-addicted mothers may continue to show irritable or restless behaviour for a number of months after birth.

Management of neonatal abstinence syndrome

Infants born to drug-addicted mothers should be carefully monitored for withdrawal symptoms. About 30% of infants with drug withdrawal can be managed conservatively. Methods include swaddling, frequent feeds and decreased sensory stimulation. Breastfeeding should be encouraged, as the small amount of opiate excreted in breast milk may help alleviate symptoms.

If severe signs of withdrawal are present, drug treatment is necessary and the first line treatment is to give opiates such as oral morphine syrup. Seizures should be treated with intravenous morphine followed by anticonvulsants if the seizure continues. Non-specific sedatives such as phenobarbitone, diazepam or chlorpromazine have been used for neonatal abstinence syndrome (NAS) but the evidence for their use is not strong. As second line treatment phenobarbitone or clonidine may be added to morphine replacement for those babies with polydrug exposure.

Screening for hepatitis B and C and HIV infection is important. If mother has active hepatitis B the baby must be given immunoglobulin and vaccinated (see Chapter 10).

Prognosis

This depends at least in part on the socioeconomic background of the family. Infants exhibit behavioural and physical features reflecting central and systemic dysfunction. These infants are at increased risk of SIDS, and they and their families require intensive follow-up after discharge by medical and community health and social services. Many will require foster parenting.

Cocaine use in pregnancy

Perinatal cocaine or 'crack' cocaine use is a major problem in the USA and elsewhere. Cocaine is a potent vasoconstrictor affecting the uteroplacental bed as well as the fetal vessels. It causes maternal and fetal tachycardia and severe hypertension. Cocaine abuse causes first-trimester abortion, placental abruption and premature birth. Malformations include hydronephrosis, cryptorchidism, skeletal defects with delayed ossification, exencephaly and eye anomalies. Cerebral artery infarction due to the vasoconstriction is most likely to occur in the second and third trimesters.

Neonatal symptoms from cocaine exposure are often seen early, while drug levels are high. They include jitteriness, irritability, disturbed sleep–wake cycle and later neurodevelopmental impairment. Breastfeeding should be avoided if the mother continues to take cocaine.

Acute alcohol withdrawal in the neonate

Neonates born to heavily alcoholic mothers (see above) can show early withdrawal at 3–12 h with hyperactivity, irritability, excessive crying and poor feeding. Extreme tremulousness and seizures may occur and can be controlled with phenobarbitone. Withdrawal occurs independently of fetal alcohol syndrome.

CLINICAL TIP: The easiest way to confirm which substances may be causing neonatal withdrawal symptoms (if there is doubt) is ask the mother to provide a urine sample for toxicology. Urine and meconium from the baby within 72 h of birth can also be analysed. Hair samples from the baby can be forensically analysed for drug exposure during the preceding 2–3 months, although in practice this is rarely necessary.

Neonatal manifestations of maternal medical diseases

Many acute maternal conditions such as septicaemia, hypertension, seizures or collapse will have adverse effects on the fetus. These are discussed elsewhere, but this section considers the specific effects of certain chronic maternal medical conditions on the fetus and newborn. Women with these conditions need appropriate preconception counselling and often require 'shared care' between their physician and obstetrician.

 Link to *Nursing the Neonate*: Obstetric issues related to neonatal care. Chapter 2, pp. 17–20.

Diabetes mellitus

Poorly controlled maternal diabetes predisposes to increased risk of miscarriage and also to late intrauterine death. Diabetes carries a 3–5-fold increase in congenital malformations and this risk is proportional to the level of glycosylated haemoglobin (HbA_{1c}) particularly during the period surrounding conception and early embryogenesis. Malforma-tions include caudal regression syndrome (with sacral agenesis), hypoplastic left colon, renal vein thrombosis and congenital heart disease, especially transposition of the great arteries (TGA). Fetal hyperinsulinaemia (in response to high circulating glucose levels) acts as a growth hormone, causing macrosomia and hypertrophic cardiomyopathy. If the diabetic woman is well controlled on insulin and her blood sugars remain in the normal range before she becomes pregnant, the risk of congenital malformation is much reduced.

After delivery the supply of glucose to the fetus stops abruptly, but the hyperinsulinaemia may persist, leading to hypoglycaemia. Breastfeeding is protective and some mothers are even encouraged to express and store colostrum before birth, for use in the early hours after delivery. The management of hypoglycaemia is discussed in Chapter 21.

Maternal hyperthyroidism (Graves' disease)

Maternal hyperthyroidism results in transient neonatal thyrotoxicosis in approximately 10–20% of pregnancies (see Chapter 21). The best predictors are the outcome of previous siblings and assays of thyroid-stimulating immunoglobulin and thyroid receptor-binding inhibitors.

Maternal idiopathic thrombocytopenia

Anti-platelet IgG antibodies cross the placenta and can cause transient low platelets in the neonate. The risks of serious intracranial bleeding are low. This is described in detail in Chapter 20.

Maternal systemic lupus erythematosus

Vasculopathy associated with maternal systemic lupus erythematosus (SLE) strongly increases the risk of recurrent miscarriage. This can be reduced by low-dose aspirin, low molecular weight heparin and even plasmapheresis to maintain the pregnancy. Mothers with SLE have a 0.5–2% chance of having a baby affected by congenital heart block due to the presence of anti-Ro and anti-La antibodies, which can cross the placenta and permanently damage the conduction system in the fetal heart.

This may require treatment with a pacemaker (see Chapter 16).

Transient neonatal myaesthenia

Congenital myasthenia is usually inherited as an autosomal recessive trait. However, occasionally the baby may develop transient weakness due to maternal acetylcholine receptor (AchR) IgG antibodies crossing the placenta. The diagnosis is often known in the mother, but as onset occurs within hours of birth, the neonatal team must be prepared to support feeding and sometimes respiration. Admin-istration of anticholinesterase (neostigmine) leads to rapid improvement and is diagnostic. Recovery usually occurs within 2 months as the circulating antibodies wane.

Maternal epilepsy

Women with epilepsy must ensure they plan pregnancy carefully. They should be switched to an anticonvulsant that is relatively safe in pregnancy, ideally well before conception so that good control can be established with the new agent. Seizures during pregnancy can cause fetal hypoxia.

SUMMARY

A healthy uterine environment is essential for normal fetal development. Although fetuses can continue to thrive despite significant changes to the mother's environment (e.g. brief periods of malnutrition, extremes of hot and cold), they can also be permanently affected by maternal diseases or by exposure to teratogenic drugs. Whenever a baby becomes ill or shows unusual symptoms, it is very important to take a thorough maternal and pregnancy history.

Mothers with pre-existing medical conditions should consult their physicians prior to conception to plan optimal treatment before and during pregnancy. In all pregnant women, drugs should be prescribed only if they are known to be safe. Tobacco, alcohol and street drugs should be avoided altogether.

 Now visit **www.essentialneonatalmed.com** to test yourself on this chapter.

CHAPTER 5
Resuscitation at birth

Key topics

Introduction

It is important to remember that the vast majority of babies are born in good condition and do not need any intervention. However, perinatal asphyxia is the most frequent and serious preventable problem for the newborn baby. Severe perinatal asphyxia may lead to a severely ill baby with major long-term sequelae such as mental retardation, cerebral palsy, blindness and epilepsy. Good perinatal care can minimize the risks of hypoxia. Neonatal depression at birth (Apgar score ≤6 at 1 min) occurs in about 14% of all births and is often unpredictable, so all professionals who are present at deliveries should have basic life support skills. Expert help capable of advanced resuscitation must be quickly available. Perinatal asphyxia remains a major source of neonatal morbidity in developed countries, and ranks with perinatal infection as the cause of at least two thirds of neonatal mortality in developing countries. Owing to problems with definition, reported incidences in full-term neonates vary from 2 to 4/1000 live births, even more so for very low birthweight (VLBW) infants, with rates of up to 60%.

Fetal responses during labour

Every contraction during normal labour interrupts flow in the uterine arteries and may cause relative hypoxia and hypoperfusion. This can be considered 'physiological' hypoxia–ischaemia. During these episodes the fetus deploys various protective mechanisms (Table 5.1). Only if these responses become overwhelmed does the fetus suffer injury. These fetal

Essential Neonatal Medicine, Fifth Edition. Sunil Sinha, Lawrence Miall, Luke Jardine.
© 2012 John Wiley & Sons, Ltd. Published 2012 by John Wiley & Sons, Ltd.

adaptations are designed to maintain function in vital organs such as the brain and myocardium. They include relative fetal bradycardia during con-

tractions, and the 'diving seal' reflex. Transient periods of asphyxia may also induce anaerobic metabolism in the fetal brain and myocardium, with utilization of ketones and lactate as alternate fuels.

Table 5.1 Responses of the normal fetus to transient episodes of 'asphyxia' in labour	
Redirection of blood flow towards:	Brain Myocardium Adrenals
and away from:	Skin Bowel Muscles
'Diving seal reflex' comprising:	Bradycardia Increased blood pressure
Anaerobic metabolism resulting in metabolic acidosis	

Fetal and neonatal responses to perinatal asphyxia

Once the normal adaptive mechanisms to perinatal hypoxia have been exhausted, the fetus will show profound but predictable reactions to ongoing hypoxia. These predominantly affect the respiratory and cardiovascular systems and are observed in babies born immediately after an acute intrapartum asphyxial event. However, with a severe insult early in labour or a delayed delivery many of these changes will be taking place in the unborn fetus (see Fig. 5.1). In the most extreme cases this leads to still-

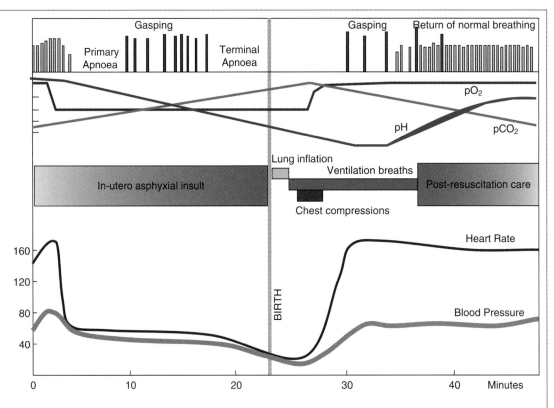

Figure 5.1 The physiological effect of acute asphyxia and the response to resuscitation. (Courtesy of Dr Sam Richmond.)

birth, but for most babies adequate resuscitation can restore the infant to a normal physiological state.

Respiratory activity

Initially there is increased respiratory activity. When the respiratory centre in the brain becomes hypoxic there is then a period of apnoea (**primary apnoea**). Secondary respiratory centres in the spinal cord (which are normally inhibited by the brain) then trigger a series of slower gasps, which eventually become less frequent until **terminal apnoea** occurs. Spontaneous recovery can only occur if the baby is able to breathe through an open airway before terminal apnoea begins. Once terminal apnoea has occurred the baby will die without active resuscitation. The precise interval between a complete asphyxial insult and terminal apnoea in the human fetus is not known as this often occurs before birth, but extrapolation from animal studies and postnatal collapse suggests newborns can withstand 10–15 min of severe asphyxia.

Cardiovascular activity

Heart rate changes occur simultaneously with the respiratory changes described above. Initially, there is tachycardia, followed by a decline to about 60 bpm. This is probably mediated by vagal stimulation and the heart is able to continue to beat by metabolising myocardial glycogen stores. Central blood pressure is maintained by peripheral vasoconstriction and by increasing stroke volume in response to bradycardia. Transient rises in heart rate and blood pressure occur when spinal gasps develop, but heart rate and blood pressure fall again as apnoea develops. This is due to myocardial anoxia, and without resuscitation the baby will die. The pulmonary vascular resistance increases dramatically with terminal apnoea, and the newborn circulation generally tends to revert to a fetal state. With effective resuscitation the oxygen level in the coronary arteries rises, the heart rate increases and the baby starts to breathe spontaneously (see Fig 5.1).

The interval between asphyxial insult and delivery is variable and the appearance of the newborn will depend on where they are on the 'physiological graph' shown in Fig. 5.1. A baby with primary apnoea will appear blue with some tone and reflex activity and the heart rate will be accelerating. The baby will usually recover spontaneously, provided the airway is open. This can be accelerated by physical stimulation.

In contrast, the baby with terminal apnoea will not recover without intervention. In this case the baby is white (vasoconstricted) or intensely cyanosed, unresponsive and flaccid; the heart rate is less than 100 bpm and perfusion is poor.

Unfortunately, in the delivery room we may not know the severity of the asphyxia and we often cannot distinguish between primary and secondary apnoea, so that prompt and effective resuscitation should be commenced in all apnoeic infants. As the baby responds it can usually be determined whether the apnoea was primary or secondary. Babies with primary apnoea have a rapidly accelerating heart rate, and will either show a few gasps or start to breathe normally. In contrast, babies with terminal apnoea will show some initial rise in heart rate in response to ventilation, start to gasp initially and then continue to do so for some time before normal, regular breaths ensue.

> **CLINICAL TIP:** The presence of gasping during recovery from apnoea is an important sign to observe and record, as it indicates a prolonged asphyxial insult.

Perinatal asphyxia

Defining perinatal asphyxia

It is vital that perinatal asphyxia is defined accurately, both from a clinical perspective, to guide appropriate treatment, and from a medico-legal point of view when establishing causation (see Box 5.1) Most asphyxiated babies will be born in a poor condition with birth depression, but conversely by no means every baby with birth depression has experienced an asphyxial insult. There are many alternative causes of birth depression (see Table 5.2).

Box 5.1 Essential characteristics needed to diagnose significant perinatal asphyxia in the newborn

- Evidence of birth depression: an Apgar score 0–3 at >5 min
- Evidence of intrapartum anaerobic metabolism:
  - Umbilical cord arterial pH <7.0
  - Umbilical cord arterial base deficit ≥16 mmol/L
- Neonatal neurological sequelae: early-onset encephalopathy characterized by hypotonia, seizures or coma)
- Evidence of multiorgan system dysfunction in the immediate neonatal period (evidence of hypoxic–ischaemic injury to other organs than the brain, such as the kidneys, heart and liver)
- Absence of an alternative aetiology (see Table 5.2)

Table 5.2 Causes of birth depression other than intrapartum asphyxia

Cause	Example	Effect
Congenital brain malformation	Lissencephaly Polymicrogyria	Encephalopathy, seizures
Intracerebral bleeding	Unexpected haemophillia A Severe thrombocytopenia	Respiratory depression Seizures
Antenatal cerebral insult	Antenatal cerebral infarction	Cystic parenchymal damage
Congenital airway anomaly	Choanal atresia Tracheal agenesis (rare) Pharyngeal cyst	Failure to establish open airway
Extreme prematurity	RDS, inadequate respiratory effort	Pulmonary insufficiency
Extrinsic lung compression	Pleural effusion, congenital diaphragmatic hernia	Pulmonary insufficiency Pulmonary hypoplasia
Oligohydramnios	Potter's syndrome, Posterior urethral valves PROM before 25 weeks	Pulmonary hypoplasia
Cardiac	Congenital heart block	Extreme bradycardia
Drugs	Anaesthetics, Opiates (as analgesia) Opiates (substance misuse) MgSO$_4$	Respiratory depression
Infection	Listeria Group B streptococcus Herpes simplex infection	Meningitis Pulmonary hypertension Encephalopathy

PROM, premature rupture of membranes; RDS, respiratory distress syndrome.

Table 5.3 The five components of the Apgar score

Sign	0	1	2
Heart rate	Absent	≤100 bpm	>100 bpm
Respiratory effort	Absent	Gasping or irregular	Regular or strong cry
Muscle tone	Limp	Reduced	Normal
Response to pharyngeal stimulation/suction[a]	None	Grimace	Cough/cry
Colour	Pale or blue	Pink with blue extremities	Pink

[a] Note: routine suction of the oropharynx is no longer recommended.

Clinical evidence of asphyxia

Virginia Apgar introduced the scoring system (see Table 5.3) that now bears her name in an attempt to describe the condition of the infant shortly after birth. Although she did not intend it to refer to asphyxia, it has nevertheless become widely used for that purpose, and in some centres asphyxia is defined (incorrectly) on the basis of a low Apgar score alone. Using an Apgar score of 3 or less at 5 min as the criterion, the incidence of asphyxia is 3–9/1000 full-term infants. If asphyxia is defined as the requirement for intermittent positive-pressure ventilation for more than 1 min, then 5/1000 full-term infants had this condition. If it is defined by hypoxic–ischaemic encephalopathy the rate drops to 1/1000 births.

Medico-legal evidence of significant asphyxia

Most cerebral palsy is not asphyxial in origin and most perinatal hypoxic–ischaemic cerebral injury (90% of cases) originates well before labour, with only a small component being solely attributed to intrapartum events. However, since children damaged by potentially preventable intra partum asphyxia have expensive ongoing care needs, their families may seek financial redress though the legal process. The legal criteria required to establish liability are summarized in Box 5.2.

CLINICAL TIP: The terms 'birth asphyxia' and 'perinatal asphyxia' were previously loosely used to describe depression at birth, but because of the potential medico-legal implications stringent criteria must now be satisfied for their use. To state objectively that there was a likelihood of a prolonged acute hypoxic–ischaemic event in labour causing permanent brain injury to a previously healthy fetus one also needs:

1 Evidence of a major 'sentinel' hypoxic event, e.g. a ruptured uterus, antepartum haemorrhage, cord prolapse or amniotic fluid embolism; i.e. something that significantly changes normal fetal oxygenation in labour. Clear evidence of a sentinel event is not always present at the time of delivery.
2 Evidence of possible fetal compromise ('distress') from the time of the sentinel event, e.g. major changes in the fetal heart rate and/or fetal acidosis on fetal blood sampling.
3 Evidence that encephalopathy is not due to other causes, such as infection, metabolic diseases and intracranial problems (e.g. intracerebral haemorrhage or congenital brain malformation) (see Table 5.2).

Communication between obstetricians or midwives and the neonatal team is best served by replacing the term 'fetal distress' with 'non-reassuring fetal status', followed by a further description of what is abnormal; e.g. 'repetitive variable decelerations' or 'fetal bradycardia of 60 bpm'. Similarly when describing resuscitation it is much more helpful to document the condition of the baby, the actions taken and the clinical response rather than merely the Apgar scores. The generic term 'birth depression' should be used until an asphyxial aetiology is established.

Causes of perinatal asphyxia

The perinatal events most associated with hypoxic–ischaemic injury are listed in Table 5.4. Those events which present with birth depression and can mimic intrapartum asphyxia are shown in Table 5.2.

Prevention of perinatal asphyxia

The prevention of perinatal asphyxia involves the following:
• recognition of high-risk pregnancies
• recognition of IUGR and placental insufficiency
• accurate assessment of gestation and the use of antenatal steroids
• appropriate management of postmaturity
• assessment of fetoplacental function, e.g. Doppler ultrasound, fetal movements
• appropriate intrapartum fetal heart rate monitoring
• treatment of fetal distress *in utero*, e.g. mother in left lateral position, expedite delivery
• ensuring that all birth attendants are trained in basic life support
• good communication between maternity and neonatal teams
• ensuring that a person with advanced resuscitation skills is available for high-risk deliveries or where there is an anticipated problem (see Table 5.5)

Assessment of the infant at birth

Traditionally, Apgar scores (see Table 5.3) have been used to assess a baby's condition at birth, 1 min and 5 min. Unfortunately the Apgar score has limited prognostic significance and is difficult to assess once medical intervention has started. Many infants can be successfully resuscitated despite an Apgar score of 0 at birth, and may sustain no long-term neurological damage.

In view of the subjective nature of the Apgar score it is considered more appropriate to assess the infant's condition in terms of heart rate, breathing, colour and tone. These assessments can be made at birth at regular intervals during resuscitation (see Table 5.6).

Stabilization at birth

Most babies, even those from a high-risk pregnancy, are born in good condition and do not need active resuscitation. Attendants should dry the baby and

Table 5.4 An approach to the aetiology of perinatal hypoxia–ischaemia

Cause	Example	Major effect on fetus/newborn
Antenatal		
Chronic placental insufficiency	PET Severe IUGR Maternal diabetes with vasculopathy	Growth restriction and reduced glycogen stores leads to poor tolerance of physiological intrapartum hypoxia or pathological asphyxia
Acute placental failure	Placental abruption Maternal cardiac arrest	Hypoxia, acidosis
Haemorrhage	Placenta previa Vasa previa (cord runs through membranes) Fetomaternal haemrrorhage	Hypovolaemia, shock, poor oxygen delivery
Uterine	Hyperstimulation of the uterus (oxytocin) Uterine rupture (previous caesarian section)	Hypoxia and acidosis
Umbilical cord	Cord prolapse Cord tight around neck (rare) True knot in cord	Interruption of blood supply (hypoxia and ischaemia)
Infection	Prolonged PROM Chorioamnionitis Group B streptococcal infection Maternal H1N1 influenza infection	Does not cause asphyxia but may render fetus vulnerable to further insult and presentation may mimic asphyxia
Postmaturity	Placental deterioration Passage of meconium	Hypoxia–ischaemia and poor tolerance of labour Meconium aspiration and PPHN
Delivery		
Mechanical	Breech with head entrapment Shoulder dystocia	Hypoxia ± birth trauma
Prolonged 2nd stage	Failure to recognize and manage abnormal lie/ presentation/ cephalo-pelvic disproportion	Hypoxia due to delayed delivery
Trauma	Precipitant delivery Difficult instrumental delivery	Intracranial haemorrhage mimics HIE Cervical cord injury presenting as HIE
Postnatal		
Complications of out-of-hospital delivery (especially if concealed pregnancy)	Failure to maintain open airway or deliberate smothering (very rare) Cold environment Failure of normal adaptation at birth	Hypoxia Extreme hypothermia Hypoglycaemia and PPHN
Acute postnatal collapse	Accidental overlaying Airway obstruction whilst at breast	Hypoxia
Iatrogenic	Accidental oesophageal intubation Inappropriate "blind" suction Excessive ventilation Poorly clamped cord	Hypoxia Vagal bradycardia Pneumothorax – hypoxia Haemorrhage – ischaemia

Table 5.5 Situations where advanced resuscitation may be needed and should be anticipated

High-risk pregnancy	Rhesus isoimmunization Moderate to severe pre-eclampsia Severe IUGR Insulin-dependent diabetic Antepartum haemorrhage Prolonged rupture of the membranes
Abnormal labour	Fetal distress, prolapsed cord Deep transverse arrest Cephalopelvic disproportion
Abnormal delivery	Emergency caesarean section Heavy meconium staining of liquor Rotational forceps delivery
Abnormal presentation	Breech, face, brow, compound, shoulder
Abnormal gestation	Preterm delivery
Abnormal fetus	Severe oligo- or polyhydramnios Known congenital abnormality Multiple births

Table 5.6 Assessment during resuscitation

	Heart rate	Breathing	Colour	Tone	Action
Good condition	>100	Crying	Pink	Normal	Dry and give to mother
Moderate birth depression	<100	Some respiratory effort	Mild cyanosis	Reduced	Open airway, consider inflation breaths
Severe depression	<60 or absent	Gasping or no breathing	White	Floppy	Call for help, open airway and begin immediate resuscitation

wrap it in a warm towel, then make the assessments described above, while ensuring that the airway is open (head in neutral position). There is no place for routine suction of the nasopharynx as normal liquor and lung fluid does not cause airway obstruction. If the baby is breathing, pink, with good tone and a normal heart rate then he/she should be given to the mother to hold or placed on her chest for skin-to-skin contact. The baby should be observed carefully and his/her condition documented at 1 min and 5 min.

Link to *Nursing the Neonate*: Normal adaptation to the postnatal environment. Chapter 3, p. 48.

CLINICAL TIP: Skin-to-skin contact (kangaroo care) immediately after birth can promote successful breast feeding and, especially in developing countries, is an effective way to maintain normothermia.

Resuscitation

Preparation

If the need for resuscitation is anticipated (see Table 5.5) the right team should be assembled. You should prepare for delivery by:
- introducing yourself to the parents
- rapid review of the history (discussion with midwife or review of notes) including any analgesia given
- switching on the overhead radiant warmer and checking equipment (see Box 5.3)

Initial assessment

The baby should be placed on the Resuscitaire and quickly dried and wrapped in warm towels, taking care to keep the head in the neutral position. In very preterm babies thermoregulation is particularly important and the baby should be placed (without drying) into a plastic bag or wrap under a radiant heater (see Fig. 24.2, Chapter 24).

The need for resuscitation should be determined by a rapid assessment of heart rate, breathing, colour and tone. Heart rate can be established by listening at the apex or by palpating umbilical pulsations. If resuscitation is required, a standard algorithm should be followed (see Fig. 5.2).

Establishing an open airway

The head should be kept in the neutral position. In a floppy baby there may be airway occlusion due to the tongue dropping back and the posterior pharyngeal wall flopping forwards, which is best treated by jaw thrust or two-person airway control, or use of an oropharyngeal airway. Occasionally, however, failure to establish adequate breathing movement in the newborn is due to obstruction of the airway with mucus, blood or meconium. The baby should then receive pharyngeal suction **under direct vision** with a large-bore suction catheter (size 12 or larger) or a paediatric Yankauer sucker. If there has been heavy meconium staining of the liquor and the baby is floppy, the pharynx should be suctioned under laryngoscopic vision. There is

Box 5.3 Resuscitation equipment on Resuscitaire

- Warm dry towels
- Plastic bag/wrap (preterm <32 weeks)
- Pressure-limited inflation device or self-inflating bag
- Gas supply (preferably air–oxygen mix)
- Suitably sized masks
- Large-bore (Yankauer) suction device
- Oropharyngeal (Guedel) airways
- Appropriate sized laryngoscope with bright light
- Endotracheal tubes (2.5–4 mm) and fixators
- CO_2 detector and stethoscope
- Drugs: adrenaline (1:10 000), sodium bicarbonate (4.2%), glucose (10%)

no role for routine suction of the baby's nasopharynx at the perineum.

> CLINICAL TIP: The relatively large occiput in babies tends to make the head flex forwards. Placing a folded towel under the baby's shoulders will help keep the head in the neutral position, keeping the airway open.

Resuscitation of the infant with moderate depression

If a baby does not breathe at birth, despite the airway being open, then the baby should be given five inflation breaths (2–3 s) at a pressure of 30 cmH_2O (25 cmH_2O in a preterm baby). A response (heart rate increasing or chest movement) should be seen by the fourth or fifth breath. If neither happens, assume that the airway is not open (reposition and consider use of jaw thrust or oropharyngeal airway). After reassessment, if the baby is responding, ventilation breaths at lower pressure may be necessary for a while until the baby is breathing regularly (reassess every 30 s).

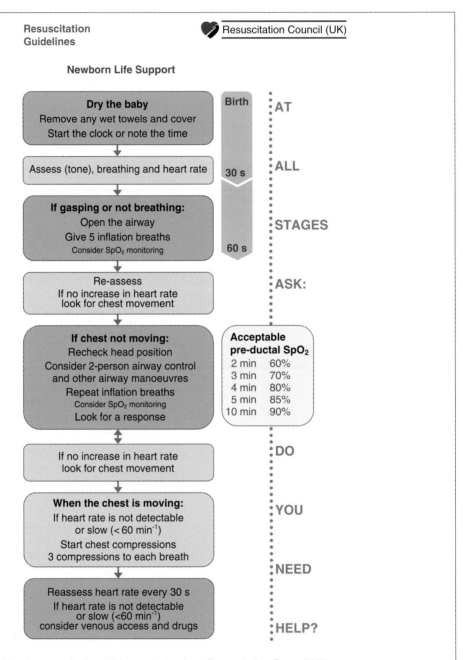

Figure 5.2 Algorithm for resuscitation. With permission from Resuscitation Council UK.

Ventilation

All medical, midwifery and nursing staff who work in a delivery suite should be proficient in providing basic lung inflation with either a pressure-regulated T-piece/mask circuit or bag–valve–mask. The technique of mask ventilation is described in Chapter 29. A soft face mask should be selected which should fit snugly around the bridge of the nose and chin, and not obstruct the nares or protrude over the orbits or the lower jaw. The jaw should be held forward as the operator ventilates at a rate of about 30 breaths/min. The chest should be observed for adequate inflation. Heart rate and colour should be continuously reassessed. The T-piece circuits allow a set pressure (including PEEP) to be delivered, whereas self-inflating bags have a blow-off valve (usually at $40\,cmH_2O$). Transiently the latter can reach very high pressures if the bag is squeezed very quickly. If chest rise is unsatisfactory, a two-handed jaw thrust or pharyngeal airway may be needed. It should be possible to ventilate all infants adequately until more experienced help arrives (see Fig. 5.3).

There is now evidence that for term babies, resuscitation in room air (21% oxygen) is preferable to resuscitation in 100% oxygen. If the baby is not responding despite good chest movement then the oxygen concentration should be increased. A portable oxygen saturation monitor can help guide the amount of oxygen required and can also provide an accurate continuous reading of the pulse. Note that

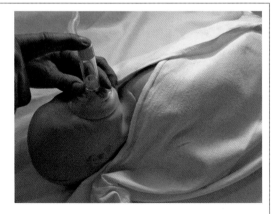

Figure 5.3 Mask inflation with the head in the neutral position.

babies can take up to 10 min to achieve saturations greater than 90% (see Fig 5.2)

Intubation and positive-pressure ventilation

If good basic airway skills are employed, intubation will rarely be required (<1 in 500 normal deliveries). However, it is indicated in prolonged resuscitation to stabilize the airway (see Fig 5.2) and may be undertaken electively for conditions such as prematurity (to deliver surfactant) or diaphragmatic hernia (to avoid distension of the bowel). Emergency intubation should be orotracheal with an appropriately sized tube (usually 3.5 mm for a term baby). Once inserted the correct tube position should be confirmed by seeing symmetrical chest rise, listening for equal air entry (at the axillae) and for an absence of breath sounds over the stomach. If there is any doubt about the tube being in the trachea this can be quickly confirmed by using a colour-change CO_2 detector in the circuit. Intubation is described in detail in Chapter 29.

External cardiac massage

If the baby has a heart rate less than 60/min despite adequate ventilation (i.e. visible chest rise), then external cardiac massage must be commenced. Both hands are placed around the infant's chest with the fingers on the back and the thumbs over the mid-sternum, and the thumbs are pressed down at a rate of 100/min. The compressions should be alternated with effective ventilation breaths at a rate of three compressions for each breath.

Drugs in resuscitation

If basic life support is undertaken promptly and effectively then drugs are rarely necessary. However they are occasionally needed in the most severely asphyxiated newborn infants, when cardiopulmonary resuscitation (CPR) has not led to an increase in heart rate. These drugs should be given centrally via an umbilical venous catheter followed by a flush of 0.9% saline (Box 5.4). The order in which they should be given is not proven. If drugs are genuinely

---

Box 5.4 Drugs used in resuscitation

- *Adrenaline:* as IV bolus. It may also be effective if given via an endotracheal tube but there is no trial evidence to support this.
- *Sodium bicarbonate* (4.2%) is given via a central vein to reverse myocardial acidosis.
- *Glucose* (10%): Following prolonged asphyxia the baby may be hypoglycaemic. If blood can be obtained direct near patient testing is available. Otherwise 10% glucose may be given empirically.
- *Naloxone:* This should only be administered once effective ventilation is being given. It is indicated to reverse severe respiratory depression secondary to recent maternal opiate administration, although prolonged ventilation is also acceptable. If naloxone is indicated, a full dose should be given IM and the baby must be monitored for several hours afterwards. Naloxone should not be given without evidence of neonatal opiate depression and must not be given to the baby of an opiate-dependent mother as this may cause acute and severe withdrawal seizures.

---

required despite good CPR then the outlook is very likely to be poor.

Postnatal collapse

Very occasionally babies are found in a collapsed state in the hours or days after birth. There are many causes for this including undiagnosed sepsis, metabolic disorders or duct-dependent congenital heart disease. As many as a third may have suffered accidental airway occlusion. The approach to resuscitation is essentially the same as that at birth.

When to stop resuscitation

As mentioned above, babies born apparently dead can be resuscitated and survive without significant neurodevelopmental sequelae. Vigorous resuscitation should be attempted on all infants who were believed to be alive immediately prior to delivery. Infants whose Apgar score remains zero at 1 and 5 min, but who survive following vigorous resuscitation, either subsequently die (80%) or are moderately to severely disabled. Most recent published data suggest that if there is no cardiac output after 10 min of witnessed effective life support then resuscitation should be abandoned.

The return of breathing is a much less robust prognostic sign. One study shows that, in infants who did not breathe for more than 20 min, about two thirds of survivors are without major handicap.

There are other possible reasons for a delay in establishing spontaneous respiration; we advise that if there is doubt as to whether to continue resuscitation, and if a senior experienced doctor is not available, the baby should be taken to the neonatal unit for further care until more detailed assessment can be undertaken.

'Brain death' cannot be diagnosed in the neonatal period. Organ donation is therefore not possible, other than heart valves. A condition referred to as 'irreversible brain injury' is a better concept. In many cases those babies with a massive brain insult sufficient to cause permanent, severe brain damage can be identified within the first 24 h of life.

Postresuscitation care of the asphyxiated infant

The sequelae of birth asphyxia may be divided into early and late.

Early sequelae

The intensive care management of early sequelae (multiorgan failure) is briefly outlined in Box 5.5.

Late sequelae

The long-term outlook depends on the severity of the asphyxia. The clinical severity of hypoxic–ischaemic encephalopathy (HIE) is a better predic-

Box 5.5 The intensive care management of early sequelae

1 **Metabolic**:
- Metabolic acidosis: correct with sodium bicarbonate
- Hypoglycaemia, due to exhausted glycogen stores: commence 10% glucose infusion
- Inappropriate antidiuretic hormone secretion (SIADH): consider fluid restriction

2 **Respiratory**:
- RDS: acidosis/hypoxia in the perinatal period increases the severity of RDS, support respiration and consider surfactant if preterm
- Transient tachypnoea of the newborn: support respiration
- Meconium aspiration syndrome secondary to *in utero* aspiration (Chapter 13); may require ventilation or high-frequency oscillatory ventilation (HFOV)

3 **Cardiac**:
- Myocardial ischaemia, with characteristic ECG changes (flat or inverted T waves, ST segment depression, abnormal Q waves): echocardiography may show a poorly contracting myocardium; treat hypotension with inotropes. Avoid fluid overload
- Persistent pulmonary hypertension of the newborn (PPHN): supportive care ± nitric oxide (see Chapter 16)
- Patency of ductus arteriosus: monitor and treat if significant (see Chapter 16)

4 **Renal impairment** (see Chapter 18): 20% of asphyxiated infants develop significant renal compromise and almost all will demonstrate oliguria, proteinuria, haematuria and elevated serum creatinine secondary to acute tubular necrosis; careful fluid management and careful monitoring of gentamicin.

5 **Haematological**: disseminated intravascular coagulation (see Chapter 20) or other coagulopathy may occur; correct with FFP, vitamin K and platelets as appropriate

6 **Gastrointestinal**: necrotizing enterocolitis (Chapter 17) may occur following a prolonged hypoxic insult; delay enteral feeding and encourage expression of breast milk

7 **Central nervous system**: The presence of coma, abnormal reflexes and sometimes onset of seizures at 6–12 h of age following an acute intrapartum asphyxial insult suggest hypoxic–ischaemic encephalopathy (HIE). This can usually be confirmed by CFM/EEG. There is now clear evidence supporting treatment of moderate to severe HIE with early therapeutic hypothermia (33.5°C for 72 h) to reduce secondary cytotoxic brain injury. Following acute intrapartum asphyxia, those infants who meet certain criteria (see Box 5.6) should commence passive cooling immediately after resuscitation. This can be achieved by switching off the overhead heater and leaving the baby exposed. Temperature must be monitored continuously with a low-reading rectal thermometer. Avoidance of hyperthermia is also crucial. If encephalopathy is confirmed then active cooling can commence. The management of HIE is discussed in detail in Chapter 22.

Box 5.6 Criteria for early passive cooling

- Evidence of asphyxial insult during labour
- pH <7.0 or base excess >−16
- Need for ongoing resuscitation at 10 min
- Abnormal neurology suggestive of encephalopathy

tor of long-term outcome than Apgar scores or cord blood arterial pH. Neuroimaging and EEG in the first days of life can give important prognostic information. An isoelectric or severely abnormal EEG/cerebral function monitoring at 6 h, together with a repeat 'flat' EEG and abnormal cerebral artery Doppler at 24 h, will predict a severe adverse outcome, which can be described to parents as representing 'irreversible brain injury'.

SUMMARY

Most babies are born healthy. Most can cope with the physiological stress of even a prolonged labour by utilizing alternative fuels and diverting blood to vital organs. When these mechanisms are exhausted the baby may suffer asphyxial damage to a variety of organs, most importantly the brain. For the first time, therapeutic hypothermia offers the prospect of an effective rescue therapy.

Normal transition after birth, and avoidance of further complications, can be facilitated by stabilization and resuscitation where necessary. Honest communication between perinatal teams and the parents is vital to ensure an accurate understanding of the likely prognosis for the infant and to explain the aetiology of any insult.

Now visit **www.essentialneonatalmed.com** to test yourself on this chapter.

CHAPTER 6
Examination of the newborn

Key topics

Introduction

The birth of a baby is a time of great excitement and sometimes trepidation. The parents will always want to know the sex of the baby and be reassured that 'everything is OK'. Most mothers will carefully scrutinize their newborn baby and will sometimes be anxious about minor features that they discover. Major congenital anomalies will often be obvious to the parents or the midwife and may need immediate explanation. Careful examination of the newborn by a trained professional is also an opportunity to pick up abnormalities before they are symptomatic and to discuss general concerns with the baby's parents.

Essential Neonatal Medicine, Fifth Edition. Sunil Sinha, Lawrence Miall, Luke Jardine.
© 2012 John Wiley & Sons, Ltd. Published 2012 by John Wiley & Sons, Ltd.

The newborn examination as a screening test

In most developed countries newborn babies are formally examined soon after birth. In the UK this occurs within the first 72 hours and again by the family doctor or health visitor at 6–8 weeks of age. The purpose of these examinations is partly to reassure parents about any minor abnormalities, but also to detect anomalies which may cause significant harm if left undetected. The conditions for which the newborn examination acts as a 'screening test' are

- developmental dysplasia of the hips (DDH)
- congenital heart disease (CHD)
- congenital cataract
- undescended testes (in males)

In the UK these four conditions are now part of the national newborn screening programme, along with newborn blood spot screening and newborn hearing screening.

Who should perform the newborn examination?

Historically the newborn examination was done in hospital, often by the most junior members of the paediatric team. All newborns are examined soon after birth by the attending midwife to check there is no major congenital anomaly and to establish the sex of the baby. The formal first newborn examination can be done by a variety of professionals – midwives, advanced nurse practitioners, paediatricians or neonatal doctors. With early discharge home it is increasingly done by community midwives or general practitioners. There is evidence that trained practitioners who specialize in newborn examination are better than very junior paediatric doctors at detecting anomalies and also offer a more holistic approach, addressing parents' concerns about feeding, sleeping and general well-being.

Link to *Nursing the Neonate*: Congenital conditions. Chapter 10, pp. 152–171.

CLINICAL TIP: It is important to realize that because the circulation is still in transition, an examination on day 1 may not be able to detect certain conditions, especially duct-dependent heart defects and left-to-right heart shunts. For this reason in the UK and in Australia a second check is performed in the community at 6 weeks of age. This can also address feeding and growth and any parenting concerns.

Approach to the newborn examination

Before examining, review any relevant family or obstetric history, including any abnormalities on antenatal ultrasound scan. The mother should be present during the examination and you should ask if she has any concerns about the baby. After careful hand washing, the baby should be undressed completely and examined on a warm surface ideally with an overhead heater. It is easiest to approach the examination in a structured 'head to toe' manner (see Fig 6.1), but some elements may need to be performed opportunistically (e.g. fundoscopy while the eyes are open, auscultation while the baby is quiet). The examination should never interrupt breastfeeding.

Growth measurement

- The **birthweight** and **head circumference** should be noted and plotted on a standard growth chart appropriate to the infant's gestational age and sex. The maximum occipito-frontal circumference (OFC) is recorded to the nearest millimetre after three readings.
- **Length:** the crown–heel measurement is recorded; this is only reliable if performed on a neonatal measuring board (e.g. Harpenden neonatometer), which requires two people: one to secure the infant's head at the top of the board and a second to extend the legs so that the foot board firmly touches the infant's soles. For this reason this is not usually part of the routine newborn examination, but should be checked if a skeletal dysplasia is suspected.

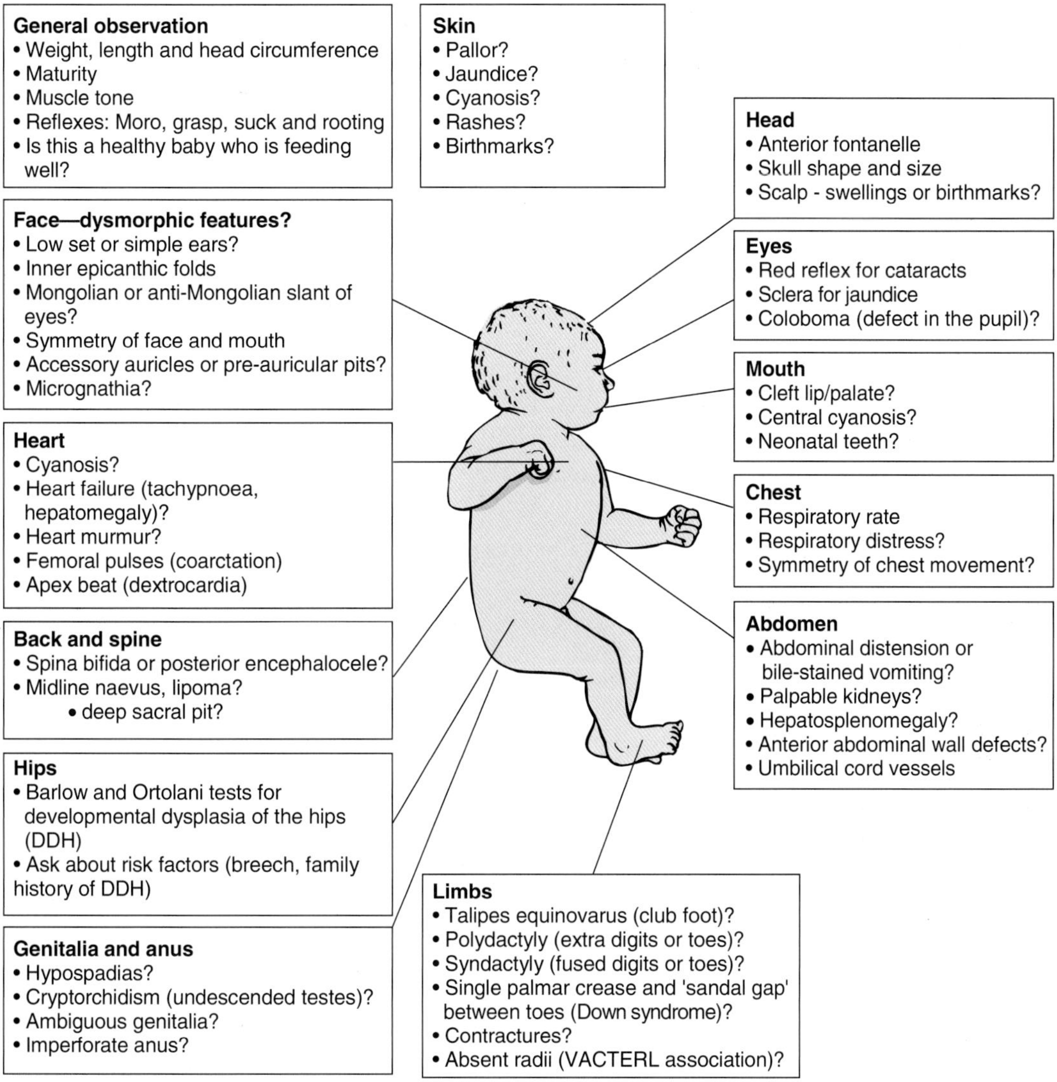

General observation
- Weight, length and head circumference
- Maturity
- Muscle tone
- Reflexes: Moro, grasp, suck and rooting
- Is this a healthy baby who is feeding well?

Skin
- Pallor?
- Jaundice?
- Cyanosis?
- Rashes?
- Birthmarks?

Head
- Anterior fontanelle
- Skull shape and size
- Scalp - swellings or birthmarks?

Face—dysmorphic features?
- Low set or simple ears?
- Inner epicanthic folds
- Mongolian or anti-Mongolian slant of eyes?
- Symmetry of face and mouth
- Accessory auricles or pre-auricular pits?
- Micrognathia?

Eyes
- Red reflex for cataracts
- Sclera for jaundice
- Coloboma (defect in the pupil)?

Mouth
- Cleft lip/palate?
- Central cyanosis?
- Neonatal teeth?

Heart
- Cyanosis?
- Heart failure (tachypnoea, hepatomegaly)?
- Heart murmur?
- Femoral pulses (coarctation)
- Apex beat (dextrocardia)

Chest
- Respiratory rate
- Respiratory distress?
- Symmetry of chest movement?

Abdomen
- Abdominal distension or bile-stained vomiting?
- Palpable kidneys?
- Hepatosplenomegaly?
- Anterior abdominal wall defects?
- Umbilical cord vessels

Back and spine
- Spina bifida or posterior encephalocele?
- Midline naevus, lipoma?
  - deep sacral pit?

Hips
- Barlow and Ortolani tests for developmental dysplasia of the hips (DDH)
- Ask about risk factors (breech, family history of DDH)

Genitalia and anus
- Hypospadias?
- Cryptorchidism (undescended testes)?
- Ambiguous genitalia?
- Imperforate anus?

Limbs
- Talipes equinovarus (club foot)?
- Polydactyly (extra digits or toes)?
- Syndactyly (fused digits or toes)?
- Single palmar crease and 'sandal gap' between toes (Down syndrome)?
- Contractures?
- Absent radii (VACTERL association)?

Figure 6.1 Head to toe examination sequence. From Miall, L. The Newborn Examination. Paediatrics at a Glance, 3rd ed., 2009. Wiley-Blackwell.

CLINICAL TIP: Measuring the head circumference can sometimes upset a baby. It may be worth leaving this until the end of the examination.

General appearance

Colour

The infant should be uniformly pink, but acrocyanosis (blueness of the hands and feet) is not abnormal. Central cyanosis, pallor, jaundice, plethora, bruises and petechial haemorrhages are abnormal and should be investigated further.

Posture

At term the normal position is with the hips abducted and partially flexed, the knees flexed, and the arms adducted and flexed at the elbow. Limited movement, exaggerated or asymmetrical movements, hypotonia or stiffness must be noted (see below).

Skin appearance

This varies with gestation; lanugo hair and relatively red skin in preterms and mild cracking and peeling in post-mature babies. Abnormal appearances, rashes, pigmentation and naevi are described on page 64. African and Asian babies may show little generalized pigmentation at birth, except for the genitalia.

Head and neck

Face

There are many recognizable patterns of abnormalities based on facial features. A dysmorphology database or reference book can be useful. Many are rare, but chromosomal disorders such as trisomy 21, 18 and 13 should be recognized (see Chapter 8). In addition, the following are often obvious: fetal alcohol syndrome (see Fig. 4.2, p. 29), Crouzon syndrome, Treacher–Collins syndrome and Potter's syndrome. Always compare with the parents' facial appearance. The shape of the face should be assessed from the front and the side.

Cry

This should be vigorous, but it should be possible to console the infant by cuddling. A cry that is weak, high-pitched or hoarse is abnormal. A cat-like cry, with microcephaly and hypotonia, is suggestive of cri-du-chat (5p-) syndrome.

Skull shape

• **Moulding** (elongated skull shape with overlapping skull bones) and **caput succedaneum** (oedematous thickening of the scalp due to passage through the birth canal) are normal and disappear within 2–3 days.
• **Plagiocephaly** (parallelogram head) is usually seen as a flattening of the occipital region on one side. It is thought to be due to the position the infant has been lying in *in utero* and has no pathological significance. It usually improves with age. Plagiocephaly seen in older infants suggests torticollis (see below). Advice on positioning and physiotherapy can help.
• **Scaphocephaly** (long head with flattened temporo-parietal regions) occurs commonly in premature infants and becomes less obvious with age. It can rarely be due to sagittal synostosis (Fig. 6.2).
• **Cephalhaematoma** occurs when bleeding over the outer surface of a skull bone elevates the periosteum, causing a soft fluctuant swelling confined to the limits of the bone (see Fig. 7.2, p. 72). It may be bilateral.
• **Fontanelles:** the anterior and posterior fontanelles are very variable in size and are normally soft and flat. Visible pulsation of the anterior fontanelle is normal. Bulging of the fontanelle may be due to raised intracranial pressure and is always abnormal. A large fontanelle is seen in hypothyroidism, severe IUGR and Down's syndrome. Separated sutures in

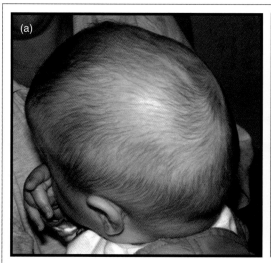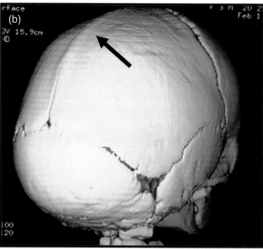

Figure 6.2 Ridged sagittal suture (3D CT scan shows sagittal synostosis).

the presence of a large OFC should raise suspicion of hydrocephalus.

• **Craniosynostosis:** this term refers to the (rare) premature fusion of one or more of the skull bones. Any bones may be affected, but the sagittal suture is most commonly involved. Facial bones may be affected and cause dysmorphism, such as is seen in Crouzon's syndrome. On examination of the head, the anterior fontanelle is usually small and the suture is ridged on palpation (Fig. 6.2). Craniosynostosis causes abnormal head growth, the pattern depending on the affected suture. Radiography or CT scanning will confirm the synostosis.

• **Craniotabes (ping-pong ball skull)** refers to the softening of the skull bones, and with pressure the skull may be momentarily indented before springing out again. It is more common in preterm infants but also occurs in full-term babies. It usually has no significance, but congenital rickets, osteogenesis imperfecta or congenital hypophosphatasia may cause craniotabes.

Eyes (see also Chapter 23)

Site

The position of the eyes should be noted. If they are too far apart (hypertelorism) or too close together,

(hypotelorism), this may be part of a generalized syndrome. Short palpebral fissures (eye openings) are a feature of fetal alcohol syndrome. Prominent epicanthic folds may be familial or seen in trisomy 21.

Conjunctiva

This is usually clear, but subconjunctival haemorrhages are not uncommon in otherwise normal infants. Jaundice may be visible first in the sclera. **Purulent conjunctivitis** is a serious symptom and infection (e.g. gonococcus, chlamydia) must be excluded. Excessive lacrimation may be associated with a blocked nasolacrimal duct.

Cornea, iris and pupil

The cornea should be clear and a red reflex elicited using an ophthalmoscope. The pupils should constrict to light. A dark shape or 'oil-drops' across the red reflex suggests a cataract and needs prompt referral to ophthalmology. A white reflex can be the only sign of congenital retinoblastoma. A keyhole-shaped pupil (coloboma) needs further investigation. Asian babies may have a pale appearance to the red reflex. In preterm babies the presence of the tunica vasculosa lentis (a network of capillaries in the lens) may give a streaked appearance to the red reflex.

CLINICAL TIP: Persuading a baby to open his/her eyes can be difficult. Be opportunistic and perform this test immediately if they are already open. Cradling the baby's head in your hand and talking to the baby may make them open their eyes. Hold the ophthalmoscope to your own eye and at a distance from the baby's face to get the red reflex. Never force the baby's eyes open.

Eyelids

Mild lid oedema may be present following a long labour, particularly in a face or brow presentation. Colobomas or clefts of the eyelid are rare.

Ears

Position

The top of the pinna should be at or above a horizontal line from the inner and outer canthi of the eye. Low-set ears are seen in a variety of conditions, including Potter's syndrome.

Shape

There is a wide familial variation. Very simple, floppy ears are seen in trisomy 21. Extreme 'bat ears' can be improved by taping down in the neonatal period but this is controversial. Check there is a patent auditory meatus.

Preauricular skin tags or sinuses are common. The tags should not be tied off, but referred to a plastic surgeon. If multiple, consider Goldenhar syndrome (hemifacial microsomia). Ear malformation may be part of Treacher–Collins syndrome.

Nose

Patency

Choanal atresia should be suspected if the baby has respiratory distress which improves with crying (when the mouth is open). It can be excluded by gently passing a feeding catheter through both nostrils. Atresias may be bilateral or, more commonly, unilateral, and may be membranous or bony. Consider CHARGE syndrome.

Mouth

Lips

Unilateral or bilateral cleft lip is a common congenital abnormality (1/1000 births). An absent philtrum (groove in the upper lip) and thin lips are seen in **fetal alcohol syndrome** (see Fig. 4.2, p. 29). 'Sucking blisters' may occasionally be seen on the lips.

Palate

- **Epstein's pearls** (small inclusion cysts in the midline of the hard palate) are normal and eventually disappear.
- **Cleft palate:** Use a torch to examine the mouth for cleft palate, bifid uvula or high arched palate. A submucosal cleft palate can only be diagnosed by inserting a clean finger into the mouth to feel for a mucous membrane-covered bony cleft. Symptoms of cleft palate include difficult feeding and milk coming down the nose.

Tongue

If the tongue is large and protruding consider hypothyroidism (see Chapter 21), Down's syndrome (usually accompanied by a small mouth); and Beckwith–Wiedemann syndrome. **Tongue tie**, due to a short frenulum, should not be cut unless causing severe feeding difficulties and rarely causes speech problems.

Primitive reflexes

- **Suck and gag reflex:** These should be present from 34–35 weeks' gestation and fully developed by term. It is always abnormal when absent after this age.
- **Rooting reflex:** as the cheek is touched the head turns to the stimulus and mouthing movements commence.

Jaw

Micrognathia (small, underdeveloped jaw) is seen in a variety of syndromes including Pierre Robin syndrome (see Chapter 14) sometimes with cleft palate. Severe micrognathia can cause obstructive apnoea due to tongue prolapse and occasionally needs treatment with a nasopharyngeal airway or rarely a tracheostomy (see Fig. 6.3)

Teeth

Natal teeth, mostly lower incisors, are not uncommon and if loose should be removed to prevent aspiration.

Mucous membranes

White patches suggest **candidiasis**, which needs to be distinguished from milk curd. Bluish mucous gland retention cysts on the floor of the mouth (ranulae) usually require no treatment.

Saliva

Drooling suggests an inability to swallow. Oesophageal atresia, or a neuromuscular disorder, should be excluded.

Neck

- **Sternomastoid tumour:** torticollis or limitation of lateral rotation, suggests shortening of the sternomastoid muscle due to haemorrhage. Sternomastoid 'tumour' occurs in the middle third of that muscle and is best treated with physiotherapy. The term 'tumour' is best avoided when talking to parents as it is confused with malignancy.
- **Turner's syndrome** and **Down's syndrome** (see Chapter 8) are associated with redundant skin at the back of the neck. A low hairline is seen in Turner's syndrome.
- **Klippel–Feil syndrome** is associated with a short neck with limited movement. It is rare.
- **Cystic hygroma:** swelling of the side of the neck, which usually transilluminates brilliantly (Fig. 6.4). Branchial clefts may give rise to a branchial cyst, a branchial sinus or branchial fistula.
- Goitre may be present at birth and is always in the midline. Check thyroid function.

Chest

Respiratory

- The features of **respiratory distress** are tachypnoea (>60 breaths/min), retraction, cyanosis, grunting and flaring of the nostrils. Chest retractions (sternal, substernal, intercostal or subcostal) suggest pulmonary disease.
- **Stridor** (see Chapter 14) indicates upper airway obstruction. An inspiratory stridor implies extrathoracic obstruction, whereas biphasic noise implies intrathoracic obstruction. Other signs of upper airway obstruction include suprasternal retraction, croupy cough and a hoarse cry.
- **Breath sounds:** auscultate with the diaphragm of the stethoscope for symmetry of air entry and

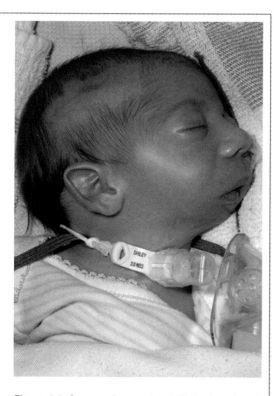

Figure 6.3 Severe micrognathia (with tracheostomy). Patient has cerebro-costo-mandibular syndrome.

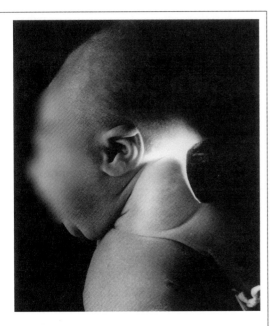

Figure 6.4 Cystic hygroma of the neck (transluminated).

adventitial breath sounds (if unilateral, suspect pneumothorax or diaphragmatic hernia). Crepitations may be normal in the first hours of life.

Shape and size

- The chest should be symmetrical in shape and move equally on respiration. A **small chest** occurs in infants with hypoplastic lungs and in a variety of rare syndromes, but is difficult to diagnose objectively.
- **Breast engorgement** occurs commonly in both sexes and is due to maternal oestrogen effect. 'Milk' may be secreted from the nipple and is not abnormal. Supernumerary nipples are a common finding.

CLINICAL TIP: More information can usually be obtained by observing the chest carefully than by listening with a stethoscope. Take time to watch the pattern of respiration and observe for intercostal recession and symmetry of chest rise.

Cardiovascular

Pulses

The normal heart rate varies between 90 and 160 beats per minute. The cause of tachycardia and bradycardia is discussed in Chapter 16. The brachial and femoral pulses should be palpable. Generally reduced peripheral pulses suggest hypoplastic left heart or cardiogenic shock, and absent femorals suggest coarctation of the aorta. Collapsing or bounding pulses are a feature of a patent ductus arteriosus (PDA)(see Chapter 16).

Apex beat

This should be localized to the fourth intercostal space in the midclavicular line. A right-sided apex beat may due to left-sided pneumothorax, left diaphragmatic hernia or true dextrocardia.

Auscultation

A triple or gallop rhythm is always abnormal. Systolic flow murmurs may be normal in the first 24 h of life. CHD is discussed in Chapter 16. Auscultation of a heart murmur in systole is ascribed as 1/6 → 6/6 according to intensity. Site of maximal intensity and any radiation should be noted. Even large septal defects may be inaudible in the first days as the right and left ventricular pressures are balanced and the shunt volume small.

Saturation screening

Many centres now use saturation monitoring to screen for duct-dependent CHD. A single postductal reading of less than 95% requires further evaluation of the baby. Respiratory disorders and sepsis can sometimes be coincidentally detected by this method. A drop in S_AO_2 from preductal (right arm) to postductal (either foot) of more than 3% is also suggestive of duct-dependent CHD.

CLINICAL TIP: The preductal oxygen saturation should never be lower than the postductal saturation. If it is, consider complex CHD such as transposition of the great arteries or double outlet right ventricle.

Abdomen

Distension suggests **intestinal obstruction** or an intra-abdominal mass. A scaphoid abdomen suggests diaphragmatic hernia. A lax abdominal wall with much redundant skin is seen in the 'prune-belly' syndrome. **Divarication** of the rectus muscles may produce a midline bulge in the abdominal wall. No treatment is required and the condition disappears with age.

Liver

This is normally palpable up to 1 cm below the costal margin. Hepatomegaly may be due to lung hyperinflation, cardiac failure, sepsis, hepatitis, intrauterine infection or haemolysis.

Spleen

The tip can be palpated in about a quarter of normal infants. Splenomegaly suggests infection (prenatal or postnatal) or haemolysis.

Kidney

May be palpable normally, particularly if the baby is relaxed. Moderate kidney enlargement may be due to hydronephrosis, dysplastic or cystic kidneys or rarely a Wilms' tumour. An adrenal mass (e.g. haemorrhage or neuroblastoma) is difficult to distinguish from a renal mass.

Anus

Check for normal position and patency. Imperforate anus is usually associated with a fistula into the vagina or in males, the bladder. An anterior anus may be associated with passage of 'toothpaste'-like stool due to sphincter dysfunction.

Umbilicus

Vessels

Normally two thick-walled arteries and a thin-walled vein are seen, surrounded by clear Wharton's jelly. In 1–2% of infants there is a single umbilical artery, sometimes with other congenital malforma-tions. If a single umbilical artery is found and the fetus has had a normal prenatal anomaly scan, no further investigations are required. If not, a renal ultrasound should be undertaken.

Stump

• The cord usually separates by 10 days, leaving a yellow or greenish eschar. A red flare around the base of the cord may reflect early sepsis and should be taken seriously. Discharge and cellulitis are also signs of infection. Discharge of urine or meconium from the stump suggests a patent urachus or patent omphalomesenteric duct, respectively. Exomphalos and gastroschisis are discussed in Chapter17.
• **Umbilical granuloma** (a small red fleshy swelling at the stump) is due to excessive granulation and *if symptomatic* can be treated by the application of a silver nitrate stick on one or two occasions. Protect the surrounding skin with barrier cream. Regular wiping with alcohol wipes can also act as an effective sclerosant. Most resolve spontaneously.
• **Umbilical hernia** at the base of the umbilicus is particularly common in African babies or those born prematurely, and usually develops in the first month or so of life. These hernias require no treatment, and usually regress by 18 months. They do not strangulate.

Genitalia

Establish that the baby has passed urine. This should occur within 24 hours of birth. If in doubt a 'urine bag' can be attached over the genitalia.

Testes

The testes are present in the scrotum in 98% of full-term male infants. Failure to descend by 6 weeks after term is abnormal. Ectopic testes or arrest in the line of normal descent should also be referred for surgical opinion. Retractile testes that come down when the baby is relaxed and warm do not need referral.

Penis and urethra

• The **foreskin** in infants is not retractable. The urethral meatus normally opens at the tip of the glans penis.

• **Hypospadias** occurs if the meatus opens on the ventral surface of the penis, and is most commonly glandular.

• **Epispadias** occurs when it opens on the dorsal surface of the penis. Advise against circumcision as the foreskin may be needed for reconstructive surgery.

Scrotum

• A **hydrocoele** transilluminates brilliantly. It may extend upwards along the spermatic cord. Most disappear spontaneously during the first year of life and require no treatment other than reassurance.

• **Inguinal hernia** rarely presents at birth but is common in premature infants due to a patent processus vaginalis. The scrotal swelling can usually be reduced. Surgery is required in all cases to prevent complications.

• **Testicular torsion:** a swollen, tender or red scrotum suggests either strangulated inguinal hernia or testicular torsion. Both require an urgent surgical opinion.

Pink nappies

Occasionally, urates may react with the urine in the newborn period, leaving a pinkish-red stain on the napkin that may be confused with haematuria. The is self-limiting and only occurs in the first few weeks of life.

Hymen

Hymenal skin tags are common in the female babies and are due to protrusion of redundant vaginal mucosa. No treatment is required and they usually regress spontaneously in a few weeks.

Vagina and vulva

• The size of the **labia majora** depends on gestational age, but by term they should completely cover the labia minora. In preterm or IUGR girls the labia minora and clitoris can appear very prominent.

• **Labial fusion** occurs in the adrenogenital syndrome, and **labial adhesions** are also not uncommonly seen in otherwise normal infants.

• **Mucoid vaginal discharge** occurs in most mature female infants shortly after birth. It is normal and may continue for 2–3 weeks. **Vaginal withdrawal bleeding** may occur in normal girls.

• **Hydrometrocolpos** describes a bulging imperforate hymen, caused by the accumulation of secretions.

Clitoris

This is variable in size. If large, consider adrenogenital syndrome, a maternal progesterone effect or an intersex state. Ambiguous genitalia are discussed in Chapter 21.

Back

It is essential to examine the back. This is best done by placing one hand over the baby's chest and one over the upper back and then turning the baby prone to rest on your hand and forearm. This 'ventral suspension' is also an opportunity to assess muscle tone.

Spine

Run your finger all the way down the spine, looking and feeling for any defects. Spina bifida is usually detected antenatally but any lump, hairy patch or naevus over the midline warrants a spinal ultrasound as these can be a marker of underlying spinal anomaly.

Scoliosis

Severe curvature of the spine (scoliosis) is usually due to hemivertebrae or failure of segmentation. It is often found incidentally on a radiograph. Orthopaedic consultation with regular follow-up is necessary. Congenital genitourinary malformation occurs in 20% of babies with congenital scoliosis and should be excluded by a renal ultrasound scan.

Sacrum

Sacral 'dimples' are very common. If they are shallow (i.e. you can clearly see the base by pulling the skin laterally on either side) then they do not need further investigation. If the natal cleft is deviated or there are any surface markings then arrange spinal ultrasound.

Extremities

This is a good point to assess movement, tone and primitive reflexes. The baby should be awake but settled in order to gain an accurate impression. A hungry, crying baby cannot be assessed accurately.

Posture

The posture depends on the gestational age (see 'Assessment of maturity', Chapter 11). A **hypotonic** baby will tend to be in the 'frog position' with reduced spontaneous movement. A **hypertonic** baby may be in a state of predominant flexion or extension. A baby with cerebral irritation may have extensor posturing with arching of the back, opisthotonus, scissoring of the legs, and thumbs tightly adducted in the cortical position.

Movements

The quality and quantity of spontaneous movements are observed. Absence or reduction of movements may occur in one limb only, two limbs on the same side of the body, or both legs. The absence of spontaneous movements is often suggestive of a systemically unwell baby and only very rarely a sign of a paralysed baby. Observe the quality of movements; are they smooth (normal) or jerky? Note any abnormal movements such as tremors, jitteriness or convulsions. Tremulousness or jitteriness must be distinguished from convulsions (see Chapter 22).

Assessment of tone

Limb tone is assessed by posture and resistance to passive movement. Gently flex, extend and rotate the limbs on each side. Compare the two sides of the body and the upper and lower limbs. The head must be in the midline to prevent eliciting the 'asymmetric tonic neck reflex' (see Chapter 22). **Hip adductor** tone is assessed by the hip angle when passively abducted. **Neck tone** is assessed with the arms held in traction and by observing the head

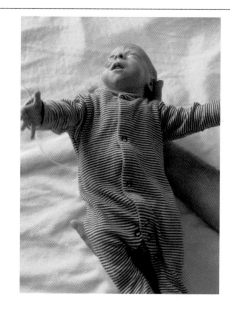

Figure 6.5 Eliciting the Moro reflex.

control when the baby is held in a sitting position. **Truncal tone** is assessed with the baby held in ventral suspension.

Primitive reflexes

- **Moro reflex:** elicited by placing one hand under the infant's shoulders and the other under his/her head and then suddenly dropping the head by several centimetres. A full response consists of abduction and extension of the arms, followed by adduction and flexion (Fig. 6.5). Asymmetry suggests a brachial plexus palsy or a bone injury (See Chapter 7).
- **Palmar grasp:** apply pressure to the palm of the hand, resulting in flexion of the fingers and a firm grasp. If traction is then applied the infant should lift his/her head off the bed so that head lag can be assessed.

Upper limbs

Assess movement, tone and reflexes as above. The fingers and palms should be examined for abnormalities. A single palmar crease may be present in

Down's syndrome but also in 15% of the normal population.

Fingers

There are a variety of common patterns of finger anomaly.
- **Clinodactyly:** a lateral curvature of the fifth finger which may be familial or associated with various syndromes.
- **Syndactyly:** fusion of the fingers – may be partial (webbing) or complete. Fusion of the third and fourth fingers can be associated with cardiac arrhythmias.
- **Polydactyly:** additional digits. These most often occur postaxially (on the ulnar aspect of fifth finger) and may or may not contain bone. They should be referred to plastic surgery for removal and not tied off. Preaxial polydactyly is associated with syndromes.
- **Cleft hand:** one, two or three central rays are missing, often leaving just a thumb and opposing digit. The term ectrodactyly or 'lobster claw hand' should no longer be used.
- **Symbrachydactyly:** Shortened or absent fingers, with preservation of the thumb. Sometimes the distal part of each finger is present just above the metacarpals.

Thumbs

Abnormal thumbs can be associated with a variety of haematological disorders:
- **TAR syndrome:** thrombocytopenia with absent radii
- **Aase's syndrome:** triphalangeal thumb and congenital anaemia
- **Fanconi's syndrome:** radial hypoplasia, pancytopenia
- **Diamond–Blackfan anaemia**

Lower limbs

Examine the legs and feet carefully, including the toes. Then complete the examination by checking for dislocatable or dislocated hips (see below). This is left to the end of the examination as it may cause the baby to become upset, although it should never cause pain.

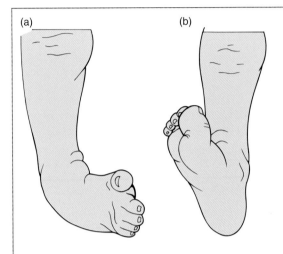

Figure 6.6 Talipes: talipes equinovarus (a) and talipes calcaneovalgus (b).

Feet

Lower limb abnormalities are common and are often associated with intrauterine compression due to oligohydramnios or neurological conditions leading to reduced fetal movement. They may vary from a mild postural problem to severe talipes.

Talipes equinovarus (clubfoot) occurs in 1/1000 births and is 10 times more common than talipes calcaneovalgus (see Fig. 6.6). When either is seen, other asociated congenital abnormalities (e.g. dislocation of the hip and myelomeningocele) should be sought. If the foot can be passively corrected to the position opposite the deformity, it is considered to be mild and requires only simple passive exercise treatment by a physiotherapist and the parents. More severe deformities will require physiotherapy, splinting, and very occasionally surgical correction. There is good evidence that serial stretching, casting and bracing (the Ponseti method) is as effective as surgery.

Toes

Polydactyly and syndactyly can occur in the toes. Syndactyly of the second and third toes is very common and often there is a familial history.

Knees

Genu recurvatum

This is rare (1 in 100,000). The knees are hyperextensible and can bend forwards. In severe cases there may be dislocation of the knee joint, and splinting may be necessary. The cause is multifactorial, with mechanical and genetic elements. Recurvatum at the knee sometimes exceeds 90°. A radiograph shows the tibia anterior to the femur.

Femoral retroversion

This is sometimes seen at follow-up of premature infants. It should be preventable by good developmental care and positioning (see Chapter 24). The child lies or stands with his/her legs externally rotated at 90° ('Charlie Chaplin' gait). This condition often causes distress to the parents but they should be strongly reassured as it rapidly corrects within a year of the child learning to walk. It is, however, important to exclude congenital dislocation of the hip as the cause of the external rotation.

Congenital abnormalities of the hips and limbs

Developmental dysplasia of the hip

Developmental dysplasia of the hip (DDH), previously known as congenital dislocation of the hip, is an important asymptomatic congenital condition that should be detectable during newborn examination. The consequences of missing DDH can be considerable. Hip dislocation occurs in 1–2/1000 newborns. The left hip is dislocated four times more commonly than the right, due to the fetal position. Risk factors for DDH are shown in Table 6.1.

Examination

Examination of the hip should start with observation for signs of established dislocation, such as unequal leg length and asymmetry of the thigh creases. The physical examination should be undertaken in two parts:

Table 6.1 Risk factors for developmental dysplasia of the hips

Risk factor	Comment
Familial history (polygenic inheritance)	DDH recurs in families at a rate of about 1/30
Breech presentation	10 times increased risk. Incidence of DDH in singleton breech delivery is 14%
Female sex	Female: male ratio is 6:1
Racial/cultural factors	Increased in Italy and in Inuit population Reduced in China and Africa
Neuromuscular disorders	Spina bifida Hypertonia (including cerebral palsy) Congenital hypotonia Congenital arthrogryposis
Trisomy 13, 18	
Multiple congenital anomalies	
Severe oligohydramnios	Due to lack of room for fetal movement

DDH, developmental dysplasia of the hips.

Ortolani's (reduction) test

This assesses whether the hip is already dislocated. With the baby relaxed on a firm surface, flex the hips and knees to 90°. Grasp the baby's thigh with the middle finger over the greater trochanter and lift it to bring the femoral head from its dislocated posterior position into alignment with the acetabulum. Simultaneously, gently abduct the thigh, lifting the femoral head over the posterior lip of the acetabulum. In a positive test the examiner senses reduction by feeling a 'clunk', and there is forwards movement of the head of the femur (Fig. 6.7).

Barlow's (dislocation) test

This test assesses whether the hip is dislocatable and is really a reversal of Ortolani's test. With one hand

(a)

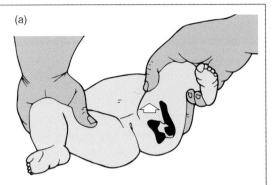

(b)

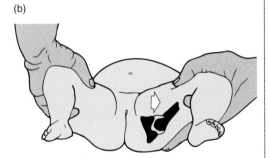

Figure 6.7 Ortolani's test. The hip cannot be abducted because of posterior dislocation of the femoral head. The hip is pulled upwards (a) and the head clunks into the acetabulum, permitting abduction (b).

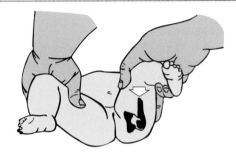

Figure 6.8 Barlow's test. The adducted hip is pushed downwards and laterally to see whether it is dislocatable.

stabilizing the pelvis, the other holds the baby's thigh and adducts it gently backwards and downwards. Dislocation is palpable as the femoral head slips over the posterior lip of the acetabulum (Fig. 6.8).

It is known that infants may have normal hips at birth that can dislocate some time later. For this reason, the hips should be examined at a 6–8 week assessment. Failure of the hip to abduct fully is a very significant sign. Shortening of the leg and asymmetrical skin creases may not be reliable clinical signs of a dislocated hip.

Following examination the hips should be described as:

• **Stable:** there is no abnormal movement of the joint. Both hips fully abduct.

• **Clicking:** the hips are stable but a 'click' is heard or felt during examination. This is probably normal if there is no excessive movement of the femoral head in the joint. Clicking occurs as a result of ligamentous laxity and is found in up to 10% of newborn infants.

• **Dislocatable:** the femoral head is in the joint (the hip can be fully abducted) but the hip dislocates posteriorly with Barlow's manoeuvre. This requires imaging and careful follow-up.

• **Dislocated:** the hip is out of joint at birth, with Ortolani's test abnormal. This requires imaging and treatment to relocate the femoral head in the acetabulum and keep it there. Without this, the acetabulum does not develop and a pseudo hip joint will be formed where the femoral head rubs against the pelvis.

Imaging

In the first 6 months of life ultrasound is the best modality. There is no place for radiographic examination for the assessment of hip dislocation until ossification occurs in the femur at about 4 months. Ultrasound clearly defines the hip anatomy and allows evaluation of the shape of the acetabulum. Routine ultrasound screening of the hips of all babies is not recommended in most countries as it leads to excessive splinting with the associated small risk of femoral head necrosis.

For when selective ultrasound examination is indicated, see Box 6.1

Box 6.1 Indications for selective ultrasound examination

- Clinical instability or highly suspicious examination
- Family history of DDH
- Breech presentation
- Associated lower limb abnormality (e.g. talipes, spina bifida)

Management

The principle is to keep the hip immobilized in an abducted position for 2–3 months to allow the acetabular rim to develop and the hip ligaments to strengthen. Several varieties of splint are used, including the Aberdeen and Von Rosen splints and the Pavlik harness. There is no place for treatment with 'double nappies'. After 3 months the splint may be removed and, if the hip is clinically stable, check radiographs are taken usually at 6 and 12 months of age. Fixed dislocations of the hip, failure to respond to treatment and late-diagnosed dislocated hips will require individual orthopaedic management. The success of treatment depends on accurate and early diagnosis of the condition.

Limb malformations

These can affect the arms or legs and be unilateral or bilateral. The main types are:
- **Amelia:** absence of one or more limbs
- **Ectromelia:** gross hypoplasia of one or more limbs
- **Phocomelia:** partial deficiency of the proximal segment with preservation of the distal parts (e.g. hands can appear to arise from the shoulder)
- **Hemimelia:** rudimentary formation of the distal part of a limb with normal proximal development
- **Amniotic band amputations:** these occur *in utero* and cause a linear amputation which does not follow a normal embryological developmental pattern
- **Absent radius:** This is seen in the VACTERL sequence and TAR syndrome (see Chapter 20) and leads to a curved forearm with radial deviation of the hand

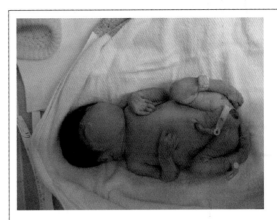

Figure 6.9 Arthrogryposis multiplex.

Arthrogryposis multiplex

This term describes multiple joint deformities involving more than one limb (Fig. 6.9). It is caused by restriction of joint movement *in utero* and there may be a variety of underlying causes:
- neuromuscular – congenital dystrophy, spinal muscular atrophy
- connective tissue disorders
- oligohydramnios
- bicornuate uterus
- genetic syndromes (<30%)

All require orthopaedic referral and intense physiotherapy. An underlying neuromuscular, connective tissue or genetic problem should be considered. Investigations are described in Chapter 22.

Neonatal dwarfism

Dwarfism may be proportional (the whole body is short but in proportion) or be due to skeletal dysplasia (disproportionate shortening of the limbs and trunk). Examples of proportional dwarfism syndromes include Russell–Silver, Cornelia de Lange, Conradi, Seckel's bird head, Cockayne, leprechaunism and progeria. These children are extremely small for gestational age (SGA) at birth.

Skeletal dysplasia

An underlying skeletal dysplasia should be suspected in any baby who is SGA with other congenital abnormalities and who has disproportionate shortening of the limbs and trunk.

Skeletal dysplasias may present simply as short stature or a disproportionate body, but a variety of other anomalies, such as hydrocephalus, craniostenosis, cleft lip and palate, polydactyly, syndactyly, dislocated hips and dysmorphic facial features, may coexist.

There are many classifications of the more than 100 distinct syndromes. The most commonly recognized syndromes in the newborn are:
• achondroplasia
• osteogenesis imperfecta types I–V
• asphyxiating thoracic dystrophy
• thanatophoric dwarf (Fig. 6.10)
• osteopetrosis (marble bone disease)
• diastrophic dwarfism
• Ellis–van Creveld syndrome.

Achondroplasia

This is the most common skeletal dysplasia with short limbs. The proximal segment (i.e. humerus and femur) is more involved than the lower seg-

ments (i.e. radius and ulna or tibia and fibula). The head is typically enlarged, the trunk appears normal. It is inherited as an autosomal dominant trait but approximately 80% are new mutations.

Osteogenesis imperfecta

This is an inherited connective tissue disorder. In its milder form, affected infants have increased susceptibility to fracture and hearing loss in later childhood, but at its most severe it is lethal and perinatal death is common. These babies often have blue sclerae and their bones fracture *in utero*, presenting at birth with short, deformed limbs. Mild forms may respond to treatment with bisphosphonates.

Skin disorders

Cutaneous lesions are present at birth in 8% of newborn infants. They are usually immediately obvious and may cause considerable concern. Sometimes they are part of a neurocutaneous syndrome where they may be skin markers of neurological disorders. Examples include Sturge–Weber syndrome, neurofibromatosis and incontinentia pigmenti.
• Cutaneous lesions in the newborn can be classified in the following major groups:
  • vascular birthmarks
  • epidermal naevi
  • pigmented birthmarks
  • ichthyotic disorders
  • blistering and bullous disorders
  • miscellaneous.

Vascular birthmarks

Vascular birthmarks can be either haemangiomas (neoplastic proliferation of vascular endothelium) or vascular malformations (abnormally sited or connected capillaries, veins or arteries). Older descriptive terminology, such as 'cavernous', 'strawberry' and 'naevus flammeus' is confusing and should be avoided.

Haemangiomas

These vascular proliferation tumours are characterized by rapid endothelial growth followed by slow

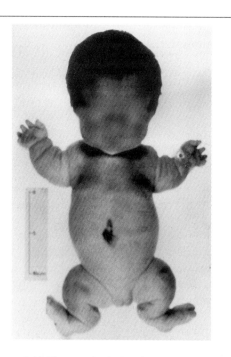

Figure 6.10 Thanatophoric dwarf.

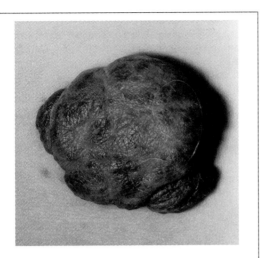

Figure 6.11 Vascular haemangioma.

involution. Approximately 30% are present at birth as a blanched or telangiectatic patch. The majority appear during the first month, and grow rapidly over the next 5 months (Fig. 6.11). Slow involution subsequently occurs over the next 5–10 years. They are much commoner in preterm infants and in girls. They were previously referred to as 'strawberry naevi'. Superficial haemangiomas deep in the dermis, subcutaneous fat or muscle produce a bluish colour in the overlying skin.

The majority of haemangiomas do not require treatment. Indications for treatment include lesions near the airway or eyes, those associated with high cardiac output failure, and extensive facial lesions. Oral corticosteroids commenced during the rapid growth phase are effective in slowing growth and hastening resolution but recent evidence suggest beta-blockers (propranolol) can have a dramatic effect with less side effects. Bleeding is rarely a problem, even after trauma, but large lesions can be associated with thrombocytopenia, intravascular coagulation and severe bleeding (Kasabach–Merritt syndrome).

Vascular malformations

These represent structural anomalies, are present at birth, grow in proportion to the infant's growth, and in general do not resolve with time. They can affect any kind of blood and lymphatic vessel and sometimes cause Kasabach–Merritt syndrome or contain arteriovenous shunts which may cause heart failure.

Capillary malformations

Fine capillary malformations, which are deep red in colour and blanch with pressure, occur on the glabella, upper eyelids, upper lips and nape of the neck. They are of no significance and tend to fade during the first 6 months. They were previously referred to as 'naevus flammeus' or 'stork marks'

Larger, flat, deep, purple-red ('port-wine') lesions may occur on any part of the body. Those in the distribution of the trigeminal nerve can be associated with retinal and intracranial vascular malformations, requiring ophthalmological follow-up. Association of this type of lesion with vascular malformation of the ipsilateral meninges and cerebral cortex is termed the Sturge–Weber syndrome. It can be associated with epilepsy. The skin manifestations may be treated with cosmetic cover creams or by pulsed dye laser in later infancy.

Epidermal naevi

These birthmarks presenting at birth or in the first few months of life represent proliferation of keratinocytes or skin appendage cells. They are rare lesions that may involve any area, including the oral cavity. On the scalp and face they are often yellowish because of a prominent sebaceous gland component. Trunk and limb epidermal naevi are scaly, flat or raised, varying in colour from black or brown to pale grey, with plaque or linear streak distribution. Excision may be indicated for small and linear lesions and for irritating and cosmetically troublesome naevi.

Hyperpigmented and hypopigmented birthmarks

These must be differentiated from the skin lesions of generalized disorders, such as neurofibromatosis and tuberous sclerosis (neurocutaneous syndromes), which usually appear **after** birth.

Congenital hyperpigmented patches

These common pale or dark-brown macular or flat hypermelanotic patches may be solitary or extensive, involving large areas of the trunk or limbs. They must be differentiated from the café au lait spots of classic neurofibromatosis.

Congenital melanocytic naevi

These are collections of melanocytes in the epidermis or dermis. When present at birth they appear as raised lesions of various shades of brown to black (Fig. 6.12). They vary in size and may have blue or pink components, often growing long black hairs. They grow in proportion to the infant. Controversy exists about the risk of malignant change. Lesions over the lower spine may be associated with a tethered spinal cord. Large or multiple lesions may be associated with benign or, rarely, malignant proliferation of melanocytes in the leptomeninges, dem-

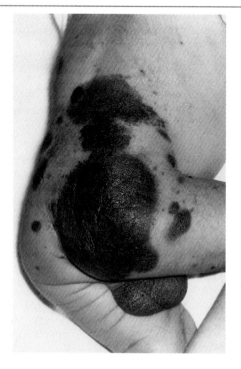

Figure 6.12 Congenital melanocytic naevus involving the buttock and loin.

onstrated by MRI. Small lesions are easily removed surgically; for larger lesions staged surgery may be possible.

Mongolian blue spots

These are flat, blue or slate-grey lesions comprising collections of melanocytes in the dermis. They are seen in the majority of oriental and black infants. In white infants there is usually a Mediterranean ancestry. Single or multiple, they occur particularly in the lumbosacral area, less often on the shoulders or back and tend to fade with age. These lesions should be documented so they are not confused with non-accidental bruising in the future. They do not require any intervention other than reassurance.

Congenital hypopigmented patches

These are pale areas of reduced melanin varying in size from a few centimetres to large areas covering the trunk and limbs. They do not involute. Similar lesions occur in incontinentia pigmenti, a rare genetic neurocutaneous condition affecting females and associated with multiple abnormalities, especially of the eye, skeleton and central nervous systems.

Ichthyotic disorders

These are a rare group of skin disorders where the skin at birth is dry and scaly. There are several varieties.

Ichthyosis vulgaris

This is an autosomal dominant disorder (1: 250) and there may be a family history of atopy. It rarely causes problems in the newborn and is treated with moisturizer.

Recessive X-linked ichthyosis

This condition only affects males and is associated with placental sulphatase deficiency. Unrecordable oestriol measurements during pregnancy should alert the clinician to this possibility in male infants.

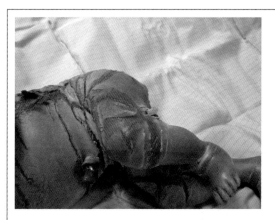

Figure 6.14 Harlequin ichthyosis with severe deep skin cracking.

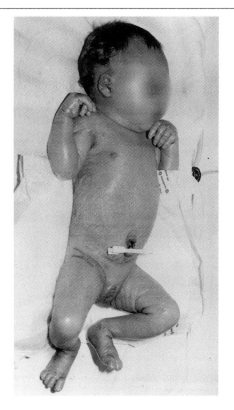

Figure 6.13 Newborn infant with collodion skin. Six weeks later the skin appeared entirely normal.

Table 6.2 Classification of blistering and bullous disorders affecting the neonate	
Transient	**Chronic**
Erythema toxicum	Epidermolysis bullosa:
Congenital candidiasis	Non-scarring
Congenital herpes	Scarring
Impetigo neonatorum	
Toxic epidermal necrolysis	
Transient neonatal pustular dermatosis (melanosis)	

Collodion baby

The mildest form of this group of disorders is the collodion baby (Fig. 6.13). At birth the infant looks as if it is covered in a dry plastic-like membrane, which cracks easily. These infants often later develop lamellar ichthyosis, but some may have no persistent skin abnormality. The more severe **harlequin icthyosis** shows severe hyperkeratosis, everted eyelids and deep skin cracking and is due to a mutation of the *ABCA12* gene (Fig. 6.14). Treatment with retinoic acids is indicated and in the most severe forms palliative care is sometimes discussed.

Blistering and bullous disorders

These constitute a wide group of unrelated disorders characterized by blistering of the skin. They can be divided into transient and chronic disorders (Table 6.2).

Erythema toxicum

These extremely common lesions (70% of term babies) appear in the first few days of life as multiple vesicles. The vesicles are differentiated from infection by the fact that they 'come and go' and the baby is completely well. Each has a macular red surround and the presence of multiple eosinophils within the vesicular fluid. No treatment is necessary.

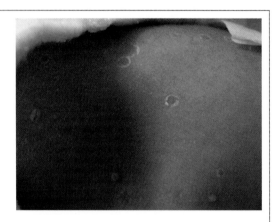

Figure 6.15 Transient neonatal pustular melanosis.

Transient neonatal pustular melanosis

Unlike erythema toxicum these lesions are present *at birth*. The pustules are fragile; the top easily wipes off leaving a halo. There is no surrounding erythema. In pigmented skin a dark hyperpigmented area is left as the pustule resolves. This is non-infectious and needs no treatment (see Fig. 6.15).

Candida vesicles

These are usually associated with oral candidiasis but can occasionally be present at birth. Diagnosis is by the identification of hyphae or budding spores from the blister. Treatment is by topical nystatin or miconazole.

Congenital herpes vesicles

A 'crop' of vesicles on the vertex of the baby can very rarely represent congenital herpes infection from contact with cervical lesions. Confirmation is by HSV RNA analysis (PCR method) of the vesicle fluid. This needs to be treated aggressively with aciclovir to prevent disseminated herpes infection (see Chapter 10).

Impetigo neonatorum

This term is used to describe staphylococcal bullous lesions appearing on the second or third day of life. The pustules develop on an erythematous base and are often seen in moist areas (neck, axillae or groin). The infant may show signs of systemic infection. Intravenous flucloxacillin should be given while culture from the pustules is awaited, as the condition may spread quickly.

Toxic epidermal necrolysis (scalded skin syndrome)

This is characterized by generalized erythema accompanied by fever and irritability, followed within a few hours by the formation of flaccid bullae filled with serous fluid. Sheets of epidermis can be stripped away with minimal shearing force, revealing a raw, oozing surface (Nikolsky's sign). This is most commonly associated with a *Staphylococcus aureus* infection (phage type 50 or 71) which produces toxins. Treatment is with systemic flucloxacillin. The large denuded areas of skin must be treated like a severe burn, requiring isolation to prevent secondary infection, and careful fluid and electrolyte management.

Epidermolysis bullosa

This describes includes a group of conditions in which blistering or bullous eruptions occur at birth or are in the first week of life after mild trauma. They can be divided into non-scarring and scarring forms.

Non-scarring (epidermolysis bullosa simplex)

This is a relatively mild form and is autosomal dominant. The soles, toes and fingers are most often affected. Blisters may be present within minutes of delivery. A more severe form, inherited as an autosomal recessive condition, may heal to leave atrophic areas. Differentiation is only possible on electron microscopy. The non-scarring types tend to improve by puberty, but lesions frequently become secondarily infected.

Scarring (dystrophic) forms

These conditions may be inherited as either autosomal dominant or recessive disorders. The blisters occur early and are deep. The recessive form is usually more severe and the gastrointestinal tract may be involved. The scarring is often extremely destructive, with loss of nails, the formation of ugly scars and contractures, fusion of digits, and sometimes digit or limb amputations.

Management will depend on the individual case, but the parents should be encouraged to ensure that the child's lifestyle is as normal as possible. Nevertheless, the avoidance of mechanical trauma, hot baths and high temperatures is important. Genetic counselling is advised.

Miscellaneous

Cutis marmorata

This represents a normal physiological reaction to cold commonly seen in the neonate and young infant. The bluish mottling usually exhibits a characteristic reticulated pattern on the trunk and extremities. It is symptomless and transient, requiring no treatment.

Cutis aplasia

This presents as a focal absence of skin at birth. Most often the lesions are on the scalp in the midline, but they can occur on the trunk or extremities. It is associated with trisomy 13. The combination of cutis aplasia and cutis marmorata is seen in Adams–Oliver syndrome (Fig. 6.16). Prevention of infection in cases of ulceration and surgical skin grafting (for larger defects) may be required.

Subcutaneous fat necrosis

A firm, woody, red nodule is felt, often over the arms, thighs, shoulders or face. This can occur after mild perinatal asphyxia or in babies who have become cold or who have received therapeutic hypothermia. It resolves spontaneously over many weeks but if extensive can be associated with significant hypercalcaemia.

Cutis laxa

Congenital cutis laxa is inherited. Affected infants have diminished resilience of the skin, which hangs in folds. This condition is not associated with joint laxity and bruising as seen in cases of Ehlers–Danlos syndrome. In Ehlers–Danlos the skin is hyperelastic

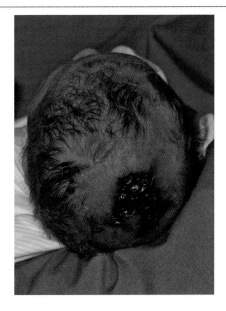

Figure 6.16 Adams–Oliver syndrome with cutis aplasia and cutis marmorata telangiectasia.

but snaps back to normal and does not hang in folds.

Harlequin colour change

This refers to a unilateral colour change commonly seen during the first few days of life in preterm but also in term infants. It occurs with axial rotation: when the infant is lying on one side the upper part of the body is paler than the lower half, which is normal or reddish in colour. It may last for seconds or minutes and requires no treatment.

Neonatal eczema (atopic dermatitis)

Eczema is a common problem after 2 months of age but is unusual in the newborn. Management consists of avoiding potential allergens and plentiful use of emollients and moisturizer.

Seborrhoeic dermatitis (cradle cap)

This inflammatory condition appears after a few weeks. There is crusting and greasy yellow scales on an erythematous base, usually over the scalp. It may spread to the face, neck, behind the ears, axillae and napkin area. Treat with olive oil, followed by gentle brushing to remove the scales. Severe cases respond to coal tar shampoo and steroid or antifungal creams.

Ectodermal dysplasia

This is an abnormality affecting the skin, sweat glands, hair and nails. Infants have sparse hair, hypoplastic nails and may develop peg-like teeth. Sweating may be abnormal.

Communication with parents

At the end of the examination it is important to document your findings carefully, either in the hospital record or in a parent-held child health record. If everything is normal then parents should be reassured. It is always sensible to ask if they have any other concerns about their baby's health at this time. If minor abnormalities have been found these should be explained carefully and also communicated to the family doctor. If more significant anomalies have been identified these should be explained carefully and appropriate follow-up arranged. Parents must be left with a clear plan and ideally with written information about the condition. Many parents will turn to online resources and it is useful to point them in the right direction of support groups and reliable websites.

SUMMARY

Carefully examining every newborn baby provides an opportunity to reassure parents about trivial congenital anomalies and to explain more significant ones. Examination of the heart, hips, eyes and testes (in boys) forms part of the newborn screening programme. It is important that examinations are performed in a thorough and systematic manner and to be familiar with normal variants and the common patterns of abnormality. Communication with parents is very important at this time- they need to know what the problem is, whether anything needs to be done and what is going to happen next.

 Now visit **www.essentialneonatalmed.com** to test yourself on this chapter.

CHAPTER 7
Birth injury

Key topics

Introduction

Despite skilled obstetric care, injuries may be sustained either during labour or during delivery. Injuries can also occur as a result of inappropriate use of excessive force. Sometimes bony injury may be an unintended consequence of saving the baby's life when there is severe shoulder dystocia. Preterm babies are particularly susceptible to injury, either at delivery or after admission to the neonatal intensive care unit (NICU) where they are vulnerable to preventable iatrogenic injuries.

The decreased incidence in birth trauma over recent years has been attributed to changing trends in obstetric management, such as caesarean section instead of difficult vaginal delivery. Despite the falling incidence, birth injury is still a cause for concern to the obstetrician and neonatologist. Parents sometimes attribute birth injury to obstetric mismanagement, and this may result in litigation. Unfortunately, such events encourage the practice of defensive obstetrics, and a high caesarean section rate may be a consequence of this. There is evidence that the presence of senior experienced obstetricians on the delivery suite can reduce the caesarean section rate.

Where iatrogenic or preventable injury has occurred it is best to be honest and explain the nature of the circumstances of the injury carefully to parents. However, injury, especially brain injury, can occur even after normal labour and delivery and mismanagement should not be implied without evidence.

Table 7.1 lists the major causes of birth injury and their incidence.

Essential Neonatal Medicine, Fifth Edition. Sunil Sinha, Lawrence Miall, Luke Jardine.
© 2012 John Wiley & Sons, Ltd. Published 2012 by John Wiley & Sons, Ltd.

Table 7.1 The commoner types of birth injury and their incidence

Cephalhaematoma	1:100
Brachial plexus injury	0.5–1:1000
Facial nerve palsy	1:500
Bony (non-skull) fracture	1:1000
Skull fractures	Rare
Subaponeurotic haemorrhage	1:1250
Major subdural haemorrhage	1:50 000
Spinal cord injuries	Very rare
Overall incidence	7:1000 births

Table 7.2 Risk factors for birth injury

Fetal condition	Prematurity Small for gestational age Multiple pregnancy Fetal distress
Malpresentation	Breech presentation (see Table 7.3) Brow, face, compound presentation
Malposition	Unengaged head Occipitoposterior arrest Deep transverse arrest
Cephalopelvic disproportion	Macrosomia, e.g. infant of diabetic mother, hydrops fetalis Macrocephaly Previous pelvic fracture
Shoulder dystocia	
Prolonged labour	Delay–cervix not fully dilated Delay–cervix fully dilated
Precipitate labour	
Maternal factors	Nulliparity Short stature Obesity
Inexperienced obstetrician or midwife	

Risk factors for birth injury

The effect of changing patterns of obstetric practice on birth-associated mechanical injuries is difficult to evaluate. However, a number of risk factors for birth injury have been identified, especially vaginal breech delivery (Tables 7.2 and 7.3).

Injuries to the scalp, skull and brain

Caput succedaneum

This is benign swelling of the subcutaneous tissue of the scalp from prolonged delivery or ventouse cup. It usually resolves within a few days, occasionally with bruising.

Erythema, abrasions and lacerations

Erythema and abrasions may be seen following forceps and vacuum delivery and with cephalopelvic disproportion. Lacerations to the scalp or face can occur during episiotomy, uterine incision at caesarean section, and scalp electrode monitoring (Fig. 7.1).

Cephalhaematoma

This occurs in about 1% of newborn infants and is due to bleeding between the periosteum and the cranial bones (usually parietal, less commonly occipital) as a result of shearing or tearing of communicating veins during delivery. The extent of the swelling is limited by the underlying skull bone and does not cross suture lines (see Fig. 7.2). It is due to buffeting of the fetal skull against the maternal pelvis, which is seen especially in prolonged labour. It may also occur following a forceps or vacuum delivery. Subperiosteal bleeding is slow and may not appear until the second day of life. Enlargement may occur during the first week and the swelling may persist for several weeks.

Box 7.1 lists complications associated with a cephalhaematoma.

Table 7.3 Injuries more likely to occur in infants delivered by breech	
Haemorrhage	Subdural tears due to tentorial rupture Rupture of intra-abdominal viscus (usually liver or kidney) Occipital osteodiastasis with cerebellar haemorrhage
Orthopaedic	Dislocation: shoulder, cervical vertebrae, hip, knee Fracture: clavicle, humerus, femur Damage to sternomastoid muscle
Neurological	Asphyxia secondary to cord prolapse Cervical brachial plexus injury: Erb's or Klumpke's paralysis Facial nerve palsy
Soft tissue injury	Extensive bruising, particularly genitals

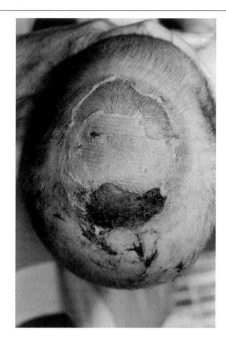

Figure 7.1 Scalp lacerations and bruising following vacuum delivery.

Subaponeurotic haemorrhage (subgaleal haemorrhage)

On rare occasions haemorrhage may occur beneath the aponeurotic sheet joining the two portions of the occipitofrontalis muscle of the scalp. This is seen particularly in black infants. It may be the consequence of trauma during delivery, especially with vacuum extraction, or may indicate the presence of a coagulation defect. The scalp becomes fluctuant ('hot water bottle' sign) and enlarges rapidly with a marked drop in haemoglobin. The severity of blood loss may be underestimated, and ensuing shock may be life-threatening. Affected babies require rapid diagnosis and appropriate transfusion with volume expanders or blood.

Skull fractures

Generally, linear fractures require no specific treatment. Depressed fractures are usually associated with forceps application or head compression produced by the maternal sacral promontory. Large fractures may be associated with cerebral contusion, and neurosurgical consultation may be necessary. Depression of the skull may remain for many months after birth (Fig 7.3)

Intracranial haemorrhages

Although mostly related to hypoxic–ischaemic injury, some forms of intracranial haemorrhage can result directly as a consequence of trauma. These often present with encephalopathy or seizures and are described in Chapter 22.

Bone and joint injuries

Traumatic fractures of bones during birth are relatively rare and present with the classic signs of pain on handling, avoidance of movement, swelling, deformity and crepitus. Fractures of the upper limb

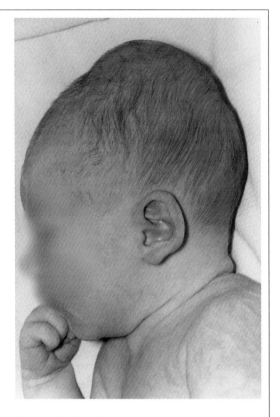

Figure 7.2 Cephalhaematoma.

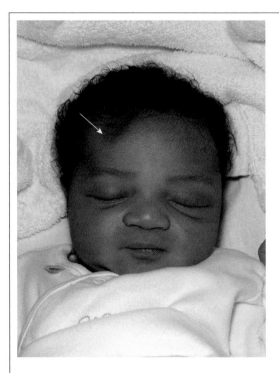

Figure 7.3 Right frontal depressed skull fracture, see arrow.

Box 7.1 Complications associated with a cephalhaematoma

These may include:

- Underlying linear skull fracture
- Jaundice due to haemolysis
- Calcification at its edge, which may occur some weeks later during the resorption process; this should not be confused with a depressed skull fracture
- Intracranial haemorrhage may rarely be associated with cephalhaematoma

---

bones may be suspected by an asymmetrical Moro reflex or failure to move one arm spontaneously. Fractures heal very fast in newborn babies, and the considerable bone remodelling that occurs almost invariably leads to resolution of normal anatomy.

Clavicle

This is the bone most frequently fractured during the birth process. It may be associated with impacted shoulders, especially in the infant of a diabetic mother or a difficult breech delivery. Specific treatment is not required. Simple analgesia should be offered if the baby seems in pain.

Humerus

Fracture of the humerus generally involves the upper third of the shaft and there is usually considerable deformity. Radial nerve injury sometimes also occurs. Treatment consists of an immobilizing plastic backslab or immobilization with a binder to the chest.

Femur

Fracture of the femur occurs rarely during breech extraction, either vaginally or at caesarean section. It occurs predominantly in the breech birth with extended legs as flexion occurs. Treatment consists of immobilization in a plaster case, traction, and a Thomas splint.

Multiple or unusual fractures

Multiple fractures are rare and should raise the possibility of osteogenesis imperfecta. Any fracture in an infant who has been home should always raise the question of non-accidental injury.

Dislocation of joints and separation of epiphyses

These are difficult to diagnose and require specialized orthopaedic assessment. Congenital dislocation of the knee joint is not due to trauma (see Chapter 6).

Peripheral nerve injuries

Nerve injuries in the newborn infant may be due to stretching, compression, twisting, hyperextension or separation of the nervous tissue. They may be classified pathologically as:
• **neuropraxia** (swelling of the nerve, with total recovery)
• **axonotmesis** (complete peripheral degeneration, may be partial recovery)
• **neurotmesis** (complete division of nerve and nerve sheath).
    Nerve conduction studies and MRI can distinguish a neuropraxia from a neurotmesis. The following nerve injuries occur in the newborn.

Facial nerve palsy

This may be due to an upper or lower motor neuron lesion, but clinical distinction between these is difficult. Lower motor neuron (LMN) facial palsy usually occurs due to oblique application of the forceps blade. The nerve may also be damaged by prolonged pressure on the maternal sacral promontory. Upper motor neuron lesions are much less common and are due to brain injury or nuclear agenesis (Möbius syndrome).
    The lesion is recognized clinically by an inability to close the eye and a lack of lower lip depression on crying, both on the affected side (Fig. 7.4). The

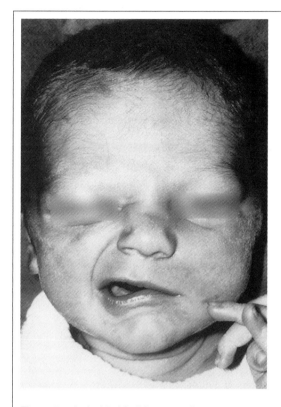

Figure 7.4 Left-sided facial nerve palsy.

nasolabial fold is absent on the affected side. In most cases complete recovery occurs by 6 weeks; only rarely is permanent facial palsy seen. If the eye cannot be closed, patching and 'artificial tear' eyedrops should be used to prevent corneal damage.

CLINICAL TIP: Lower motor neuron facial nerve palsy must be distinguished from 'asymmetrical crying facies' syndrome, where there is an absence of the depressor anguli oris muscle. In this condition eye closure is normal but there is failure of the mouth to move downwards and outwards on the affected side when the infant cries. Asymmetry usually remains into adult life but becomes less obvious with time. It often runs in families.

Obstetric brachial palsy

The majority of babies with obstetric brachial palsy (OBP) are thought to have sustained birth trauma, but a very few cases cannot be explained in this way and a prenatal causation has been proposed for these. Trauma to the brachial plexus may be due to excessive lateral flexion, rotation or traction upon the neck. Such trauma may be seen with normal delivery, with impacted shoulders or during delivery of the aftercoming head of a breech. There is a strong association with shoulder dystocia.

Three types of brachial plexus injury can be described:
• **Erb's palsy (C5–6)** (Fig. 7.5). In this lesion the fifth and sixth cervical nerve roots are injured and the arm will be held in adduction, with the elbow extended and the forearm pronated with the wrist flexed. This is traditionally known as the 'waiter's tip' position. Note that the fingers can still move.
• **Klumpke's paralysis (C7–T1).** In this uncommon lesion the seventh and eighth cervical and first thoracic segment nerve roots are injured: this involves the small muscles of the hand, with localized wrist drop and flaccid paralysis of the hand. The grasp reflex will be absent. This is especially associated with difficult delivery of the head following preterm breech delivery.
• **Total paralysis of the arm (C5–T1).** Where all trunks of the brachial plexus have been damaged there will be complete paralysis of the arm, with flaccidity and often cutis marmorata due to vasomotor disturbance. Spinal injury should be suspected when paralysis is bilateral. It may or may not be associated with Horner's syndrome.

Mild injuries recover within a few days, and more severe lesions can be expected to largely recover in 2–4 months. However, complete recovery only occurs in 50% of affected babies, and partial recovery in another 48%. Absence of any recovery is very rare.

Management requires physiotherapy in all cases. Specialist assessment at 3 months allows a decision to made as to whether early nerve reconstructive surgery is needed, but this remains controversial. Achieving function of the shoulder and elbow is crucial.

Radial nerve injury

Rarely radial nerve paralysis may result from fracture of the humerus, as may occur when there is difficulty in delivering the arm during breech extraction. The use of the 'deltoid region' as a site for intramuscular injection is now avoided as this was associated with radial nerve injury.

Sciatic nerve injury

Misplacement of the needle tip during intramuscular injection into the buttock region carries with it a risk of injuring the sciatic nerve.

Phrenic nerve injury

This is caused by injury to cervical nerve roots C3, C4 and C5, and is generally associated with brachial

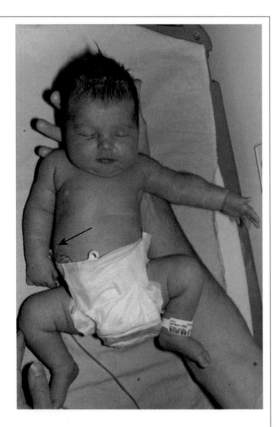

Figure 7.5 Right-sided Erb's palsy showing the typical 'waiter's tip' position of the hand. Note the unilateral moro reflex on the left.

plexus palsy. As the newborn infant predominantly breathes with the diaphragm rather than the intercostal muscles there is often respiratory distress. The clinical diagnosis is confirmed by chest radiograph, which shows an elevated hemidiaphragm, and radiography or ultrasound scan shows an immobile diaphragm.

Recurrent laryngeal nerve

This is a rare cause of laryngeal stridor and may be due to birth injury associated with excessive lateral traction of the neck. Occasionally trauma to the recurrent laryngeal nerve occurs during cardiac surgery. The diagnosis is made by microlaryngoscopy, and treatment is expectant.

Spinal cord injury

This is rare and usually associated with difficult breech deliveries involving internal version and breech extraction; rarely it may occur with shoulder dystocia. The injury is due to stretching of the cervical spinal cord and occasionally due to complete severance with fatal consequences. There are three modes of clinical presentation:
• Poor condition from birth, respiratory depression, shock and hypothermia leading to death.
• Normal at birth but later develops respiratory depression, paralysed legs and urinary retention.
• Paralysis from birth; the extent of the paresis depending on the spinal level involved.

The investigation of choice is spinal MRI. Neurosurgical decompression is necessary for a large haematoma in the spinal canal. Infarction of the spinal cord is also reported as a complication of hypoxic–ischaemic insult and as the result of embolic infarction associated with an umbilical arterial catheter (UAC) or extravasation of parenteral nutrition into lumbar plexus veins from a misplaced peripherally inserted central catheter (PICC) line.

Soft tissue injuries

Traumatic petechiae

Traumatic petechiae occur over the head, neck and upper chest following a difficult delivery can be mistaken for cyanosis. Oxygen saturation testing will be normal. They often occur with breech presentation and in infants born with the umbilical cord tightly around the neck. They may be related to a sudden increase in intrathoracic pressure during passage of the chest through the birth canal. These petechiae usually fade within 2–3 days and require no treatment other than parental reassurance. Traumatic petechiae must be clearly distinguished from generalized petechiae associated with coagulopathy or low platelets.

Ecchymoses (bruising)

Bruising may be seen with traumatic deliveries, precipitate labour, preterm infants, poorly controlled deliveries, abnormal presentations (e.g. face, brow, breech) or with thrombocytopenia.

Subcutaneous fat necrosis

This term is applied to well-demarcated indurated areas in the skin occurring where pressure has been applied (e.g. forceps blades on the face).

Sternomastoid tumour

Often associated with torticollis, this benign fibroblastic swelling is described in Chapter 6.

Organ injuries

Liver and spleen

Subcapsular haematoma of the liver can occur after a breech extraction or following external cardiac massage. It may also result from 'atraumatic' vertex deliveries. Rupture of the liver or spleen is more likely to occur where there is hepatosplenomegaly (rhesus haemolytic disease, diabetic mother).

Adrenals

Adrenal haemorrhages may occur with breech extraction, although they are usually a postmortem finding and are unsuspected in live infants. They are more commonly associated with overwhelming bacterial infection and disseminated intravascular coagulopathy.

Table 7.4 Iatrogenic injury occurring in newborns, often on the NICU	
Skin lesions	Fetal scalp electrode lacerations Burns from transcutaneous CO_2 and O_2 monitors Injury from saturation monitor pressure (Fig 7.6) Calcified heel nodules from repeated heel-pricks Chemical burns from skin antiseptics (Fig 7.7) Extravasation lesions due to leakage of intravenous solutions
Visual deficit	Retinopathy of prematurity secondary to oxygen toxicity (see Chapter 23)
Hearing deficits	Gentamicin toxicity Incubator noise (especially CPAP circuits)
Necrotizing enterocolitis	Inappropriate escalation of feeds Excessive osmolality of feeds
Rib or limb fractures	Severe osteopenia of prematurity (chapter 21)
Direct trauma from catheters, tubes and needles	Digit damage, nerve palsies, amputation, retained foreign bodies
Vascular injury	Thrombotic or ischaemic injury following misplaced or inappropriate insertion of arterial lines (e.g. into an end-artery; see Chapter 29). Inappropriate infusion via an arterial line (e.g. inotropes)
Respiratory injuries	Nares can be damaged by pressure on NG tubes or poorly fitting CPAP nasal prongs Subglottic stenosis from excessively large endotracheal tube Aspiration of milk from misplaced NG tube (prevent by testing for gastric acid with pH paper prior to every feed) Bronchopulmonary dysplasia secondary to oxygen toxicity
Postural deformities	Can be minimized by good positioning and developmental care (see Chapter 24) Scaphocephaly External rotation of hips and feet
Metabolic disturbance	Over-infusion of intravenous fluids Infusion of wrong fluids or medication Intravenous infusion of milk feeds (now largely prevented by use of unique connectors)
Nosocomial infection	Poor infection prevention and control measures Poor hand-washing or asepsis technique Overcrowding in the NICU

Kidneys

Ruptured kidneys may occur very rarely during delivery in breech preterm infants.

Testicles

Testicular bruising and haemorrhage are commonly seen in breech presentations. No treatment other than simple analgesia is necessary.

Injuries sustained in the neonatal intensive care unit

An increasing number and range of traumatic lesions are due to iatrogenic insults sustained in the modern NICU. These lesions predominantly occur in preterm infants and relate to the invasive procedures and technology used to treat increasingly small and fragile infants (Table 7.4, Figures 7.6 and 7.7). Most of these are preventable and good risk management processes should be put in place to ensure their occurrence is minimized or prevented. Honest explanation to the parents and urgent appropriate treatment can mitigate the adverse effects. Superficial extravasation injuries can be treated by urgent flushing with large volumes of subcutaneous saline (see Chapter 29).

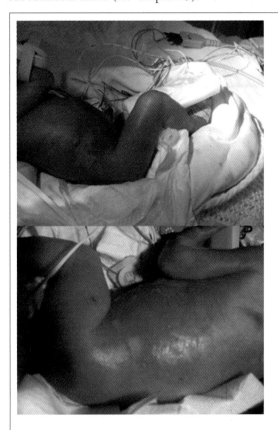

Figure 7.7 Chemical burn from aqueous 2% chlorhexidine used prior to UAC insertion in an extreme preterm baby. Reproduced from *Arch Dis Child Fetal Neonatal Ed*, Lashkari, H P et al., 2011 with permission from BMJ Publishing Group Ltd.

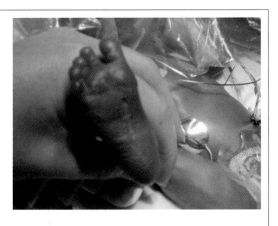

Figure 7.6 Bruising to the foot from S_AO_2 probe.

Injury to a newborn baby, whether it occurs during natural birth, during operative delivery or on the NICU, is always a tragedy for the parents, especially if it is easily preventable. An open and honest approach is required – parents will want a careful explanation of what happened, what injury has occurred and how it will be treated. Some injuries may be an expected complication of treatment and some will remain unexplained, even after extensive investigation. It is vital that perinatal and neonatal services put in place risk reduction systems to prevent injuries occurring.

SUMMARY

CHAPTER 8
Genetic disorders

Key topics

Introduction

Human genetics is a rapidly expanding field in almost all fields of medicine. The list of genetic loci and mutations that may cause genetic disease is ever expanding and are catalogued in the Online Mendelian Inheritance in Man website (http://www.ncbi.nlm.nih.gov/entrez/query.fcgi?db=OMIM). It is now possible to sequence an individual's DNA, thereby identifying risk factors for the development of future disease. There is an increasing recognition of polygenic diseases, where a number of genes interact to increase the risk of disease. A detailed discussion of all the causes and types of mutations that may occur is beyond the scope of this book. For further information the reader should refer to specific texts on the molecular basis of genetic disease.

Gene structure

Every cell in the body normally contains 2 sets of 23 chromosomes (the haploid number). Therefore there are 46 chromosomes (the diploid number) in every cell, 2 are sex chromosomes (either XX in females or XY in males) and 44 are autosomes. A chromosome contains a double strand of DNA tightly wound together. During meiosis the chromosomes separate and align themselves around the centre of the cell, and half migrate into each

daughter cell. Fertilization requires fusion of the maternal oocyte (containing 23 chromosomes) and the paternal sperm (containing 23 chromosomes). Mitochondria also have their own distinct genome. Mitochondria are passed only through the ova and therefore all mitochondrial DNA comes from the mother.

DNA consists of two strands of very long sequences of nucleotides (see Fig. 8.1). A nucleotide consists of a five-carbon ringed sugar, a

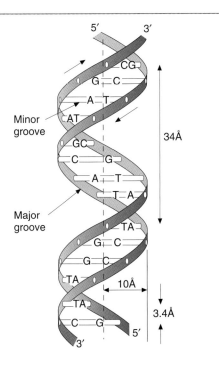

Figure 8.1 Diagram of a DNA double helix.

Box 8.1 Tissue specimens suitable for genetic testing

- Blood: lymphocytes (collected in a heparinized tube), ideally from a patient who has not recently ingested alcohol, antibiotics or drugs of addiction
- Bone marrow
- Embryo
- Skin (fibroblast culture): useful up to 2 days after death
- Desquamated cells in amniotic fluid
- Chorionic villus sample

and other non-coding sections which have poorly understood functional properties but do not translate into proteins.

Commonly used investigations

Genetic testing can now be undertaken prior to conception (e.g. test parents for gene), in vitro (e.g. test embryo preimplantation), during gestation (e.g. perform chorionic villus sampling or amniocentesis) or after birth. For any genetic investigation, a specimen containing genetic material is required. Various tissues can be sampled or cultured, depending on the timing and urgency of the diagnostic test being undertaken. Commonly used tissues are listed in Box 8.1

Chromosome analysis

A Giemsa (G) stain gives the overall appearance of the karyotype. G-banding of the chromosomes gives detailed information about more subtle abnormalities. Chromosomes are grouped according to banding characteristics, size of chromosomes and centromere position. The larger chromosomes are designated by the lowest numbers, and each chromosome is divided by the centromere into a short arm (p) and a long arm (q) (see Fig. 8.2). Karyotype analysis should be available in 24–48 h but banding can take up to 14 days.

triphosphate (attached to the 5 carbon), a hydroxyl group (attached to the 3 carbon), a hydrogen group (attached to the 2 carbon) and one of four bases (attached to the 1 carbon): adenine (A), cytosine (C), guanine (G) and thymidine (T). The other strand of DNA (also called the **antisense** strand) contains the complementary bases, wherever there is an A the opposite strand has a T (and vice versa), and wherever there is a G the opposite strand has a C (and vice versa). In RNA, thymidine is replaced by uracil (U). A series of 3 nucleotides makes a codon (e.g. UAA, AUG, UGA) and each is a specific instruction for either stopping transcription or insertion of a specific amino acid. In total there are 64 possible codons for the 20 amino acids.

The total amount of chromosomal DNA codes for about 3 billion base pairs. However, only 1.5% contain codes for genes (of which there are approximately 23,000). This coding DNA is subsequently translated into proteins. The remainder is RNA genes, sections involved in gene regulation,

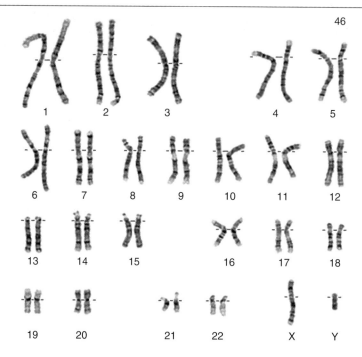

Figure 8.2 Normal chromosome pattern and number after Giemsa staining. This is an example of a male karyotype. The hashed horizontal line is at the centromere and divides the chromosome into short (p) and long (q) arms.

Polymerase chain reaction

Although it is not itself a genetic test, the development of the polymerase chain reaction (PCR) technique has proved incredibly useful for providing genetic material for other investigations. This technique allows for rapid amplification of small fragments of DNA. It is extremely sensitive, to the point that DNA from a single cell can be amplified a million times in only a couple of hours. This technique is relatively inexpensive and is performed in most laboratories.

Fluorescence in-situ hybridization

The fluorescence in-situ hybridization (FISH) technique allows more careful examination of chromosomes for very small abnormalities of which the DNA sequence is already known. The DNA is initially denatured and then a specific sequence of DNA with a fluorescent marker is added and the culture is incubated to allow hybridization. The DNA is then washed removing any unbound sequences. If the marker has bound to its complementary sequence it will be detectable on fluorescence microscopy examination. It can be used for rapid diagnosis of conditions such as trisomy 21, trisomy 13 and trisomy 18 as well as others such as velocardiofacial syndrome. See Fig. 8.3 for an example.

Microarrays

Microarray testing is a method of analysing whether or not a number of specific genes are being expressed in cells. A microarray works by measuring the amount of sample mRNA molecules bound to a specific template of the gene. By using an array of

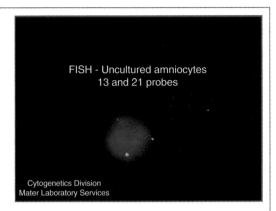

FISH - Uncultured amniocytes
13 and 21 probes

Cytogenetics Division
Mater Laboratory Services

Figure 8.3 Image showing FISH probes for chromosome 21 (red) and chromosome 13 (green). There are three red signals (abnormal) and two green signals (normal); this patient therefore has trisomy 21.

Box 8.2 Possible indications for genetic testing

- Recurrent unexplained first-trimester pregnancy loss
- High risk of genetic abnormality on antenatal testing (e.g. increased risk of chromosomal disorder on triple test or abnormalities on ultrasound)
- Fresh stillbirth with physical abnormalities
- Infant with previous chromosomal disorder
- Known genetic disorder in family
- Neonate with dysmorphic features

hundreds or thousands of gene templates, the amount of mRNA bound to each site on the array can be measured. This process generates a profile of gene expression in the cell and can accomplish many genetic tests in parallel.

Indications for investigations

While it is now much easier to perform many of the above investigations, there are still a number of important issues that need to be considered before they are ordered. Some of these include: purpose of test (e.g. diagnosis versus screening), tissue sample required to get the result, length of time before results will be available, cost of the investigation and ethical implications for child/siblings/parent/relatives. Consultation with a clinical geneticist may be required. Some possible indications for genetic testing are listed in Box 8.2.

Genetic variation

Changes in the genome account for our individuality but can also impact on the normal function of cells and organs. There are three basic categories for genetic variation:

- structural changes or changes in large segments of DNA that affect more than one gene
- changes in the DNA sequence
- multifactorial changes.

These changes can lead to gene deletions, gene duplications, gene fusions, abnormal proteins and abnormal cell functions.

Structural changes

The commonly found structural changes include:

- changes in the number of chromosomes
- deletions or additions of segments of chromosomes
- translocations of chromosomes

Other changes such as inversions and ring chromosomes have also been reported.

Changes in chromosome number

Aneuploidy is defined as an abnormal number of chromosomes (either too many or too few). One extra chromosome is called **trisomy** and one chromosome deletion is called a **monosomy**. These abnormalities may occur with autosomes or sex chromosomes. Some commonly found examples are listed in Table 8.1. Most monosomies are incompatible with life and cause spontaneous abortion; one commonly encountered exception is Turner's syndrome where only one of the X chromsomes is present (labelled 45,XO – see Table 8.1). **Polyploidy** is a multiple of the haploid number. For example, the triploidy 69 karyotype usually results in abortion, stillbirth or early neonatal death.

Table 8.1 Specific chromosomal abnormalities

	Trisomy 21 (Down's syndrome, Fig. 8.5)	Trisomy 13 (Patau's syndrome)	Trisomy 18 (Edward's syndrome, Fig. 8.6)	45,XO syndrome (Turner's syndrome, ovarian dysgenesis)	XXY syndrome (Klinefelter's syndrome)
Incidence	1 in 600 births	1 in 5000 births	1 in 3500 births (females predominate)	1 in 2500 of live female births (however, majority abort in first few prenatal months)	1 in 500 male births
Karyotype	94% result from non-disjunction, 3.5% translocations, 2.5% mosaicism	75% non-disjunction, 20% translocation, 5% mosaicism	85–95% non-disjunction, 5% mosaicism	60% 45,XO. Remainder – great variety including mosaics, deletions	80% XXY, 10% mosaic, 10% XXYY or XXXY
Maternal age	Important. 1 in 1500 incidence with maternal age 15–29 years, 1 in 50 at 45 years	Older maternal age seems to be important. Mean maternal age approx. 31 years	Mean maternal age 32	No apparent influence	Average maternal age slightly increased
Clinical features	Hypotonia, flat facies, slanted palpebral fissures, small ears, etc.	Large 'onion nose', defects of fusion of eyes, nose, lip and forebrain (holoprosencephaly), polydactyly, microcephaly, single umbilical artery;	Triangular face, hooked flexion deformity 2nd finger, rocker bottom feet, single umbilical artery, short sternum	Short stature (length), 'shield-like' chest. Widely spaced nipples, neck webbing, lymphoedema of hands and feet	Appear normal male baby. Usually diagnosed at puberty with failure of appearance of secondary sex characteristics; tall stature. Small testes post puberty
Associated major abnormalities	Congenital heart disease (common A-V canal), duodenal atresia	Congenital heart disease, scalp defects	Heart disease, kidney malformation	Coarctation of aorta, horseshoe kidneys	

Table 8.1 (*Continued*)

	Trisomy 21 (Down's syndrome, Fig. 8.5)	Trisomy 13 (Patau's syndrome)	Trisomy 18 (Edward's syndrome, Fig. 8.6)	45,XO syndrome (Turner's syndrome, ovarian dysgenesis)	XXY syndrome (Klinefelter's syndrome)
Survival	This will depend on associated malformation. Usually good	Majority die in early infancy	Majority die within first 3 months	Normal except for those with serious cardiac and renal problems	Normal
Recurrence risk	Depends on maternal age. Overall approximately 1 in 100 for non-disjunction type. In translocation depends on karyotype of parents	Low in non-disjunction type. Higher in translocation type depending on karyotype of parents	Less than 1 in 100 recurrence risk	No significant risk	No increased risk

CLINICAL TIP: Mosaicism occurs when there is more than one distinct cell line, one line usually being normal and the other abnormal. Thus, only a percentage of the cells will have the abnormal chromosomes. Approximately 2% of Down's syndrome babies are mosaics, and these usually have less obvious stigmata and often higher intellectual ability than in the more common trisomy 21.

Deletions or additions

Deletions of large sections of chromosomes are labelled according to the position on the chromosome where they occur, e.g. cri du chat syndrome is secondary to a deletion of the short arm of chromosome 5 (labelled 5p-). A long-arm deletion would be labelled (q-). Additions are rare and normally only compatible with life if the addition is small. One exception is triplet repeat expansions. In these cases a gene has an abnormal repeated number of copies of certain base triplets (up to 100), and the greater the number of repeats, the more severely affected is the person. Examples of a triplet repeat expansion disorder seen in neonates include myotonic dystrophy and fragile X syndrome

Translocations

A translocation refers to the breakage of two non-homologous chromosomes with rejoining of the broken pieces in new ways. When there is significant alteration of genetic material (addition or deletion), the translocation is said to be **unbalanced** and the individual is phenotypically abnormal. Where there is a normal amount of genetic material, the individual has a **balanced** translocation and is phenotypically normal.

CLINICAL TIP: Individuals with a balanced translocation convey a considerable risk to their offspring of spontaneous abortion or unbalanced translocation (risk of unbalanced translocation is 4/6). Alternatively, the infant may inherit the same balanced translocation (risk of balanced translocation is 1/6) or be completely normal (chance of being normal is 1/6).

CLINICAL TIP: Chromosome disorders are complex, but in general

- Aneuploidy is better tolerated than polyploidy.
- Additions of chromosomes are better tolerated than deletions (i.e. trisomy is better than monosomy, p+ better than p-).
- Abnormalities of sex chromosomes are better tolerated than abnormalities of autosomes.
- The higher the chromosome number, the better tolerated is the abnormality e.g. trisomy 21 is better than trisomy 13).

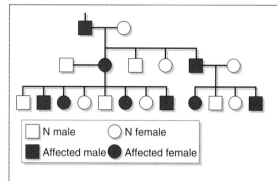

Figure 8.4 A family pedigree showing autosomal dominant inheritance.

Box 8.3 Features of autosomal dominant inheritance

- Males and females are affected in equal proportions
- Marked variation in expressivity (e.g. osteogenesis imperfecta may range from blue sclerae or deafness to severe bone fragility)
- Inherited from one parent
- Half the offspring of an affected parent can be expected to have the disorder
- New cases commonly arise as spontaneous mutations, and are more common with advanced paternal age

Changes in DNA sequence

Changes can occur to the DNA sequence in a variety of ways including:
- change in single nucleotide (called a **single nucleotide polymorphism** if common in the population or a **point mutation** if uncommon)
- insertion or deletion of a codon or a nucleotide (leading to a 'frame shift') which alters the protein structure and function
- short tandem repeats
- copy number variations.

Many of these changes can be inherited from parents by mendelian modes of inheritance. These are single-gene defects or abnormalities, caused by a defective gene occurring either on autosomes (**autosomal disorders**) or on sex chromosomes (**sex-linked, X-linked disorders**). They usually exhibit obvious and characteristic pedigree patterns.

Autosomal dominant disorders

An example of a pedigree showing autosomal dominant inheritance is in Fig. 8.4. Some features of this group are listed in Box 8.3.

The mutation may be present in only one chromosome of a pair (matched with a normal allele on the homologous chromosome) or on both. In either case the cause is a single critical error in the genetic information.

Autosomal dominant disorders include:
- major malformations: polycystic kidneys
- minor malformations: finger anomalies – shortening, fusion, additions

- central nervous system (CNS) disorders: Huntington's disease, tuberous sclerosis, neurofibromatosis
- mesenchymal disorders: osteogenesis imperfecta, achondroplasia, Marfan's syndrome
- tumours: retinoblastoma, colon polyposis
- haematological: hereditary (congenital) spherocytosis.

Autosomal recessive disorders

An example of a pedigree showing autosomal recessive inheritance is shown in Fig. 8.5. The features of this group are listed in Box 8.4.

The commonest severe autosomal recessive disease in Europe is cystic fibrosis. The carrier rate in the community of cystic fibrosis is 1 in 25, so that the chance of two carriers mating is 1 in 625. One in four of their offspring will be affected, so that the incidence of cystic fibrosis in the community is 1 in 2500.

Other autosomal recessive disorders include:
- haemoglobinopathies: thalassaemia syndromes, sickle-cell disease
- storage diseases: glycogen storage, e.g. type I (von Gierke), type II (Pompe); other, e.g. Hurler's syndrome
- CNS degenerations: white matter, e.g. metachromatic leukodystrophy; grey matter, e.g. Tay–Sachs, hepatolenticular degeneration (Wilson's disease)
- treatable inborn errors of metabolism: phenylketonuria, galactosaemia, adrenogenital syndrome
- neuromuscular: spinal muscle atrophy (Werdnig–Hoffman).

X-linked recessive disorders

An example of a pedigree showing X-linked recessive inheritance is shown in Fig. 8.6.

An X-linked recessive trait is caused by an abnormal gene on the X chromosome. The pattern of X-linked inheritance depends on the fact that females have two X chromosomes, whereas males have only one. Thus males are said to be 'hemizygous' with respect to X-linked traits, and any gene on the male's single X chromosome is expressed. The 'carrier' female is protected from the effects of the recessive gene by the normal gene on her other X chromosome.

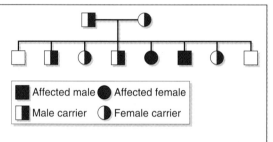

Figure 8.5 A family pedigree showing autosomal recessive inheritance.

Box 8.4 Features of autosomal recessive disorders

- The disorder is inherited from both parents, each of whom is a heterozygote (carrier)
- The recurrence risk is 1 in 4
- Males and females are equally affected
- If both parents are heterozygous for the condition, two-thirds of the unaffected offspring can be expected to be heterozygotes and only 1 in 4 of the offspring will be genotypically normal
- Relatively few recessive disorders arise as mutants
- Consanguinity increases the likelihood of carriers of rare genes mating, thereby increasing the incidence of affected individuals

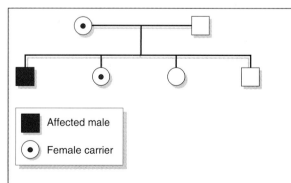

Figure 8.6 A family pedigree showing X-linked recessive inheritance.

Box 8.5 Features of X-linked recessive disorders

- Predominantly males are affected.
- The female carries the trait (rarely the female carrier may be mildly affected)
- Half the male offspring of a female carrier are affected
- Half the female offspring of a carrier will themselves become carriers
- All the female offspring of an affected male will be carriers
- Often expressed as a new mutation, making genetic counselling difficult (probably 33% of all cases of lethal X-linked recessive diseases)
- Many X-linked recessive diseases are lethal (muscular dystrophy, X-linked agammaglobulinaemia, Lesch–Nyhan syndrome), so that the disorder can only be handed on by the carrier female. However, in glucose 6-phosphate dehydrogenase (G6PD) deficiency and colour blindness the disorder may be passed on by the affected males to daughters but not to sons

The features of this group are listed in Box 8.5. X-linked recessive diseases include:
- haemophilia A, haemophilia B (Christmas disease)
- Duchenne muscular dystrophy
- agammaglobulinaemia
- G6PD deficiency
- colour blindness.

CLINICAL TIP: The Lyon hypothesis refers to the random inactivation of one X chromosome in a female (either maternal X or paternal X) at a stage during cell division. This enables heterozygous females to exhibit some features of an X-linked recessive disease, for example, elevated creatinine phosphokinase in Duchenne muscular dystrophy.

X-linked dominant inheritance

These conditions are rare, with the only clinically important disorders being vitamin D-resistant rickets, incontinentia pigmenti and pseudohypoparathyroidism. Some X-linked dominant disorders appear to be lethal to the male, so that only females are affected (e.g. incontinentia pigmenti).

CLINICAL TIP: Genomic **imprinting** is the phenomenon in which the expression of certain genes is determined by whether the gene is inherited from the female or male parent. In neonatal practice the best example of this is expression of the Prader–Willi syndrome if the gene is expressed on the paternal allele, or Angelman's syndrome associated with expression of the maternal allele.

Multifactorial inheritance

Many congenital abnormalities may be caused by the interaction of multiple factors, both genetic and environmental. These disorders do not exhibit the characteristic patterns of mendelian inheritance, although their recurrence within families is greater than that predicted for the general population. Some of the associations can be explained by number of genes involved, gene interaction, penetrance and phenotypic expression. Other environmental factors (e.g. exposure, timing of exposure, dose) may also play important roles. Some examples of diseases with evidence of a genetic basis include:
- anencephaly
- spina bifida
- cleft lip
- cleft palate

- clubfoot (talipes equinovarus)
- congenital dislocation of the hip
- congenital heart diseases
- Hirschsprung's disease
- pyloric stenosis.

Some diseases that present later in life, such as diabetes mellitus, schizophrenia and hypertension, are also examples of multifactorial inheritance.

The genetic basis of many of these diseases is increasingly being described.

Epigenetics

Epigenetics refers to changes in the non-coding structure of the DNA. Although they cause no change in the DNA code, these epigenetic changes still influence gene expression. DNA methylation, which suppresses gene expression, is a commonly identified epigenetic change. The changes may continue with future divisions of that cell and remain for multiple generations.

Approach to the dysmorphic neonate

In some instances the suspected cause of dysmorphism in a neonate may be obvious from classic clinical features, such as with trisomy 21. In others the cause may be more subtle, with single or multiple birth defects, some of which may appear unrelated. Box 8.6 provides a systematic approach to diagnosis, which may identify treatment options and help with prognosis.

Prevention of congenital abnormalities

Birth defects are a major cause of perinatal and postnatal mortality and morbidity, which have a significant impact on family life and the community as a whole. It is therefore important to have an approach to preventing such defects and identifying causes when they occur.

Strategies used to prevent birth defects include:
- rubella immunization of adolescent girls
- preconceptual counselling in families with known genetic conditions (e.g. cystic fibrosis) or maternal

---

Box 8.6 Approach to the dysmorphic infant

The following steps are required:

1 A detailed medical history to obtain information about the pregnancy and the possibility of exposure to teratogens. A family pedigree should be obtained when a genetic disorder is suspected.
2 A detailed clinical examination should be carried out and all abnormalities documented.
3 Investigations, which initially include:
   - chromosomal analysis
   - metabolic studies on blood and urine in suspected inborn errors of metabolism
   - radiology, including head, renal ultrasound and radiographs to distinguish bone dysplasia; autopsy if the infant dies
4 Consultation with specialists: radiologist, geneticist, biochemist, ophthalmologist, neurologist, etc.
5 Database consultation may aid in the diagnosis of multiple birth defects, e.g. OMIM, London Dysmorphology Database.

---

conditions that increase the risk (e.g. insulin-dependent diabetes mellitus)
- avoidance of drugs known to be teratogens (see Table 4.4)
- administration of folic acid for at least 1 month before conception in planned pregnancies and in the early months of pregnancy to reduce the incidence of neural tube defects (see Chapter 22). Some countries, such as Australia, have legislated to make folate supplementation mandatory in some food products (e.g. bread).
- avoidance of maternal exposure to known chemical teratogens and irradiation (see Chapter 4)
- community education in the avoidance of harmful practices and the use of potential teratogens, including smoking, alcohol and cocaine during pregnancy
- prenatal diagnosis using ultrasound, chorionic villus sampling, amniocentesis, maternal serum,

fetal blood sampling and fetal biopsy, as early pre-natal diagnosis will provide an opportunity for counselling and possibly termination of pregnancy
• neonatal screening for the early detection and treatment of diseases or conditions before perma-nent damage is incurred, e.g. phenylketonuria, galactosaemia, hypothyroidism, cystic fibrosis and congenital dislocation of the hip.

SUMMARY

Genetics is a complex and rapidly expanding field. The genetic basis of many diseases has now been identified. Investigations which help to identify genetic disease include clinical examination, family history, specific genetic investigations (e.g. chromosome analysis and microarray) and metabolic investigations.

Early diagnosis of a genetic disease has a number of benefits including prognosis, initiation of appropriate treatment to prevent or minimize damage, possible termination of pregnancy or palliative care of affected infants, and prevention of reoccurrence in future pregnancies.

Now visit **www.essentialneonatalmed.com** to test yourself on this chapter.

CHAPTER 9
Infant feeding and nutrition

Key points

Introduction

Besides meeting nutritional requirements and promoting growth, early nutrition has biological effects on the individual with important implications for their later life as an adolescent and adult. Over the last decade or so, it has also been shown that human infants, like other species, are 'programmed' by early nutrition for long-term outcomes such as effect on blood pressure (hypertension) insulin resistance (diabetes), tendency to obesity, allergies and neurodevelopmental outcomes including cognitive function. Thus it makes sense that these findings are factored into the design of modern nutritional strategies.

The ideal food for healthy full-term infants is breast milk. If the baby is born growth restricted, the volume of milk required is higher than for a normally grown baby of the same age (see below). Premature infants have different nutritional requirements from full-term infants and need to be fed either directly into the bowel (enteral feeding) or intravenously (parenteral nutrition).

Essential Neonatal Medicine, Fifth Edition. Sunil Sinha, Lawrence Miall, Luke Jardine.
© 2012 John Wiley & Sons, Ltd. Published 2012 by John Wiley & Sons, Ltd.

Specific nutritional requirements

Fluids

Water is the major constituent of infants, but its proportion varies with maturity (Fig. 9.1). Newborn infants, especially preterm ones, have a higher percentage of total body water than children and adults, but the proportion decreases with age as ability to conserve water increases. For this reason, the daily requirement of the newborn is relatively higher than that of older children, and that of the premature infant is higher still. Mechanisms for conserving water are often poorly developed in immature infants, and their requirements depend on conceptual age, postnatal age and environment.

A healthy breastfed infant will consume as much fluid as is required, given ready access to the breast. Healthy bottle-fed infants will also 'know' how much fluid they need and should be allowed to consume milk when they want it, to the volume that satisfies them. Unfortunately, many mothers feel that their baby should take all the milk at every feed, and overfeeding may become a problem. In addition, ill or premature babies need to be given their requirements as they cannot be relied upon to take what they need. For these reasons, recommended feeding schedules have been devised (Table 9.1). These fluid requirements will be maintained up to 3 months of age, and then slowly reduced to 100 mL/kg/day by the age of 1 year.

Infants who have suffered intrauterine growth restriction should be fed to an expected weight as if they had grown normally *in utero*. Ill preterm infants, particularly those with lung disease, may tolerate fluids poorly and develop worsening lung disease, patency of ductus arteriosus and oedema. Some very immature infants may lose large amounts of water through their kidneys or skin. In such cases a significantly higher fluid intake may be required.

For these reasons, recommended feeding schedules are of little value in sick infants: the fluid intake must be tailored to the infant's requirements and state of hydration. Clinical assessment of hydration is made by skin turgor, fontanelle tension, moistness of the mucous membranes and urine output. In practice, clinical methods for assessing fluid requirements are unreliable: laboratory investigations are more helpful. Serum sodium, potassium, creatinine, osmolality and haemoglobin (haematocrit) should be measured. In addition, urinary osmolality or specific gravity (SG) is an important measurement. Daily weighing is a most valuable assessment of hydration and growth.

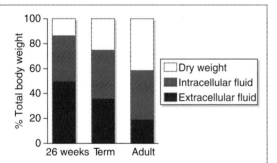

Figure 9.1 Total body water and extracellular fluid expressed as percentages of body weight. Redrawn from Dear (1984), with permission from Reed Business Publishing.

Table 9.1 Recommended feeding schedules (fluid volume mL/kg according to day of life)

	Day of life						
	1	**2**	**3**	**4**	**5**	**6**	**7**
Term infant	30–60	60	90	120	130	140	150
Preterm infant	60	80	100	120	140	160	160–180
'Sick' preterm infant	60	70	80	90	100	110	120

Add 20 mL/kg for open radiant heat source incubator and for phototherapy.

Serum osmolality may be affected by hyponatraemia, hyperglycaemia or uraemia, and may be unreliable under these circumstances. Similarly, glycosuria or proteinuria may affect urinary SG. In practice we aim to keep the urinary SG between 1005 and 1010, increasing the fluid volume if the urine becomes more concentrated, and consider fluid reduction in the presence of very dilute urine.

Inappropriate antidiuretic hormone (IADH) secretion is a relatively common condition in both premature and full-term infants with severe lung or cerebral disorders. It may also be seen following neonatal surgery. The hallmark is dilute serum (low serum sodium and osmolality) with concentrated urine. Peripheral oedema is often present. The treatment is fluid restriction until the serum osmolality returns to the normal range (270–285 mmol/L). If serum sodium is dangerously low (<118 mmol/L), careful correction with hypertonic saline infusion may be needed to avoid complications such as cerebral oedema (water intoxication)

Energy and macronutrients

Energy requirements for optimal growth depend on the baby's birthweight, gestational age and state of health. Ill babies are likely to be more catabolic and will have greater energy requirements. In addition, the smaller the infant the greater are the requirements per kilogram, and this is particularly so in infants who have suffered intrauterine growth restriction. Table 9.2 gives the energy requirements of various groups of infants for optimal growth. Of the recommended 120 kcal/kg per day of energy for the preterm infant, only 25 kcal/kg per day are for energy storage for growth.

Table 9.2 Energy requirements for optimal growth at the end of the first week of life

	Daily energy requirement	
	(kcal/kg)	(kJ/kg)
Premature infant	120	516
Small for gestational age	140+	602
Term infant	100	403

Carbohydrate

The carbohydrate of human milk is predominantly lactose (90–95%) with small amounts of oligosaccharides (5–10%). Lactose (a disaccharide made up of glucose and galactose) must be metabolized to glucose for energy utilization in the brain and other organs. Approximately 40% of the infant's total energy requirement comes from the carbohydrate in milk.

Fat

Fat in milk provides approximately half of the infant's energy requirements. Human milk fat is better absorbed than cows' milk fat. The mature infant absorbs about 90% of the fat in human milk, but infants weighing less than 1500 g absorb only 75–80% of fat from human milk, and less from artificial milk. Unsaturated fatty acids are better absorbed than saturated fatty acids, and medium-chain triglyceride better than long-chain triglyceride. Infants require 4–6 g fat/kg per day.

Considerable interest has developed in the role of long-chain polyunsaturated fatty acids (LC-PUFAs) in milk and their role in brain development. LC-PUFAs are present in human but not bovine milk. As accumulation of fetal LC-PUFAs is increased up to five times in the last trimester, prematurely born infants are thought to be particularly at risk of deficiency. All ready-to-feed preterm formulas are supplemented with LC-PUFAs. The predominant polyunsaturated fats are omega-6 (linoleic acid) and omega-3 (alpha-linolenic acid [ALA]), which are required for production of arachidonic acid and docosahexanoic acid respectively.

Protein

Approximately 10% of the infant's energy requirements is provided by protein. The recommended daily intake is 2.5–3.5 g/kg per day for full-term infants and 3.0–3.8 g/kg per day for very premature infants; ESPGHAN now recommend 4–4.5/kg per day for infants less than 1000 g. Milk protein is divided into curd (mainly casein) and whey (predominantly lactalbumin). Human milk contains more whey, and cows' milk considerably more curd.

Table 9.3 Recommended enteral intake of minerals for term and VLBW infants		
	Enteral mineral intake (mmol/kg per day)	
	Term infant	VLBW infant
Sodium	2.5–3.5	3.0–4.0
Potassium	2.5–3.5	2.0–3.0
Chloride	5.0	1.5–4.5
Phosphorus	1.0–1.5	1.9–4.5
Calcium	1.2–1.5	3–5.5
Magnesium	0.6	0.3–0.6

Source: Koo and Tsang (1993).

Table 9.4 Recommended daily enteral intake of some trace minerals		
	Daily requirement	
	(mmol/kg)	(µg/kg)
Zinc	7.7–12.3	500–800
Copper	1.9	120
Manganese	0.01	0.75
Chromium	0.001	0.05

Source: Ehrenkranz (1993).

There are also important differences in the amino acid profile of human and cows' milk.

Minerals

The recommended minimal mineral requirements for optimal nutrition are shown in Table 9.3. In sick infants, particularly those receiving intravenous nutrition, it is important to monitor serum levels of these minerals and adjust intakes accordingly. Extra sodium may be required by the very-low-birthweight (VLBW) infant, as there may be a high urinary loss for the first weeks of life. Potassium should not be given until adequate renal function has been established.

Trace elements

Recommended enteral requirements of trace elements are shown in Table 9.4. Copper and zinc have been shown to be essential trace elements for newborn infants. Other trace elements thought to be essential are chromium, manganese, iodine, cobalt and selenium. Breast milk and modern formula feeds contain some of these elements.

Iron

Both preterm and term infants born to healthy mothers have sufficient iron stores at birth to double

their haemoglobin mass. Depletion of these stores occurs at 3 months in premature and 5 months in term infants. If the baby is not receiving adequate iron in the diet by this age, iron deficiency anaemia will develop. Although the iron content of breast milk declines from 0.6 mg/L at 2 weeks to 0.3 mg/L at 5 months, breast milk provides sufficient iron for a term infant up to 6 months of age. Preterm infants (irrespective of which milk they receive) should be monitored for iron deficiency anaemia and supplemented with oral iron if needed. Some units routinely provide iron supplement without the need for blood tests.

Vitamins

The daily vitamin requirements for the newborn and young infant are shown in Table 9.5. The fat-soluble vitamins A, D, E and K are stored in the body and large doses may result in toxicity. Excess doses of water-soluble vitamins are readily excreted. The preterm infant probably requires more vitamin D (1000 IU/day). This is discussed in the section on rickets of prematurity (see Chapter 20). There is no good evidence that routine supplementation with vitamin E prevents late anaemia, or bronchopulmonary dysplasia. Vitamin K is the only vitamin in which the normal breastfed infant may become seriously deficient; deficiency of this vitamin may cause haemorrhagic disease of the newborn (see Chapter 20). Despite controversies regarding the best dose and route of administration, all breastfed babies should be given vitamin K supplementation except

Table 9.5 Recommended daily dosage for vitamin supplementation	
Vitamin A	500–1500 IU
Vitamin D	400 IU
Vitamin E	5 IU
Vitamin C (ascorbic acid)	35 mg
Folate	50 μg
Niacin	5 mg
Riboflavin	0.4 mg
Thiamine	0.2 mg
Vitamin B_6	0.2 mg
Vitamin B_{12}	1 μg
Vitamin K	15 μg

for those who have already received intramuscular injection of vitamin K because of either their prematurity or sickness.

Breastfeeding

Breastfeeding brings many benefits to both mother and baby (see Box 9.1).

In 1991 UNICEF and the World Health Organization (WHO) introduced the global baby-friendly hospital initiative to improve breastfeeding programmes. The '10 steps' to successful breastfeeding are intended as a standard of good practice (Box 9.2).

Physiology of lactation

During pregnancy there is a marked increase in the number of ducts and alveoli within the breast in response to oestrogens, progesterone and placental lactogen. In the third trimester, prolactin secreted by the anterior pituitary sensitizes the glandular tissue with the secretion of small amounts of colostrum. The flow of milk after birth is under the control of the **let-down reflex**. The baby rooting at the nipple causes afferent impulses to pass to the posterior pituitary, which secretes oxytocin. This stimulates the smooth muscle fibres surrounding the alveoli to

Box 9.1 Benefits of breastfeeding

For the baby

- It provides a source of nutrition that changes with the baby's changing metabolic needs
- It confers an advantage in intellectual attainment (see below)
- It is anti-infective (see below)
- It is antiallergic. The avoidance of foreign proteins in formula feeds reduces the risk of asthma and eczema in infants predisposed to these conditions
- It provides protection against various illnesses (e.g. gastroenteritis), although apparent protection against SIDS probably relates to maternal education, socioeconomic status and birthweight, rather than to breastfeeding per se
- Reduced likelihood and severity of cows' milk protein allergy
- Decreased incidence of infant obesity and subsequently type 2 diabetes, hypertension and hyperlipidaemia

For the mother

- Successful breastfeeding brings a sense of personal pride and achievement
- It promotes a close mother–baby relationship, which provides security, warmth and comfort to baby
- Lactation helps the mother lose weight acquired in pregnancy
- Convenience – there is no preparation of formula. Breast milk can also be simply expressed, stored and given to the baby by others
- Lactational amenorrhoea remains the world's most important contraceptive by delaying the return of ovulation
- Oxytocin release during breastfeeding contracts the uterus and helps its involution
- Financial benefit, as breastfeeding does not cost
- It is possible to continue breastfeeding if a mother needs to return to paid work
- Breastfeeding confers some health advantages on the mother, as there appears to be some protection against ovarian and premenopausal breast cancer and osteoporosis

Box 9.2 The '10 steps' to successful breastfeeding

Step 1 Have a written breastfeeding policy that is routinely communicated to all healthcare staff

Step 2 Train all healthcare staff in the skills necessary to implement this policy

Step 3 Inform all women (face to face and with leaflets) about the benefits and management of breastfeeding

Step 4 Help mothers initiate breastfeeding shortly after delivery

Step 5 Show mothers how to breastfeed and how to maintain lactation (by expressing milk) even if they may be separated from their infants

Step 6 Give newborn infants no food or drink unless 'medically' indicated (no promotion of formula milks)

Step 7 Practise 'rooming-in'; all mothers should have their infant's cots next to them 24 h a day

Step 8 Encourage breastfeeding on demand

Step 9 Give no artificial teats or pacifiers ('dummies') to breastfeeding infants

Step 10 Foster the establishment of breastfeeding support groups and refer mothers to them

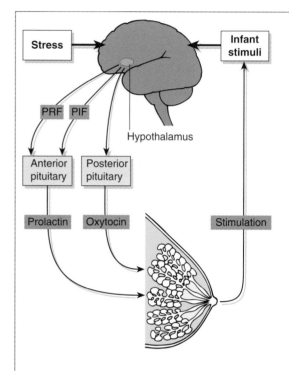

Figure 9.2 Hormonal maintenance of lactation. PIF, prolactin inhibiting factor; PRF, prolactin releasing factor.

• **Endogenous (maternal) factors.** In the first weeks of lactation, prolactin secretion occurs in response to feeding and controls milk production.
• **Exogenous (baby) factors.** After a few weeks of successful breastfeeding the baby exerts the major control on breast milk production. The amount of milk produced is related to effective and frequent removal of milk from the breast by the baby.

Nutritional aspects

Human milk is uniquely adapted to the requirements of babies, with low levels of protein and minerals compared with the milks of other species. The energy content of human milk (67 kcal/100 mL) is provided by fat (54%), carbohydrate (40%) and protein (6%). Human milk has a very low protein content of only 0.9 g/100 mL, with a whey:casein ratio of 0.7. A larger proportion of the nitrogen in human milk is derived from non-protein sources

force the milk into the large ducts. After birth there is an increase in prolactin levels, which maintains milk production. The hormonal maintenance of lactation is summarized in Fig. 9.2.

Stress inhibits oxytocin release and may reduce milk production. This may cause the baby to cry more, thereby heightening maternal stress and further inhibiting milk production. This may be an important factor in the failure of long-term lactation (see below).

Milk production is controlled by endogenous and exogenous factors:

compared with cows' milk. Human milk contains twice as much lactalbumin as cows' milk (and is immunologically different), but no lactoglobulin, which is a significant component of the protein constitution of cows' milk. The levels of amino acids such as taurine, aspartic acid, glutamic acid and asparagine are especially high. Human milk fat is better absorbed than cows' milk fat because of the smaller size of the emulsified fat globules and the presence of lipase in human milk

The main differences between human and cows' milk are shown in Table 9.6. There is a higher proportion of unsaturated fatty acids and a lower proportion of saturated fatty acids in human milk than in cows' milk. Human milk contains more vitamins A, C and E and nicotinic acid than does cows' milk, but less vitamin B_1, B_2, B_6, B_{12} and K. The low mineral level in human milk results in a low renal solute load for the immature kidney. Although calcium and phosphate levels in cows' milk are higher than in human milk, their absorption from cows' milk is much lower.

Variations in breast milk

Early breast milk contains a higher sodium and protein concentration than milk from mothers who have fed their infants for several months. The amount of lactose in breast milk increases with postnatal age as the intestinal disaccharidase enzyme mechanism matures. Interestingly, up to 90% of milk is taken from the breast in the first 4 min of feeding; the rest of the 'feed' is largely non-nutritive. Bottle-fed infants have quite a different pattern of intake, less than 40% of the feed being taken in the first 5 min.

The milk constituents of mothers who deliver prematurely are different from those of women who deliver at full term. Preterm milk contains a higher protein and sodium content than term milk. In addition, preterm milk contains considerably more immunoglobulin (IgA) and other immune factors, and is more protective against necrotizing enterocolitis, than term milk. The composition of preterm human milk varies markedly but there is a progressive decline in energy, lactose and fat content over time. For mothers whose breast milk supply exceeds preterm requirements, feeding with energy and fat-rich 'hind milk' may increase weight gain.

Anti-infective properties of breast milk

Breastfeeding is an effective method of protection from infection while a baby's immunological system is developing. Breastfed infants are less likely to develop gastroenteritis, necrotizing enterocolitis (NEC), otitis media and other serious infections, such as septicaemia and meningitis. This is due to numerous host resistance factors in human milk, which include:

- **Immunoglobulins:** IgA is the most important immunoglobulin secreted in breast milk, and is in very high concentrations in colostrum.
- **Cells:** breast milk contains vast numbers of macrophages, polymorphs, and both T and B lymphocytes.
- **Lysozyme:** this acts to lyse the *Escherichia coli* cell membrane.

Table 9.6 Proteins in human milk and cows' milk

	Protein content (g/100 mL)	
	Human milk	Cows' milk
Total protein	0.89	3.30
Caseins	0.25	2.60
Total whey protein	0.64	0.70
α-Lactalbumin	0.26	0.12
α-Lactoglobulin	–	0.30
Lactoferrin	0.17	Trace
Serum albumin	0.05	0.03
Lysozyme	0.05	Trace
IgA	0.10	0.003
IgG	0.003	0.06
IgM	0.002	0.003
Others	0.07	0.15

Source: Reproduced from Hambraeus *et al.* (1984).

• **Lactoferrin:** this binds iron, which is necessary for some bacteria to multiply.
• **Antiviral properties**, possibly due to secretory IgA or interferon production by lymphocytes.
• **Probiotics:** the stool of breastfed babies is more acid than that of artificially fed infants. This, together with the carbohydrate bifidus factor, encourages lactobacilli to flourish, which has the effect of inhibiting the growth of *E. coli*.

Contraindications to breastfeeding

These are uncommon and most of them are only relative rather than absolute contraindication.

In the mother

• **Acute illness:** a relative contraindication, as illness is usually over quickly
• **Chronic illness:** receiving chemotherapy; mental illness (depending on medications and safety); tuberculosis (active treatment)
• **Breast infection/abscess:** management is either temporary expression of that breast or continue feeding, depending on severity
• **HIV infection in the mother** can be transmitted to the baby through the cells in breast milk. In developing countries the risk of gastroenteritis from contaminated feeds outweighs the risk of acquiring HIV infection from breast milk, but in developed countries, where clean water is taken for granted, breastfeeding by HIV-positive women is contraindicated
• **Illicit drugs and substance abuse:** breastfeeding is not an absolute contraindication. Ideally breastfeeding should occur before planned use of such drugs or substances. Mothers on prescribed methadone are still able to breastfeed and this in fact could be beneficial in reducing withdrawal symptoms in babies.

In the infant

• **Acute illness:** this may be temporary. and the expression and storage of breast milk should be encouraged
• **Mechanical problems:** severe cleft lip and/or palate

• **Metabolic problems:** galactosaemia, phenylketonuria, lactose intolerance
• **Breast milk jaundice** (see Chapter 19): interruption of breastfeeding is not necessary; usually diagnosis is made by exclusion of other pathological causes.

Excretion of drugs in breast milk

Factors that enhance the transfer of drugs in breast milk include
• **lipid solubility** of the drug
• **pH:** the pH of milk is 6.6–7.4, so that basic drugs such as antihistamines, aminophylline, opiates and antidepressants are more likely to be excreted in higher concentrations
• **degree of ionization:** unionized drugs are more likely to be excreted
• **protein binding:** drugs that are not protein bound show a greater tendency to be excreted
• **molecular weight:** drugs of low molecular weight are excreted to a greater extent.

The suitability or unsuitability of breastfeeding when a mother has to take a drug should be judged on individual basis taking into account the drug's pharmacological properties and its risk–benefit analysis.

Techniques of breastfeeding

Establishment of lactation

Preparation for breastfeeding should begin in the antenatal period.

The infant should be put to the breast as soon as possible after delivery, and the timing and duration of feeds should be responsive to the needs of the baby. Breastfeeding at night should be encouraged. Supplementing breast milk with water or glucose reduces the duration of breastfeeding with no compensating benefit, and should be strongly discouraged.

The baby should never be pulled off the breast. The jaw should be released by depressing with the finger at the corner of the baby's mouth. Feeds should be started on alternate breasts. Nipple creams and sprays are unnecessary; application of breast milk to nipples after a feed accelerates healing.

Problems with breastfeeding

Ill or preterm baby

The mother should be encouraged to express by hand within a few hours of birth, as frequent breast expression up to 8–10 times a day increases lactation. A pump should only be used if it is comfortable and convenient and the nipples are not already traumatized. Current recommendation is to commence use of an electric pump after 24 h.

Jaundiced baby

The sleepy, jaundiced baby should be encouraged to breastfeed first but may need to take expressed breast milk from a bottle, so that an adequate intake of milk may be given and documented.

Insufficient breast milk

While in hospital the mother will require a great deal of support and reassurance and continued nipple stimulation to establish an adequate supply of milk. After discharge, social and emotional problems may influence the milk supply.

Reasons for low supply include maternal anxiety, inadequate sucking stimulus due to inappropriate feeding routines and behaviours, and inadequate glandular response. The most common reason for early weaning is the mother's perception of inadequate milk production.

Milk engorgement

This can largely be prevented by demand feeding. Once breast engorgement has occurred, hot packs before feeding and cold packs after feeding are helpful. The mother should only express sufficient milk to soften the areola, to enable the baby to latch on to the breast.

Cracked nipples

Cracks are caused by incorrect positioning of the baby on the breast. Nipple soreness may be due to positional soreness, nipple fissure, infection such as candida, and dermatitis. Rarely is it necessary to take the baby off the breast, and there is little evidence that this practice accelerates healing. Nipple care with the application of lanolin or masse cream and exposure to sunlight and fresh air may help heal the cracks. Hindmilk left on the nipples to dry after a feed may aid the healing process.

Inverted or retracted nipples

There is no evidence that inverted or retracted nipples inhibit the woman's ability to breastfeed her baby successfully, or that treatment prior to birth with nipple exercises or shields improves breastfeeding rates.

Sleepy babies

Babies may be sleepy in the first day or two after delivery, and this state may relate to analgesia and anaesthesia or mild birth asphyxia. They should not be left without feed for too long because of the danger of hypoglycaemia, particularly in low-birthweight babies and those with intrauterine growth restriction.

'Fighting the breast'

This is often associated with maternal anxiety and is aggravated if there are difficulties in getting the baby to the breast. Careful support and reassurance are necessary to establish successful lactation under these circumstances.

Twin feeding

If the twins are full term and vigorous, twin feeding should be possible even from day 1. Often the twins are small and do not readily suckle at the breast, so that expression may be necessary initially. It is an individual choice as to whether the babies are fed together or separately.

Weaning (changing from breast milk to another milk)

The decision on when to wean is an individual one between mother and baby. If breastfeeding has been established for more than 4–6 months, weaning should be a gradual process over at least 2–3 weeks. The last feed to be stopped should be the evening feed. It is advisable to put the infant on a formula milk and not to start 'doorstep' cow's milk until 12 months of age.

Advice to breastfeeding mothers

If there are problems with breastfeeding after discharge from hospital, midwives and/or health visitors can provide help and support. Most countries have a wide range of community resources well equipped to deal with the mother under stress. Lactation consultants are readily available both in hospital and after discharge and so are the breastfeeding support groups.

Iron supplementation

Term infants receive sufficient supplemental iron in breast milk alone, at least until 6 months of age, and probably until 9 months. Breast milk contains sufficient vitamins for the full-term infant until solids are introduced. The preterm infant needs supplemental iron whether breastfed or not. There is, however, no generally agreed principle as to when and for how long to give iron supplements to these babies.

Breast milk banks

There are many advantages to feeding infants with breast milk, namely the nutritional balance of breast milk, its antimicrobial properties and the avoidance of foreign protein. For these reasons, milk banks have been established in order to provide breast milk for infants in whom artificial feeds may be disadvantageous. The practice of breast milk banking was put in doubt with the worldwide epidemic of HIV/AIDS, but by careful screening of donor mothers milk banking is enjoying renewed enthusiasm. Donor mothers are invariably well-established breastfeeders. The milk is collected in sterile plastic bottles and stored in the mother's own domestic refrigerator at 4°C for no longer than 48 h. It is then delivered to the milk bank and frozen (−20°C) prior to heat treatment.

Milk is not accepted from women who are HIV- or hepatitis B-positive.

Breast milk and intelligence

There has been considerable debate as to whether babies who have been breastfed subsequently have a higher intelligence quotient (IQ) than those given formula milk in the early months of life. This debate is beset with the difficulties of self-selection, as it is often women of higher socioeconomic class who elect to breastfeed, and intelligence has a major genetic influence.

Artificial feeding/formulas

If a mother fails in her attempts to breastfeed or does not wish to undertake breastfeeding, she must not be made to feel inadequate or guilty. Successful bottle-feeding is much better than unsuccessful breastfeeding. Mothers make an informed decision not to breastfeed because of early return to work, adoption and previous lack of success.

Cows' milk

Unmodified cows' milk is not recommended during the first 12 months of life because:
• its iron content is low and of poor bioavailability
• it has higher levels of protein, sodium, potassium, phosphorus and calcium compared with human milk or formula
• it has a high renal solute load
• it is lacking in vitamin C and essential fatty acids
• there is potential gastrointestinal tract blood loss, secondary to cow's milk colitis.

Cows' milk can be introduced into the infant's diet during the second 6 months of life as custard, yoghurt and cheese. Complementary feeding is not recommended until 6 months of age.

Cows' milk-based formulas

Commercially produced infant formulas that are reconstituted with water are sold as powders or 'ready-to-feed' liquids. The infant milk manufacturers produce milks that are similar to mature breast milk and are often marketed as 'breast milk substitutes'. The WHO has set down very strict criteria in the International Code of Marketing of Breast-milk Substitutes. More recently, formula feeds have been developed that are better suited to the needs of premature infants.

The milk pharmaceutical industry has modified cow's milk in attempts to mimic human milk in

Table 9.7 Modifications to cows'-milk-based formulas		
Component	**Usual form in cows' milk**	**Modification**
Protein	Casein dominant	Whey dominant protein Hydrolysates of whey, casein or amino acids Added nucleotides
Fat	LCT	Medium-chain TGs Added LC-PUFAs
Carbohydrate	Lactose	Lactose-free Lactose, sucrose- and fructose-free Added thickening agents Added prebiotics
Minerals	High Na, K, calcium, phosphate	Demineralized

LCT, long-chain triglycerides.

nutritional content (Table 9.7). These modifications increase the cost of infant formulas. Casein-dominant formulas are usually cheaper than whey-dominant ones. Formula milk now contains pre-biotic oligosaccharides that encourage a healthy gut flora.

Modification of cows' milk-based formulas

Starter and follow-on formulas
Starter formulas are suitable from birth to 1 year. Follow-on formulas have slightly higher protein and electrolyte levels and are usually casein dominant. They are often recommended from 6 months of age.

Soy formulas
These have higher levels of aluminium and phyto-oestrogens than cows' milk-based formulas but no adverse effects have been substantiated. There is no benefit over cow's milk formulas as a supplement for the breastfed infant and no proven benefit in prevention of atopic disease. Soy-based formulas have low lactose content and are suitable for treatment of infants with galactosaemia. Some are sucrose free and suitable for sucrose intolerance.

Preterm formulas
Special formulas have been developed to meet the nutritional requirement of growing preterm infants who may have ongoing and catch-up need for extra nutrients that may not be met by term formulas. Hence, preterm babies should be discharged on formulas that have nutritional content somewhere halfway between preterm and standard formula. This is particularly beneficial for babies who have chronic lung disease or who were born too early. The protein content of preterm formulas (whey based) is higher than that of term formula (2.7–3 g/100 kcal) and they also have adequate levels of vitamins and minerals.

Major nutrients in milk

Protein modification

Whey/casein
Breast milk is 60–70% whey dominant whereas cows' milk is 60% casein dominant. Infant formula can be either whey or casein dominant. Whey-dominant formulas form an easier-to-digest curd in the stomach, are more similar to breast milk and are probably more suitable for young babies.

Hydrolysates

In hydrolysed formulas the protein molecules have been partly or completely broken down to smaller molecules, which may be less allergenic. Formulas may be hydrolysed whey or casein or amino acids.

Nucleotides are present in breast milk and are progressively being introduced into formulas because of their potential to benefit the development of the gastrointestinal tract, immune system and intestinal microflora, and help iron absorption.

Fat modification

Long-chain polyunsaturated fatty acids (LC-PUFAs) are present in breast milk as omega-3 (alpha-linolenic acid → docosahexanoic acid [DHA]) and omega-6 (linoleic acid → arachidonic acid [AA]) and are major structural components of brain, retina and myelin for nerve sheaths. As preterm infants are deficient at birth in LC-PUFAs and cannot readily form DHA, LC-PUFAs are considered an essential supplement of preterm formulas. Although many formulas for term infants contain added LC-PUFAs, clinical trials are still under way to see whether they confer long-term benefits. In some modified cows' milk formulas, such as some preterm formulas and semi- and complete elemental formulas, fat content is altered from long-chain triglycerides (LCT) to medium-chain triglycerides (MCT) in order to enhance absorption.

Carbohydrate modification

Lactose intolerance (LI) results from the deficiency of the enzyme lactase and may be primary (very rare) or secondary following damage to the gut lining from conditions such as gastroenteritis, malnutrition, protein allergy, coeliac disease or inflammatory bowel disease. Lactose-free cow's milk-based formulas are usually the preferred choice for secondary LI, whereas more elemental formulas will be required for prolonged LI, especially if there is evidence of other malabsorption. Several of the soy formulas are both lactose- and sucrose-free and can be used for primary LI or lactose and sucrose intolerance.

Thickening agents

Thickening agents such as rice starch, carob bean flour or pregelatinized corn starch may be added to a standard formula or may come as an antireflux formula substituted for lactose. These formulas may stop regurgitation.

Prebiotics and probiotics

Probiotics are live microbial supplements that colonize the gut and provide benefits to the host. Common examples are bifidobacteria and lacto-bacilli. A large number of other species have also been developed. Probiotics are thought to be efficient in preventing and treating diarrhoea in children and evidence suggests that they may prevent NEC (see Chapter 17).

Prebiotics are non-digestible foods that make their way through the digestive system and help good bacteria grow and flourish. Prebiotics keep beneficial bacteria healthy. However, the scientific evidence to support their routine use in newborns is not fully established as yet.

Elemental or partially elemental formulas

These have modified protein (hydrolysates of whey or casein, or amino acids), carbohydrate (glucose polymers, lactose free) and fat (variable amounts of MCT). They are used in cases of allergy or intolerance to cows', goats' or soy protein, fat malabsorption, short gut syndrome, chylous effusions and sometimes severe infantile colic.

Other modified milks required in the management of specific malabsorption conditions are shown in Table 9.8. The management of these conditions requires the support of a metabolic physician or other specialist and the close support of an experienced nutritionist.

Techniques of artificial feeding

Volumes

The amounts as suggested in the first section of this chapter should be given.

Interval between feeds

In general, term infants weighing less than 3 kg are initially fed 3-hourly. Infants over 3 kg can be fed on demand or 4-hourly. It is reasonable to delete the night feed if the infant does not wake and is over 3 kg in weight.

Sterilization

A suitable technique for teats and bottles should be followed. One commonly used is the 'Milton method'. Water used in the preparation of feeds

Table 9.8 Adapted formulas for various malabsorptive conditions

Condition	Recommended formula
Allergy/intolerance to cows'/goats' or soy milk	Hydrolysed or partially elemental formula
Fat malabsorption (cystic fibrosis, biliary atresia, short gut syndrome)	Elemental or partially elemental formulas
Lactose intolerance	Lactose-free
Sucrose intolerance	Sucrose-free
Fructose intolerance	Special carbohydrate-modified (cows' or soy)
Galactosaemia	Lactose-free milks (cows' or soy)
Phenylketonuria	Amino acid formula (low protein)
Other inborn errors of metabolism	Other specialized milks

must be bacteriologically safe. This may be conveniently achieved by boiling the water for 10 min before it is used for feed preparation.

Preparation of feeds

Guidelines suggested by milk manufacturers for their products should be carefully followed. The preparation of overconcentrated feeds is an important cause of hypernatraemic dehydration.

Feeding the preterm infant

Growth

In utero the fetus grows at about 15 g/kg per day and this is usually the goal for preterm infants of birthweight less than 2 kg. For infants of birthweight greater than 2 kg, the expected weight gain is more than 20 g/day with growth in length of 0.7–1.0 cm/week and increase in head circumference 0.7–1.0 cm/week. The long-term goal of neonatal nutrition is to allow maximum attainment of potential growth and development.

Preterm infants have low body reserves of nutrients and high requirements compared with term infants (see Tables 9.1–9.4) because most nutrient accretion occurs in the last 3 months of pregnancy. Early undernutrition may contribute to long-term problems such as poor bone mineralization and metabolic syndrome (Barker hypothesis). The short-term nutritional goal is to mimic the growth and development that occurs *in utero*.

Feeding the very-low-birthweight infant

Few subjects in neonatal medicine generate as much controversy as the appropriate way to feed the very premature infant. Some ill VLBW infants will not tolerate milk feeds and require parenteral nutrition. For those to whom milk may safely be given there is sometimes a choice between breast milk (expressed from the infant's own mother – EBM – or banked breast milk – BBM) or a formula feed. Unfortunately, there are still insufficient human breast milk banks, even in developed countries, and pasteurization and/or freezing EBM will reduce some of its unique immunological properties. Specially adapted formula milks have been developed for the needs of premature babies that meet their nutritional requirements better than standard formula feeds.

The following are the general principles on which feeding the VLBW baby is based.

Expressed breast milk

The preferred milk for preterm and low-birthweight infants is EBM from the biological mother. Breast milk expressed from the mother who delivers preterm has many important properties that make it the milk of choice for the preterm infant. These include:
- reduced risk of infection owing to the anti-infective properties described earlier
- possible reduced risk of NEC in premature infants
- the presence of growth factors in milk, which may be absorbed intact through the baby's gut

- advantages for cognitive development
- enhanced absorption, less steatorrhoea
- contains protein of high quality and bioavailability, plus unique fats and carbohydrates.

Breast or human milk fortifiers

Although the composition of preterm breast milk is more appropriate for the nutritional needs of the preterm infant than term breast milk, it does not meet the fetal accretion rate of nutrients. Human milk fortifiers (HMFs) can be added to EBM when a preterm infant (<32 weeks' gestation) is fully enterally fed, to boost the energy, protein, sodium, calcium, phosphorus and vitamin levels. A number of fortifiers are available commercially. They have shown advantages in the short term, but long-term outcomes and safety are still not known. Recent evidence suggests very preterm infants (<1000 g) may benefit from even greater protein supplementation.

Low-birthweight formulas

Table 9.9 shows the typical contents of low-birthweight formulas compared with formulas for mature infants. The former often contain more sodium, potassium, protein and carbohydrate than breast milk or regular artificial feeds. We continue to feed the preterm infant on one of these formulas until the infant's postconceptual age is 35 weeks, and then change to a regular formula feed.

Preterm milks are available as ready-to-feed formulas, usually as 81 kcal/100 mL. They have high levels of nutrients and low osmolality (<325 mosmol/L). They are supplemented with LC-PUFAs and nucleotides, and have a high Ca:phosphate ratio and variable proportions of MCTs.

Trophic feeding

Early exposure of the baby's gut to enteral feeds, even if they are receiving parenteral feeding, has been shown to mature gut function. Low-volume hypocaloric feeds (2 mL/kg per hour) significantly reduce the time for a baby to reach full feeding compared with babies who do not have early feeding. This effect is probably mediated through the stimulation of gut hormones (priming the gut).

Practical management guidelines

There is evidence that having and following a feeding policy reduces the risk of NEC. In developing a policy for feeding the VLBW infant, the principles in Box 9.3 should be considered.

Total parenteral nutrition

Total parenteral nutrition (TPN) is not the preferred method for feeding infants and should be used only when appropriate enteral feeding is not possible. Supplemental parenteral nutrition is

Table 9.9 Typical contents of various milks fed to mature and immature infants (contents per 100 mL of milk)

	Mature human milk	Modified milk formula	Demineralized whey formula	Preterm formula
Energy (kcal)	70	65	68	80
Protein (g)	1.34	1.7	1.45	2.0
Sodium (mg)	15	25	19	35
Calcium (mg)	35	61	35	90
Phosphorus (mg)	15	49	29	50
Carbohydrate (g)	7.0	2.8	7.0	6.6–8.6
Fat (g)	4.2	2.6	3.82	4.8

Box 9.3 Principles in feeding the VLBW infant

- Early introduction of breast milk is beneficial even if the milk is given in small volumes (trophic feeding for bowel adaptation). Fresh (rather than frozen) breast milk should be used wherever possible
- Increase the volume of enteral feeds slowly in babies who are at very high risk of NEC (critically ill, severe IUGR, particularly if absent or reversed diastolic flow on antenatal Doppler studies) even though current trials do not confirm any benefit of slow feeding
- Once feeding with breast milk is established, supplement the milk with either breast milk fortifiers or low-birthweight formula. If breast milk is not available, a preterm formula should be used
- The nasogastric route is preferred; nasojejunal feeding should not be used unless there is a particular indication
- There appears to be no advantage of continuous feeding over bolus feeding, which is more physiological. In babies with GOR, continuous feeding may be more appropriate to reduce reflux

frequently practised while the preterm infant (<30 weeks' gestation) slowly adapts to increasing enteral feeds. If TPN is going to be required, it should be introduced as early as the first day.

Indications

The main indications for TPN are:
- preterm infants <30 weeks' gestation and/or <1000 g
- preterm infants >30 weeks but unlikely to receive full feeds by day 7
- severe IUGR with abnormal Doppler flow studies
- NEC
- gastrointestinal tract anomalies.

Methods of delivery

The solutions used in TPN are highly irritant and may cause severe tissue damage if subcutaneous extravasation occurs. For this reason, administration of TPN through a long peripheral or central venous line is advisable.

The TPN regimen aims to provide carbohydrate, fat, protein, electrolytes, minerals, vitamins and trace elements. TPN can be conveniently ordered and administered through standardized bags with modifications as necessary to dextrose, sodium, calcium and phosphate. Generally amino acid bags will be left connected for 48 h with a long-life bacterial filter. Lipid emulsion syringes need to be changed daily.

Carbohydrate

This is usually in the form of 5%, 7.5% or 10% dextrose, and it is to this that the electrolyte and mineral mixture is added. Dextrose is mixed with the amino acid solution in the ratio of 3:1. This combined solution is both acidic and hypertonic.

Protein

This is provided as a mixture of crystalline L-amino acids. The provision of amino acids in these solutions does not closely match the amino acid requirements of ill infants, and regular serum and urinary amino acid profiles should be measured. The rate of infusion for protein is 2.5–4.0 g/kg per day, and the protein is mixed with the dextrose–electrolyte solution before infusion. Newer protein solutions have an amino acid profile similar to cord blood including all the essential amino acids.

Fat

Fat emulsions are made from soya bean oil, egg yolk lecithin and glycerol or olive oil, and contain a high proportion of essential long-chain fatty acids. Fats are protein bound in the plasma and may displace bilirubin from albumin, hence caution with infusion is necessary in jaundiced infants. Many 20% fat emulsions have appropriate phospholipid: triglyceride ratios and are rapidly cleared from plasma. Commencement at 1 g/kg per day as early as day 1–2 of life, increasing in increments of 1 g/kg per day every day or up to 3–4 g/kg per day is recommended. Intravenous fat emulsions should be infused simultaneously with carbohydrate and protein solutions through a Y-connector distal to a bacterial filter.

Minerals

Sodium and potassium requirements are estimated daily and added to the dextrose as required. A mineral mix such as Peditrace provides the necessary trace minerals.

Vitamins

Water-soluble vitamins (e.g. Solvito 0.5 mL/kg per day) and fat-soluble vitamins (e.g. Vitialipid 1 mL/kg per day) are added to the solutions. Vitialipid is mixed with fat emulsion, but is photosensitive; the syringe to which it is added should be protected from light.

Trace elements

Trace elements such as copper and zinc are present in a number of commercial TPN products. Other trace elements (Peditrace) should be added to the TPN solution when TPN is used for more than 7 days.

Clinical management

Individual neonatal units need to develop their own clinical and laboratory monitoring of TPN. However, the following procedures play a crucial part:
• Before infusion commences take a mandatory radiograph, with radio-opaque contrast if necessary, after insertion of a long/central line.
• Observe the infusion site closely, especially when a peripheral line is used.
• Measure blood glucose regularly.
• Weigh regularly.
• Observe serum for lipaemia or measure TG levels.

Laboratory tests

Laboratory investigations for monitoring the safety of TPN should include the following:
• Full blood count (FBC), electrolytes and creatinine – every second day for 1 week and then twice weekly.

• Plasma calcium, phosphate and magnesium twice weekly.
• Liver function tests if TPN >2 weeks.

Complications

Complications from TPN have been reduced with use of newer commercial products. However, the major areas of concern are as follows:
• **Infection.** There is a constant risk of septicaemia when giving TPN. **Coagulase-negative staphylococcus** is the commonest cause of systemic infection. Regular monitoring for sepsis is required, including FBC, C-reactive protein (CRP) and blood cultures.
• **Hyperglycaemia.** Premature babies do not tolerate glucose well. Stick tests for glucose should be carried out regularly. Insulin may be necessary. Minimal enteric feeds have a glucose-lowering effect.
• **Metabolic disturbances.** Careful biochemical surveillance is essential in all infants receiving TPN (see above).
• **Cholestatic jaundice** resulting from prolonged TPN, especially due to lack of hepatic stimulation in the absence of enteral feeding.
• **Hyperammonaemia**.
• **Lipaemia and fat accumulation in the lungs.** Lipid peroxidation when exposed to light is prevented with a silver foil covering lipid infusate or addition of vitamin C. Liberated free fatty acids from lipid infusate can displace bilirubin from albumin.
• **Metabolic acidosis**.
• **Venous thrombosis** (long line).
• **Tissue injury** due to extravasation (peripheral line).

Common feeding disorders

The most frequent problems are posseting, vomiting, colic, constipation, diarrhoea and failure to thrive.

Vomiting

• **Possetting.** Many babies have small spills of feed (posset), and this is considered normal.
• **Vomiting.** This is a common symptom in the newborn and its causes may be non-organic or organic:

- **Non-organic:** overfeeding; incorrect preparation of feeds; overstimulation or excessive handling of baby; crying; air swallowing
- **Organic:** infection (urinary tract infection, gastroenteritis, meningitis, otitis media); gastro-oesophageal reflux, gastritis (meconium, blood), hiatus hernia; organic bowel obstruction, pyloric stenosis, small bowel obstruction, large bowel obstruction; transient gastrointestinal intolerance (e.g. prematurity, metabolic disorders); food allergy (cows' milk). Bile-stained vomiting must always be urgently investigated to exclude acute surgical conditions of the bowel.

Investigation

The cause of infant vomiting can usually be determined if a careful history of feeding technique, description of the vomiting, preparation of the infant formula and other symptoms are assessed. The physical examination must be complete. If still inconclusive, appropriate investigations are necessary, for example:
- abdominal radiograph (bowel obstruction)
- ultrasound examination
- contrast radiograph of upper gastrointestinal tract (hiatus hernia, gastro-oesophageal reflux)
- urine microscopy (urinary tract infection)
- septic screen including urine for microscopy and culture (infection, sepsis)
- stool cultures and microscopy (infection)
- oesophageal pH probe monitoring (gastro-oesophageal reflux.)

Management of the vomiting baby

- Identify and treat the cause wherever possible.
- Maintain fluid balance: parenteral therapy may be indicated.

Organic causes of vomiting

Gastritis

This may be due to meconium or blood swallowed before or during birth. Characteristically it is associated with mucous vomiting.

For treatment, aspiration of the stomach, and instillation of small amount of milk (trophic feeding) will usually suffice but occasionally some antacids or ranitidine may be given. Routine washout of stomach and gastric lavage with normal saline is not recommended.

Gastro-oesophageal reflux and gastro-oesophageal reflux disease

Gastro-oesophageal reflux (GOR) is a common cause of vomiting in the newborn infant. It is not necessarily a pathological entity and does not routinely require any pharmacological treatment. It results from an incompetent lower gastro-oesophageal sphincter and is particularly prevalent in preterm infants, as well as neurologically abnormal infants with severe hypo- or hypertonia. It frequently occurs following repair of diaphragmatic hernia and oesophageal atresia. The vomiting usually occurs at the end of a feed, and particularly when 'winding' the baby. Preterm infants are particularly prone to vomiting due to lax lower oesophageal sphincter tone, delayed gastric emptying and poor oesophageal contractility, all of which improve with maturity.

When GOR is associated with symptoms and complications causing harm to patients (see Box 9.4), it is called gastro-oesophageal reflux disease (GORD). Whereas GOR does not require treatment, GORD often requires further assessment and treatment:

Investigations

Infants with mild symptoms do not require investigation. In severe cases of GOR or GORD, further

---

Box 9.4 Signs and symptoms of GORD

- Persistent vomiting leading to failure to thrive
- Oesophagitis, hiatus hernia, oesophageal stricture
- Obstructive apnoea, apparent life threatening event (ALTE)
- Recurrent aspiration of milk, with the development of a brassy cough, wheeze and stridor

tests may be required including contrast video fluoroscopy of upper gastrointestinal tract (GIT) and oesophageal pH monitoring. Oesophagoscopy (upper GIT endoscopy) may be useful in a few infants.

General measures

Certain general measures can help infants with reflux.

- **Prone position** with a 30–40° head-up tilt appears to be the position of choice. However, the increased risk of sudden infant death syndrome (SIDS) with this sleep position makes it untenable. Mild cases usually improve when the infant is nursed in a more upright position.
- **Thickening the feeds** with an agent such as rice starch, carob bean flour or corn starch is usually effective, in combination with upright feeding. Antireflux milks use similar thickeners. Some formula feeds containing rice starch (e.g. Enfamil AR) are designed to thicken when in contact with warm stomach acid.
- **Acid suppression.** H_2 receptor antagonists such as ranitidine have proven to be effective, however prolonged use of acid suppressant drugs have been recognised to increase the risk of gut sepsis as they inhibit the growth of natural bacteria flora the most effective in a dose of 2 mg/kg three times a day. Antacids are not recommended in the newborn period but may reduce stomach acidity in later infancy. Proton pump inhibitors such as omeprazole are the most potent acid suppressors used after other therapies have failed, or they may be used as first line agents for selected infants with respiratory or neurological symptoms.
- **Continuous feeding** via nasogastric tube or gastrostomy or even transpyloric tube is sometimes required.
- **Surgery.** Rarely fundoplication will be necessary when medical treatment fails or when respiratory complications occur.

Pyloric stenosis

This condition usually presents after the first month of life: rarely it may occur in the first week. It is characterized by projectile vomiting, more commonly in boys, and is associated with visible peristalsis and a palpable 'tumour'. There is often a family history. The baby is usually irritable and there may be hypokalaemia, metabolic acidosis and low chloride. The diagnosis is often confirmed by ultrasound prior to surgery, which consists of splitting the muscle of the pylorus (Ramstedt's operation).

Infant colic

Some apparently healthy infants, who are feeding well and gaining weight, cry at certain times during the day, but especially in the evening around 6 pm. The infant has attacks of screaming, draws up his/her legs and cannot be comforted. The condition tends to disappear spontaneously at about 3 months. There is often no obvious cause, although many explanations have been given including overfeeding, underfeeding, milk allergy, spoiling and boredom.

Treatment includes attention to feeding techniques, posture feeding and warmth to the abdomen (e.g. baths). The removal of dairy products from the maternal diet when breastfeeding occasionally helps.

Constipation

This term means hard, dry stool without regard to the frequency. Often when mothers talk of constipation they mean an absence of stools for 2–3 days, which may be normal. Breastfed babies are unlikely to be constipated and yet may not have a stool for several days.

Aetiological factors

There are several possible causes of constipation:
- inadequate or improper feeding, e.g. a milk formula that is too concentrated
- anatomical abnormalities, e.g. anal stenosis, Hirschsprung's disease, fissure *in ano*.

Treatment

The management will depend on the underlying cause. Local anaesthetic cream (e.g. xylocaine) is used for fissure in ano. Alteration of the feeds may be indicated, e.g. dilute orange juice or extra water. The addition of a stool-wetting agent such as dioctyl sodium increases the fluid in the stools. Milk of magnesia may be used as a mild laxative. Glycerine suppositories and/or small enemas may occasionally be indicated.

Diarrhoea

This term is used to mean loose frequent stools with stool volume greater than 10 mL/kg per day. Acute diarrhoea lasts less than 10 days whereas chronic diarrhoea persists beyond 2–3 weeks. The pathological mechanisms include osmotic, secretory and inflammatory processes. Stools initially change colour from a dark green-black (meconium), through a greenish-yellow transitional stage, and attain the typical yellow colour by 4–5 days. Stools may normally be very frequent initially, especially in breastfed babies, and this situation should not be confused with diarrhoea. Infants undergoing phototherapy commonly have greenish loose stools, and these must be distinguished from diarrhoeal stools.

Management will involve treatment of the specific cause whenever possible, and attention to fluid balance as necessary. Anti-diarrhoeal drugs are not used in the newborn period.

Failure to thrive

This is a term used to describe infants whose weight gain is inadequate. Weight gain in the first year of life is not linear, but frequently occurs in spurts. Generally babies at least double their birthweight by 5 months, and treble it by 1 year. The infant who fails to thrive shows a characteristic fall-off in weight gain and linear growth. These measurements cross centile lines in a downward direction, and this is more significant than an infant whose measurements are on or below the third centile but who grows along a line parallel to the centile line. Normal head growth may continue despite poor weight gain, as brain growth is the last to fail. A broad approach to management of an infant with failure to thrive can start with classification into non-organic and organic causes:
- non-organic: inadequate parenting and poor nutrition.
- organic: failure of intake, abnormal losses or failure of utilization (malabsorption) or chronic illness.

Such babies require close follow up and detailed evaluation of the underlying cause and response to intervention.

SUMMARY

- Breast milk is the ideal food for normal babies, both term and preterm.
- The preterm infant fed unfortified human milk receives inadequate energy and nutrients to equal fetal accretion rates.
- Unmodified cow's milk is not recommended during the first 12 months of life.
- Survival reflexes of suck, swallow, cough and gag are usually not developed until 34 weeks' gestation.
- The nutritional reference standard for the term newborn is the exclusively breastfed infant.
- TPN should only be used when enteral feeding is not possible or is going to be delayed.

 Now visit **www.essentialneonatalmed.com** to test yourself on this chapter.

CHAPTER 10
Infection

Key topics

Introduction

Infection may be acquired *in utero* (congenital), during labour and delivery (intrapartum or early onset) or after birth (postnatal or late-onset). In the neonate, infection can present in many different ways and may involve almost any system in the body. Infection must be considered in almost every differential diagnosis of any condition affecting the newborn. Infection poses a significant risk of mortality and is associated with major morbidity. The incidence of infection is approximately 5 per 1000 live births, and is more common in premature infants.

The immune system

To allow growth and development, the fetal and neonatal immune system must achieve a number of important tasks, including:
- avoidance of inflammatory responses that can induce alloimmune reactions between mother and fetus
- transition between the normally sterile intrauterine environment to the antigen-rich outside world
- defence against viral and bacterial pathogens
- primary colonization of the skin and intestinal tract by microorganisms.

The immune system develops from early in fetal life, but is not functionally fully integrated until about 1 year of age. Protection is initially provided by physical and chemical barriers in the epithelial and mucous membranes. The next line of defence is provided by the immune system and can be divided into non-specific (or innate) and specific (or adaptive) components. While these components are considered separately, they are integrally related and interact with each other to enhance and fine tune the immune response.

Essential Neonatal Medicine, Fifth Edition. Sunil Sinha, Lawrence Miall, Luke Jardine.
© 2012 John Wiley & Sons, Ltd. Published 2012 by John Wiley & Sons, Ltd.

Non-specific immunity

Non-specific immunity is the first line of defence against invasive pathogenic organisms in the neonate. It can be further divided into humoral and cellular responses.

• The **humoral response** includes complement, interferons, lactoferrin and lysozymes. Complement activation causes a cascade of events that leads to lysis of cell membranes. Alpha and beta interferon are proteins produced by cells infected with virus and make other cells resistant to infection. Gamma interferon increases the immune response by increasing killing of intracellular organisms. Lactoferrin (present in human milk) binds iron and reduces growth of *E. coli*. Lysozymes (found in tears, saliva and neutrophils) have antibacterial activity.

• The **cellular response** consists primarily of phagocytic white cells (neutrophils, macrophages, monocytes, natural killer cells) which adhere to and ingest bacteria. Enzymes and free oxygen radicals are then released which kill the organism. Phagocytic cells are attracted to sites of infection by chemicals released in the acute inflammatory response.

CLINICAL TIP: Erythema toxicum neonatorum – a rash consisting of pustules surrounded by erythema develops in approximately 50% of all newborns. The exact cause is unknown, but the pustules contain eosinophils and neutrophils and may be caused by macrophages in the skin reacting to colonizing bacteria (in particular staphylococci).

Specific immunity

Specific immunity is mediated through antibodies (produced by B lymphocytes) and specific cytotoxic cells (T lymphocytes). When a foreign antigen binds to a specific receptor, either antibody or a specific T lymphocyte is produced. Activation of specific immunity results in immunological memory.

B lymphocytes

When stimulated, B lymphocytes (or B cells) transform to plasma cells and produce immunoglobulin (Ig). IgM is the first type to be produced at 15 weeks' gestation, and IgG is first produced at 20 weeks. Initially fetal levels of the three major Ig types are minimal and they remain very low at birth. IgM is normally the first antibody produced in the primary immune response. Its major role is to fix complement. Adult levels of IgM are not normally attained until 5 years of age. IgG is the only immunoglobulin that crosses the placenta. Maternal IgG starts to cross the placenta from as early as 9 weeks but maximum transfer occurs after 32 weeks' gestation and peaks at term, hence premature infants may miss out on this important antibody transfer. At birth the baby has high levels of maternally derived IgG, giving the neonate effective passive immunity, but the levels fall in the months after birth and are not detectable by 9 months of age. By 2 months of age infants are able to produce a good IgG response, but adult levels are not attained until 7–8 years of age. The physiological nadir in IgG levels occurs between 3 and 6 months of age. IgG leads to bacterial cell lysis by opsonization and complement fixation and also neutralizes viruses and toxins. IgA is produced by secretory cells and is found in mucous membranes and breast milk. Levels rise slowly and may not peak until the teenage years. Its major role is to protect the gastrointestinal tract from infection.

CLINICAL TIP: Breast milk has an important role in protection against infection. It contains all of the immunoglobulins as well as lactoferrin, lysozymes and leukocytes. Breast milk contains a number of pre- and probiotics. Preterm infants fed breast milk compared to formula have a lower rate of mortality and decreased incidence of necrotising enterocolitis (NEC). See Chapter 17.

T lymphocytes

T lymphocytes (or T cells) are produced in the fetal bone marrow and migrate to the thymus – hence the term thymus (or T)-related lymphocytes. They can be divided into T helper (TH) cells and cytotoxic T cells. TH cells are CD4+ and once switched on can develop into TH1 cells or TH2 cells. TH1 cells activate cytotoxic T cells to kill intracellular organisms. TH2 cells secrete cytokines to help B lymphocytes produce antibodies. Cytotoxic T cells are CD8+ and are responsible for killing infected cells and preventing viral replication.

> **CLINICAL TIP:** The **hygiene hypothesis** proposes that early exposure to microbial components serves to polarize the immune response towards TH1 and away from TH2 responses, thereby reducing the likelihood of allergy and/or atopy. This is supported by the finding that as the rates of common infections have dropped in developed countries, the rates of allergy and autoimmune disease have risen.

Susceptibility of the neonate to infection

A number of differences exist between the neonatal immune system and adult immune systems and these are listed in Box 10.1. In particular, the decreased production of TH1-cell-polarizing cytokines leaves the newborn susceptible to microbial infection and contributes to the impairment of neonatal immune responses to most vaccines. Exogenous factors may also predispose the infant to infection and are also listed in Box 10.1.

Congenital infection

Intrauterine infections may have devastating effects on the fetus. Maternal infection may be completely asymptomatic or have only non-specific symptoms such as fever, malaise, myalgia, headache and nausea. Maternal infection may result in vertical transmission to the fetus. Several congenital infec-

tions have a similar clinical picture, and it is convenient to think about, and investigate, the TORCH group as a whole. TORCH is an acronym derived from the first letter of the following conditions: toxoplasmosis, other (e.g. Coxsackie B virus, varicella, HIV), rubella, cytomegalovirus (CMV), herpes simplex.

Infection at the embryonic stage (first 12 weeks) may lead to multiple abnormalities (Fig. 10.1). With infection occurring later, the baby may be born with a viraemia and may have neonatal illness associated with jaundice, enlarged liver and spleen, anaemia and thrombocytopenia. The predominant features of the three most common prenatal infections are shown in Table 10.1.

The investigation of infants with suspected congenital infections should include:
• review of maternal history for immunization and exposure to infectious agents
• serological tests, including quantitative IgM and specific antibody serology for TORCH infections, and polymerase chain reaction (PCR) to amplify DNA particles
• urine for CMV PCR
• throat and nose swabs, cerebrospinal fluid (CSF) and faeces for viral culture
• cranial ultrasound and/or MRI to detect intracranial calcification in toxoplasmosis, CMV and rubella, and radiographs of long bones to show periostitis in syphilis and viral osteopathy in rubella and CMV
• ophthalmological examination to detect chorioretinitis (toxoplasmosis, CMV) and cataracts, retinitis and microphthalmia in rubella.

Cytomegalovirus

CMV is the commonest congenital infection and may affect as many as 0.3 to 2% of live births in Australia. In primary maternal CMV infection there is a 50% risk of vertical transmission and in secondary maternal infection the risk of transmission is 1–13% depending on the length of time elapsed since the primary infection (higher risk with duration <4 years). Only 10% of congenitally infected infants will develop symptoms in primary maternal infection and in secondary maternal infection less than 1% will develop symptoms. The risk

Box 10.1 Endogenous and exogenous factors that increase the risk of infection in the neonate

Endogenous factors

- Decreased numbers and function of neutrophils
- Decreased production of tumor necrosis factor (TNF) by monocytes
- Phagocytic action is less effective in the newborn
- Decreased complement levels compared with adults
- Low levels of immunoglobulins, particularly IgM and IgA
- Premature infants fail to receive normal passive IgG transfer during the last trimester of pregnancy
- Decreased levels of the IgG G2 subclass (increases risk of infection with encapsulated organisms)
- Naive T lymphocytes are harder to switch on
- Neonatal lymphocytes do not function as efficiently as mature lymphocytes owing to a reduced production of cytokines.
- T lymphocyte response is predominantly TH2 rather than TH1 which may predispose to listeria and salmonella infection (as they rely on a TH1 response).

Exogenous factors

- Breaches of the skin barrier such as long lines, cannulas and venepuncture for blood tests may allow entry of bacteria to the baby
- Fat emulsions. Agents such as Intralipid may impair the phagocytic function of the white cells
- The baby is born bacteriologically sterile, with little competition from existing bacterial flora when exposed to potential pathogens. Babies exposed to very early antibiotic use, either as newborns or as fetuses, may be predisposed to colonization with potentially pathogenic organisms
- Drugs may further impair immune function, with corticosteroids being the main offenders
- Hyperbilirubinaemia reduces immune function in several different ways

of serious adverse neurological outcome increases if primary infection occurs in the first half of pregnancy.

Signs and symptoms of congenital CMV infection include small for gestational age, thrombocytopenia, seizures, hepatomegaly, splenomegaly, pneumonia, pleural effusions, pericardial effusions, intra-abdominal calcifications, ascites, hydrops fetalis, intracranial calcifications, microcephaly, hydrocephalus, sensory neural hearing loss, and chorioretinitis. Mortality rates for symptomatic congenital CMV are 10–30%.

CMV acquired postnatally is an important source of this condition and may be contracted from caregivers, infected blood (all blood products should be screened for CMV) and breast milk.

In infants with symptomatic congenital CMV there is preliminary evidence that intravenous gan-

ciclovir started within 28 days of birth may improve neurological outcome.

Rubella

Because of high immunization rates, congenital rubella syndrome currently affects less than 50 children each year in the UK. When maternal infection occurs before 8 weeks of pregnancy, 80–90% of infants will have symptoms; this rate falls to 50% if infection occurs at 8–12 weeks and to 20% if infection occurs between 12 and 20 weeks. The risk of congenital infection is less than 1% after 20 weeks' gestation. The risk of a fetus being damaged as a result of inadvertent rubella vaccination given to a pregnant woman is very small. Clinical features of congenital rubella are highlighted in Table 10.2.

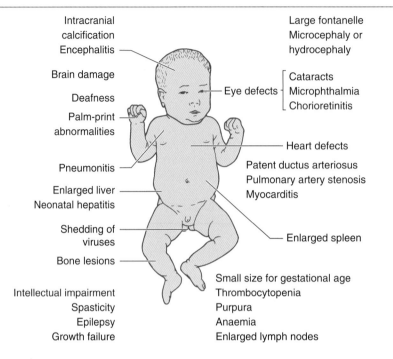

Intracranial
calcification
Encephalitis

Brain damage

Deafness

Palm-print
abnormalities

Pneumonitis

Enlarged liver
Neonatal hepatitis

Shedding of
viruses

Bone lesions

Intellectual impairment
Spasticity
Epilepsy
Growth failure

Large fontanelle
Microcephaly or
hydrocephaly

Cataracts
Eye defects Microphthalmia
Chorioretinitis

Heart defects
Patent ductus arteriosus
Pulmonary artery stenosis
Myocarditis

Enlarged spleen

Small size for gestational age
Thrombocytopenia
Purpura
Anaemia
Enlarged lymph nodes

Figure 10.1 Schematic representation of the clinical features of prenatal TORCH infections.

Table 10.1 Principles of management of congenital infection		
Organism	**Maternal treatment**	**Infant treatment**
CMV		Ganciclovir for 3 months
Toxoplasmosis	Spiramyicin and sulfadiazine or pyrimethamine + sulfadiazine	Spiramycin alternating with pyrimethamine + sulfadiazine for 1 year
Syphilis	Penicillin	Penicillin for 10 days
Hepatitis B		Vaccination at birth, 1 and 6 months
HIV	Antiretroviral treatment from 28 weeks	Oral zidovudine for 4–6 weeks Deliver by elective caesarean section Avoid breastfeeding
Varicella		ZIG and, if vesicles, start aciclovir

Toxoplasmosis

Toxoplasmas are protozoal organisms that rarely cause congenital infection in the UK and Australia; such infection is considerably more common in France. Infection may be prevented by avoiding raw/undercooked meat, washing hands after gardening and washing raw vegetables. Fetal infection after maternal seroconversion may be diagnosed by PCR or serological testing on fetal blood obtained by cordocentesis. Maternal treatment is with sulfadoxine and pyrimethamine alone or alternating with spiramycin (not before 16 weeks' gestational

Table 10.2 Relative clinical features of prenatal rubella, cytomegalovirus and toxoplasmosis

	Rubella	Cytomegalovirus	Toxoplasmosis
Eye involvement	++	++	+++
Microphthalmia	+	+	+
Chorioretinitis	+	++	++
Cataracts	++	–	–
Intrauterine growth retardation	+++	+	+
Brain	++	++	+++
Hydrocephaly	–	–	++
Microcephaly	+	++	+
Calcification	++	++	++
Deafness	+++	+++	++
Hepatosplenomegaly	++	++	++
Cardiac	++	–	+ –
Purpura	++	++	–
Pneumonitis	+	++	+
Bony involvement	++	+	–

age). Maternal infection in the first trimester has low risk of transmission (5–15%) but a high risk of damage to the fetus if it occurs (60–80%). Maternal infection in the second trimester has a 25–40% risk of vertical transmission and a 15–25% risk of damage to the baby. Maternal infection in the last trimester of pregnancy has a high risk of vertical transmission but a low risk (2–10%) of damage to the baby. The classical features are the triad of chorioretinitis, hydrocephalus and periventricular calcification. Even if asymptomatic at birth, signs and symptoms may not appear for several years.

The congenitally infected baby (even if asymptomatic) should be treated with with pyrimethamine and sulfadiazine (plus folinic acid) continuously or alternating with spiramycin.

Syphilis

The incidence of this condition has increased recently in developed countries. Congenital infec-

tion is seen if maternal infection occurs after the fourth month of gestation. Penicillin is an effective treatment for mother and fetus. Classically the infant at birth is found to have persistent snuffles, skin eruptions and widespread metaphyseal bony lesions. However, many infants show no symptoms at birth.

Interstitial keratitis is the commonest feature of congenital infection, and hepatomegaly is present in almost all cases. While treatment of maternal syphilis in pregnancy usually eradicates infection in the infant, the mother will still have positive tests for VDRL (Venereal Disease Research Laboratory), TPHA (Treponema Pallidum Haemagglutination Assay), and RPR (Rapid Plasma Reagin). The infant will also be positive as a result of passive transfer of IgG to the fetus. More specific investigations are necessary.

The fluorescent treponema antibody absorption (FTA-ABS) test should be performed for both IgG and IgM. The IgG response will remain positive for several weeks but should be negative by 6 months. The IgM response should be negative at birth. If the IgM is positive or if the VDRL/RPR titre is four times higher in the baby than in the mother, the infant should be treated for congenital syphilis with parenteral benzylpenicillin for at least 10 days. The CSF should be examined before treatment.

Hepatitis B

This is largely a disease of developing countries, but with worldwide travel it is now relatively common in the UK and Australia. Mothers who develop acute hepatitis B infection in the first or second trimester of pregnancy have a 10% risk of perinatal transmission. Mothers who develop acute hepatitis B infection in the third trimester of pregnancy have a 75% risk of the infant developing the disease, but the neonatal disease is rarely severe or fatal. More commonly, mothers who are chronically hepatitis B 'surface antigen' positive pass the infection vertically to their baby via the placenta. Forty per cent of children with persistent hepatitis B infection will die in adult life of hepatocellular carcinoma or chronic liver disease.

All women should be screened for hepatitis B at booking, with serological tests for surface antigen (HBsAg). They are at greatest risk of infecting their babies if they are also HBe antigen (HBeAg) positive. If a woman has antibody to HBe (antiHBeAb), then the risk of serious disease to her infants is very small. Therefore, women who are HBsAg positive and negative for HBeAg and have antiHBeAb, are at low risk of their infants developing severe disease. Their infants may become chronic carriers of HBsAg and are at risk of developing carcinoma of the liver. Symptoms of liver disease in the neonatal period are rare in affected babies.

Prevention of transmission is possible by immunizing infants born to women who have acute hepatitis B in the last trimester of pregnancy, or where the mother is HBsAg positive.

Treatment of the baby is with hepatitis B immunoglobulin (HBIG) and vaccination, which should be given within 12 h of birth. Further immunizations with hepatitis B should be done according to local schedules. Follow-up serology should be performed at 12 months. Women positive for hepatitis B should be encouraged to breastfeed.

Hepatitis C

Perinatal transmission of hepatitis C virus (HCV) occurs in pregnant women with anti-HCV-positive tests. Pregnant women who are anti-HCV positive should have the appropriate antibody and antigen testing. Infants born to pregnant women who are HCV RNA positive have approximately a 6% risk of acquiring the infection with the risk being proportional to the RNA load. There is no evidence that breastfeeding increases the risk of perinatal transmission. Follow-up serology should be done at 18 months. Currently women in high-risk groups, such as women with substance dependency, sex industry workers, and those with hepatitis B or who are HIV positive, are tested for HCV antibodies.

HIV

The HIV retrovirus damages the immune system and causes AIDS. HIV is an important perinatal pathogen, but with effective treatment the risk of transmission from mother to infant can now be virtually eliminated. In worldwide terms HIV/AIDS is common, with over 30 million people infected, 90% of whom live in the developing world. In the UK HIV/AIDS is relatively rare (0.9 per 1000 women), but the incidence in London is six times higher. The UK has a rapidly increasing population of asylum seekers from sub-Saharan Africa, and consequently the prevalence of women who are HIV-positive is increasing throughout the country. The incidence of newly diagnosed HIV in black Africans has, however, significantly decreased since 2004 and the majority of new HIV diagnoses are now white men. All women should be offered routine screening for HIV in early pregnancy after appropriate counselling. Most women of childbearing age with HIV are asymptomatic, and AIDS is rare in pregnancy. Women at particularly high risk of transmitting HIV to their babies are those with symptomatic HIV/AIDS, a falling or low CD4 T-lymphocyte count or high viral load (>10,000 copies/mL). It is estimated that one-third of HIV transmission occurs *in utero* and two thirds during the peripartum period.

Management

In developed countries, the risk of vertical transmission from mother to child for a non-breastfeeding woman is 15–20%, and with appropriate management and advice in pregnancy and early infancy this can be reduced to 1–12%. Management can be considered under the following headings.

Antenatal

Antiretroviral therapy from 28 weeks of gestation until delivery; zidovudine monotherapy reduces the risk of vertical transmission by 50%. Highly active antiretroviral therapy (HAART) with multiple drugs such as zidovudine together with nevirapine or lamivudine may be recommended depending on local circumstances, the presence of high maternal viral load and the health of the mother. The local specialist in HIV should be consulted in each case.

Avoid chorionic villus sampling or second-trimester amniocentesis wherever possible. If these are considered necessary, HAART may be indicated.

Intrapartum

Avoid allowing spontaneous membrane rupture by performing a planned caesarean section at 38 weeks, particularly if viral load is greater than 1000/mL. This has been shown to reduce the risk of mother–infant transmission significantly in addition to prenatal drug treatment. In women with an 'undetectable' viral load at 36 weeks, normal vaginal delivery may be offered in some centres.

Neonatal

At delivery the baby should be considered to be potentially infective. Gloves, mask and goggles should be worn. Avoid intramuscular vitamin K administration until the baby has been washed. Discourage breastfeeding as HIV may be transmitted to the infant through breast milk. It is estimated that breastfeeding causes HIV acquisition in 20–30% of breastfed infants.

All babies born to HIV-positive women should be treated with oral zidovudine within 6 hours of delivery for 4–6 weeks after birth. The precise regimen will depend on local expert advice.

The baby will require regular follow up testing (for up to 18 months) but recommendations vary between countries. Do not send cord blood as it, may be contaminated by maternal blood.

Parvovirus B19

This virus most commonly causes a mild illness known as erythema infectiosum (fifth disease). It is characterized by mild systemic symptoms, including fever and a distinctive facial rash with a 'slapped cheek' appearance. Approximately 40% of women in Australia are susceptible to parvovirus infection in pregnancy. Infection in pregnancy, which is often asymptomatic in the mother, can cause severe anaemia with resultant hydrops and fetal death, but the risk of death is less than 10% after proven maternal infection. Fetal anaemia may be successfully treated by intrauterine transfusion.

Varicella

Varicella exposure normally occurs in childhood and 90% of adults in Western countries are immune. Varicella infection in pregnancy can have various effects depending on the timing of infection. If maternal chickenpox develops before 20 weeks' gestation there is a 2–3% risk of the fetus developing congenital varicella syndrome. This consists of skin scarring, eye abnormalities (cataracts, chorioretinitis, microphthalmia), hypoplasia of limbs, cortical atrophy, microcephaly, intellectual impairment, neurogenic bladder, oesophageal dilatation and early death. Maternal chickenpox developing in the period of a week before or up to 28 days after birth predisposes the infant to a very high risk of potentially fatal varicella. Zoster immunoglobulin (ZIG) should be given immediately to infants at high risk of congenital varicella as the mortality rate may be as high as 30%. The infant is then carefully watched and, at the first sign of a vesicle, respiratory distress or the baby becoming unwell, intravenous aciclovir should be commenced for 10 days. This treatment should prevent serious infections. Varicella in the first and second trimesters rarely causes congenital defects. If the pregnant woman is not immune to varicella zoster, and the infection occurs before 20

Box 10.2 Maternal risk factors for early-onset neonatal infection

- Maternal features of sepsis or chorioamnionitis, e.g. fever ≥38°C, high white cell count, tender uterus, offensive or purulent liquor
- Preterm labour <37 weeks' gestation
- Membranes ruptured for more than 18–24h
- prolonged labour beyond 12h
- Frequent vaginal examinations
- Group B streptococcus (GBS) colonization or bacteriuria in current pregnancy
- Previous infant with early-onset GBS disease (EOGBSD)

Box 10.3 Signs and symptoms of neonatal infection

- Abnormal FBC
- Increased C-reactive protein (CRP)
- Unexpected need for resuscitation at birth
- Respiratory distress (can range from mild tachypnoea, nasal flaring, accessory muscle use, chest recession, and expiratory grunt through to severe respiratory distress requiring intubation)
- Apnoea
- Temperature instability (especially hypothermia)
- Lethargy
- Hypotonia
- Irritability
- Weak cry
- Rashes/purpura
- Poor perfusion
- Hypotension
- Renal failure
- Hypoglycaemia
- Hyperglycaemia
- Poor feeding
- Feed intolerance (vomiting, abdominal distension, increased gastric aspirates)
- Diarrhoea
- Jaundice
- Disseminated intravascular coagulation (DIC)
- Seizures
- Bulging fontanelle
- Metabolic or respiratory acidosis

weeks' gestation, then she should receive ZIG as soon as possible after contact.

Intrapartum (early-onset) infection

At birth it may be difficult to decide whether a baby is infected or not. The presence of a number of maternal factors (Box 10.2) significantly increases the risk of infection in the newborn period. Prophylactic antibiotics administered to the mother should be considered, but guidelines vary between countries. A newborn infant with early-onset infection may be initially asymptomatic or have any of the clinical signs and symptoms listed in Box 10.3.

Investigations

Ideally a blood culture (>1 mL) should be collected before antibiotics are commenced. A full blood count (FBC) should also be done. Abnormal findings can include increased white cell count, neutropenia, increased numbers of immature neutrophils (e.g. bands, blasts, myelocytes, metamyelocytes), increased immature:mature (IM) or immature:total (IT) neutrophil ratios, left shift, toxic granulation, vacuolation, Dohle bodies, intracellular organisms and thrombocytopenia. An elevated C-reactive protein (CRP) may be a marker of infection.

Lumbar puncture should be considered and is essential if the blood culture becomes positive or if the baby has signs or symptoms of meningitis.

Management

Every newborn baby is at risk of infection. Surveillance for infection includes monitoring for signs and symptoms of infection (see Box 10.3) as well as regular assessment of temperature, pulse rate and respiratory rate. Any baby at risk of infection or who is symptomatic should commence intravenous antibiotics. Antibiotics should be continued for 36–48h and blood culture results checked before the decision to cease antibiotics is made. Regimes vary according to local practices but should consist of adequate Gram-positive cover (e.g. benzylpenicillin or ampicillin) and Gram-negative cover (e.g. gentamicin). Anaerobic cover (e.g. metronidazole) may be required in some circumstances (e.g. suspected NEC).

> **CLINICAL TIP:** A normal FBC does not exclude neonatal infection. If the baby has clinical signs or symptoms suggestive of infection a blood culture should be collected and the baby should be commenced on intravenous antibiotics.

Early-onset group B β-haemolytic streptococcus

Group B β-haemolytic streptococcus (GBS) is the most common cause of early-onset sepsis. Although the prognosis has improved, it is fatal in 10–20% of cases depending on gestational age and age of onset. Vaginal or rectal colonization with GBS is found in 15–30% of pregnant women depending on the local population, and 10–20% of infants born to colonized women will themselves be colonized. Early-onset GBS infection in the neonate occurs in only 1% of colonized women. In the UK and Australia the incidence of early-onset GBS infection in the neonate is approximately 0.4–1.0 in 1000 liveborn infants. In areas that are known to have high rates of colonization (e.g. the USA), routine screening for GBS in pregnancy is often undertaken. Intrapartum prophylaxis for women with risk factors (see Box 10.2) significantly reduces the risk of early-onset infection (but does not eliminate it). Local guidelines for intrapartum prophylaxis should be used to guide treatment.

Presentation and diagnosis

Babies with early-onset GBS disease may be asymptomatic or have any of the signs in Box 10.3. Some neonates appear to be particularly susceptible to this infection if their mother has low circulating anti-GBS IgG. Premature infants are particularly poor at killing this organism.

Eighty per cent of babies who develop early-onset disease will have at least one of the risk factors identified in Box 10.2.

Most babies presenting with early-onset disease develop symptoms in the first 4–6h of life. The baby may initially develop signs of respiratory distress, which clinically and radiologically may be indistinguishable from respiratory distress syndrome (RDS). GBS infection must be considered as a possible cause of any baby presenting with early-onset illness.

Management

Early administration of intravenous antibiotic is essential, as is supportive treatment to maintain the baby in good condition and early recognition of complications of the infection. Where the diagnosis is unconfirmed, penicillin (or amoxicillin) together with gentamicin is the best choice, and these two drugs act synergistically against GBS. When the diagnosis is confirmed, antibiotic treatment with benzylpenicillin should be administered for 10–14 days.

Escherichia coli

E. coli (particularly the K1 strain), is associated with perinatal infection. *E. coli* may cause septicaemia or meningitis. The sensitivity of *E. coli* to antibiotics is variable. The incidence of *E. coli* infection appears to be increasing, due to the increasing use of antibiotics aimed at preventing GBS.

Listeria monocytogenes

This is a not uncommon perinatal pathogen and may invade the fetus through intact membranes. Characteristically, infected infants pass meconium *in utero*, and if this is seen in premature infants listeria should be strongly suspected. The organism has a predilection for the lungs and brain. Hydrocephalus is a common sequel to listeria meningitis. The organism is usually sensitive to ampicillin.

Herpes simplex virus (HSV)

Neonatal herpes simplex infection is a rare but devastating condition. The incidence in Australia is approximately 3 per 100,000 live births. Herpes simplex virus (HSV) can be classified as either type 1 or 2. Neonatal infection now occurs as a result of HSV type 1 and 2 in equal proportion. Caesarean section reduces the risk of infection if there is active maternal shedding of HSV. In most babies with neonatal HSV, there is no history of genital herpes and their mothers are asymptomatic. The virus enters the baby through skin, eye or mouth and may disseminate to the brain or other organs.

The risk of an infant being infected from a parent, nurse or midwife with cold sores is small, but not negligible. Careful hand-washing is all that is necessary to avoid this risk. Rarely, paronychia may be due to herpesvirus, and staff with this type of active infection must not handle infants.

Presentation and diagnosis

Neonatal HSV presents in one of three ways:
• **Neurological symptoms.** Approximately one-third of babies present with encephalopathic signs of meningoencephalitis, most commonly at 10–14 days.
• **Systemic symptoms.** These babies present in the first few days of life with signs of major overwhelming illness including shock, respiratory failure and often severe hepatitis and coagulation disorders. Meningoencephalitis may also develop.
• **Cutaneous symptoms**, including rash and keratoconjunctivitis, in the second week of life. These babies rarely become seriously ill.

HSV infection must be considered in the differential diagnosis of any ill baby. Rapid diagnosis is made by immunofluorescence or PCR amplification from blood and CSF. Always consider HSV infection when lumbar puncture reveals an excess of white cells that is bacterial culture negative. In babies with encephalopathy the EEG may show a characteristic appearance. Brain imaging may also show specific abnormalities.

Management

If the mother has recurrent HSV infection, or has seroconverted with primary infection well before delivery, the baby is at low risk of neonatal HSV disease. In low-risk cases, surface swabs (eye, throat, umbilicus, rectum and urine) should be collected

and processed for HSV DNA by PCR. The baby should also be monitored for signs of infection. If the swab is positive or the baby becomes unwell, a lumbar puncture should be performed and intravenous aciclovir should be commenced. If the mother has primary infection close to delivery or active primary infection at the time of delivery the baby is at high risk of neonatal HSV disease. In high-risk babies swabs should also be collected but the baby should be immediately commenced on intravenous aciclovir. Aciclovir should be administered for at least 14 days but up to 21 days if evidence of encephalitis or systemic disease. In babies with systemic disease 35–60% die, and of those with neurological disease 10–15% die. HSV-2 has a worse prognosis than HSV-1. The outcome for surviving infants is poor, with over 50% being left severely disabled. The prognosis is good for cutaneous disease, but late neurodevelopmental sequelae have been reported in up to 30%.

Chlamydia trachomatis

Chlamydia is found in the vagina of 4% of pregnant women. Up to 70% of infants born through an infected cervix will acquire chlamydia, but most show no symptoms. Chlamydia conjunctivitis and, less commonly, pneumonia occur in a relatively small proportion of infants. The conjunctivitis is purulent and is clinically indistinguishable from that of gonococcal ophthalmia. Specific culture media are necessary for this organism however diagnosis can be made by detecting DNA with PCR. Infants should be treated with tetracycline eye ointment and oral erythromycin.

Others

Pneumococcus, *Haemophilus influenzae* and anaerobic organisms may cause significant perinatal infection. Anaerobes are contracted from the birth canal and require special culture media for their identification. The first two organisms are probably haematogenously spread from maternal septicaemia. They may cause profound shock in the infant, indistinguishable clinically from group B β-haemolytic streptococci.

Postnatal (late-onset) infection

Unfortunately, the definition of late-onset infection is not universal. The most common definition is signs of infection developing at least 48 h after birth, but another definition is signs of infection developing 7 days or more after birth. The implication is that the infection has been acquired from the baby's environment or caregivers rather than vertically from the mother. It may, however, be very difficult to differentiate infections acquired during delivery from those acquired postnatally. Almost every bacterium and virus known to infect humans may cause clinical infection in the newborn. Staphylococcus species are probably the most important group of infections infants acquire in the neonatal unit.

When a nosocomial infection is suspected, the following risk factors should be reviewed:
• **Direct contamination** by the hands of medical staff or parents due to inadequate hand-washing techniques.
• **Frequently performed procedures**, such as intubation, endotracheal suction, insertion of catheters, collection of blood samples, humidification of oxygen, parenteral nutrition and blood transfusions, all predispose sick babies to infection.
• **Cross-infection:** the routes of neonatal cross-infection are illustrated in Fig. 10.2.

Clinical features

There are no pathognomonic signs of infection or any totally reliable way to make an early diagnosis in the laboratory. The doctor must have a high level of suspicion for infection and not be too reliant on blood tests to make the diagnosis. If in doubt, treat the baby. Clinical signs and symptoms are listed in Box 10.3.

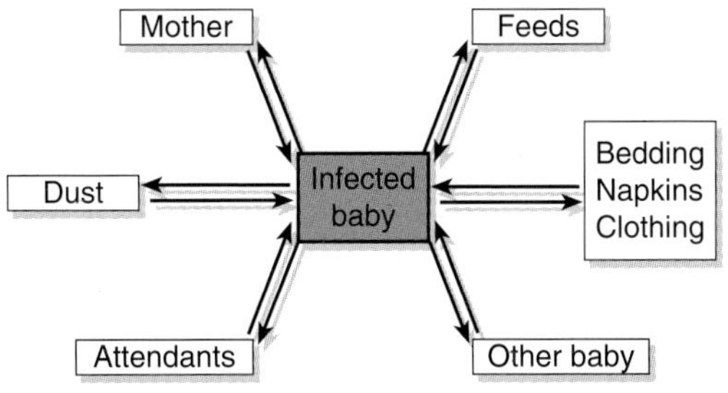

Investigations

If infection is suspected, the following investigations may be useful in finding the causative organism:
• Blood culture
• Urine for microscopy/culture and sensitivity (M/C/S). CSF for M/C/S, consider PCR for selected organisms (e.g. HSV)
• Tracheal aspirates are sent to the laboratory for microscopy, culture and antibiotic sensitivity testing
• Nasopharyngeal aspirate for M/C/S and viral studies
• Collection of skin swabs (e.g. ear, anus) may identify pathogenic organisms and help guide antibiotic choice; they are also useful in infection control by identifying possible cases of cross-infection
• FBC
• CRP
• IL-6 and procalcitonin (mostly used in research)

CLINICAL TIP: Collection of a 'bag' urine sample may be useful to initially exclude a UTI but a positive result may be due to contamination. Analysing a suprapubic sample significantly decreases the risk of a false-positive result but it is more difficult to collect.

Management

General supportive measures include monitoring of vital signs (heart rate/respiratory/blood pressure), thermoregulation, respiratory support, cardiovascular support and intravenous fluids/nutrition.

Specific therapy

The clinical dilemma is whether to treat blindly without knowing which organism is causing the infection. A best-guess policy is required, but review

Figure 10.2 Routes of neonatal cross-infection.

of all cultures taken over the previous few weeks is helpful to establish whether the infant has been colonized by potentially pathogenic organisms. It is usual to commence with two or three antibiotics until bacteriological culture and sensitivity results are obtained. Knowledge of the sensitivities of 'local' pathogens is also important in order to choose the best antibiotics. Recommendations vary according to local guidelines. Once the organism and sensitivity have been identified, only the most appropriate antibiotic should be used in an attempt to decrease the emergence of multiresistant organisms.

CLINICAL TIP: Because of the high rate of nosocomial infection in neonates with vascular access devices (e.g. umbilical catheters, central venous lines, etc.), a number of studies have looked at using prophylactic antibiotics to prevent infection. While this does decrease the rate of infection it may increase the risk of antimicrobial resistance and is not currently recommended.

Common acute acquired infections

Late-onset group B β-haemolytic streptococcus infection

Late-onset GBS infection is often characterized by meningitis, which usually develops some time after 5–7 days. The type III serotype of GBS has been more frequently associated with late-onset disease. Late-onset disease may be acquired from infected breast milk or from a caregiver other than the mother. Intrapartum or immediate postpartum antibiotic treatment for GBS does not decrease the risk of late-onset GBS disease. Recurrent neonatal GBS infection is reported in 1% of neonates.

Coagulase-negative staphylococci

Apart from perinatally acquired GBS and *E. coli*, the most common organisms to cause septicaemia in the newborn unit are coagulase-negative staphylococci. This should not be dismissed as a contami-

nant if it is both cultured from blood culture bottles and the infant is unwell; it must be treated as a pathogen. It is particularly likely to occur when parenteral nutrition is being administered, especially if a silastic catheter 'long line' is in situ. The long line should be removed when antibiotics are started if the infant is ill.

Staphylococcus aureus

S. aureus is a frequent pathogen in the neonatal unit and has a predisposition for sites such as bone and the soft tissues. Methicillin-resistant *S. aureus* (MRSA) is an emerging problem in most intensive care units and requires rigorous treatment as well as preventive measures to stop its spread to other patients.

Others

Other organisms that can commonly cause late-onset septicaemia include Pseudomonas, Proteus, Klebsiella, Serratia and Candida.

Meningitis

Meningitis is more common, and mortality and morbidity rates higher, in the first month of life than at any other age. The organisms most usually encountered are *E. coli* and group B haemolytic streptococci. In addition to the other organisms seen with septicaemia, epidemics of *Listeria monocytogenes* occur. Table 10.3 shows the most common causes of pathogens in developed countries. Many of the early clinical manifestations are non-specific. Coma, convulsions, opisthotonus, increasing head size and a bulging fontanelle are late signs of meningitis.

Investigations
1 A lumbar puncture must be done in all infants with suspected meningitis. The CSF is often turbid and cloudy, with an elevated white cell count, low sugar and high protein. Positive cultures on CSF are obtained in about 50% of cases of suspected bacterial meningitis. A premature neonate may normally have up to 12 white cells/mm^3 in the CSF and a term baby up to 5 white cells/mm^3, but if all these cells are granulocytes meningitis cannot be excluded.
2 CSF should be sent for PCR for viral RNA/DNA (e.g. HSV, enterovirus, etc.)

Table 10.3 Common causes of neonatal meningitis and outcome

Organism	Proportion (%)	Mortality (%)	Severe/moderate disability (%)
GBS	50	12	25
E. coli	20	15	25
Other Gram-positive	18	Low	30
Other Gram-negative	7	Low	25
Listeria	5	15	25

3 Blood cultures are positive in about 50% of neonates with bacterial meningitis.
4 A full blood count may reveal variable pictures of neutropenia, neutrophilia and toxic changes.

Management

Principles of management are outlined in Box 10.4. The initial therapy for suspected meningitis in or after the first week of life is a combination of ampicillin, gentamicin and cefotaxime. Always consider herpes simplex as a cause of meningitis and add aciclovir if suspected (see p. 118).

Once the organism has been identified then microbiological advice as to the most appropriate antibiotic should be sought. Be aware of local patterns of antibiotic resistance. Meropenem may be indicated where multiple-resistant Gram-negative organisms are known to be prevalent.

Rapid sterilization of the CSF is essential and it is recommended that a second lumbar puncture be performed after 48 s of therapy to ensure that the CSF is sterile.

Continue intravenous antibiotics for at least 2 weeks in GBS infection and for at least 3 weeks in Gram-negative infections. There is no evidence that intrathecal antibiotics improve outcome.

Ultrasound brain imaging should be performed in all infants with meningitis to detect progressive hydrocephalus, which may need treatment.

Box 10.4 Principles of management of neonatal meningitis

- Perform lumbar puncture if baby is at risk of meningitis or is ill
- Perform full infection screen (50% of babies will also have septicaemia)
- Start ampicillin, gentamicin and cefotaxime together
- Always consider herpes simplex and add aciclovir if in doubt
- Repeat lumbar puncture after 48 h to establish CSF is sterile
- Once sensitivities are known, stop inappropriate antibiotics
- Continue treatment for at least 2 weeks if GBS and >3 weeks if other organism
- Ultrasound imaging weekly to assess ventricular size
- If persistence of symptoms consider cerebral abscess (MRI or CT brain scan)
- Perform hearing test on recovery

Outcome

Postmeningitis hydrocephalus is a well-recognized complication, particularly in listeria meningitis. Brain abscess may occur, particularly with citrobacter and enterobacter meningitis. Deafness is a recognized complication, and a hearing test (in addition to the routine screening test) should be performed on discharge from hospital.

Approximately 50% of all babies with neonatal meningitis will show some neurodevelopmental problems at 5 years of age. The risk of severe or moderately adverse outcome is shown in Table 10.3.

Systemic candidiasis

Diagnosis of this condition depends on a high clinical suspicion for the organism. It may rarely be congenital, associated with maternal vaginitis, or acquired in a baby receiving neonatal intensive care. *Candida albicans* accounts for over 90% of infections although *C. parapsilosis* is also seen rarely.

Preterm infants undergoing intensive care are particularly vulnerable to candida sepsis. Risk factors include:
- extremely low birthweight and current weight less than 1000 g
- parenteral nutrition
- central vascular catheter
- mechanical ventilation
- course of antibiotics.

The best method of diagnosis is to identify budding hyphae in urine from a suprapubic stab. The organism may also be isolated from arterial and/or venous blood cultures. Diagnosis may also be strongly suspected by observing 'fungal balls' on renal ultrasound scan or a pathognomonic appearance on ophthalmoscopy.

Treatment is with amphotericin B, usually in a liposomal formation (AmBisome) as it is less toxic. 5-Flucytosine acts synergistically with amphotericin and may be added in severe infection. Fluconazole may be used in amphotericin resistance or increasingly as a first-line antifungal agent in sensitive cases of *C. albicans*. Central vein lines should be removed on starting treatment.

Death has been reported to occur in 40% of babies who are infected at <37 weeks' gestation.

Fungal prophylaxis

Prophylactic systemic fluconazole significantly decreases the incidence of invasive fungal infection in extremely low birthweight (ELBW) infants. There is limited information on the long-term risks associated with systemic prophylaxis. Oral/topical non-absorbed antifungals (nystatin or miconazole) are commonly used in many neonatal units for fungal prophlyaxis.

Lower respiratory tract infections

These are discussed in Chapter 13.

Urinary tract infection

This is discussed in Chapter 18.

Conjunctivitis ('sticky eyes')

Mild eye infections are very common and are referred to as 'sticky eyes'. Purulent conjunctivitis may be either a congenital or an acquired infection. Conjunctivitis is sometimes secondary to a blocked nasolacrimal duct. Usually the organisms involved are *S. aureus*, *E. coli*, *Pseudomonas* spp., *Chlamydia trachomatis* and *Neisseria gonorrhoeae*. Reddened swelling in the region of the lacrimal sac (dacrocystitis) may occur following infection of a blocked nasolacrimal duct. The term ophthalmia neonatorum is reserved for infection with *N. gonorrhoeae*.

Management

Conjunctival swabs should be taken and sent promptly to the laboratory. If ophthalmia neonatorum or *Ch. trachomatis* specific swabs for PCR testing can be performed. If maternal gonorrhoea is suspected, prophylactic treatment of the newborn's eyes with 1% silver nitrate eyedrops may prevent purulent conjunctivitis.

With mild conjunctivitis, or 'sticky eyes', frequent eye toilet with normal saline may be all that is required. More florid infections will need the frequent instillation of antibiotic drops (e.g. chloramphenicol or sulfacetamide) after cultures have been taken and eye toilet carried out. After the conjunctivitis has settled somewhat, antibiotic ointment may be used.

Treatment of gonococcal ophthalmia varies between institutions but will normally involve a combination of topical eye drops and systemic antibiotics for at least 10 days. For the treatment of chlamydia, see p. 118.

Infection of the skin and subcutaneous tissues

Omphalitis and funisitis

Infections of the umbilical cord (funisitis) and umbilical stump (omphalitis) are usually due to *S. aureus* or *E. coli*, or other Gram-negative bacteria. Infection may arise as the result of chorioamnionitis. Because of the potential seriousness of the spread of infection to the portal vein and subsequent portal hypertension, infection in this area must be treated promptly. If there are signs of spread with surrounding cellulitis, parenteral antibiotics such as flucloxacillin and gentamicin are necessary after appropriate swabs and cultures have been taken. Topical treatment with an antibiotic is also necessary.

Paronychia

Reddening of the skin in the nailfold is common and may proceed to pus formation when staphylococcal infection is present. Topical treatment consists of applications of mupirocin calcium (Bactroban) and is usually all that is necessary to eradicate minor bacterial infections. Parenteral and topical antibiotics are indicated if systemic spread is suspected with bacterial infection.

Thrush

Yeast infection is common, particularly if there has been *C. albicans* colonization of the maternal genital tract. It is also likely to occur in association with the use of broad-spectrum antibiotics and in debilitated neonates receiving total parenteral nutrition. It commonly occurs in the mouth and looks like milk curds that cannot be removed with a swab stick. The infection usually occurs towards the end of the first week of life. In the napkin area it appears as a spreading centrifugal rash. It sometimes occurs as a secondary infection following ammoniacal dermatitis. Napkin psoriasis is a rare condition that starts in the napkin area and may become widespread, usually secondary to thrush. The treatment of oral candidiasis consists of the use of nystatin drops or miconazole (Daktarin) gel and its use should be continued for at least 3 days after the lesions disappear. For the napkin area, nystatin or clotrimazole (Canesten) cream applied four times daily is usually sufficient.

Gastroenteritis

Gastroenteritis usually occurs in epidemic form in neonatal nurseries. Outbreaks have in the past been associated with enteropathogenic *E. coli*, and occasionally with salmonella and shigella, but currently the most frequent nursery pathogen is human rotavirus.

Because the neonate withstands salt and water loss poorly, dehydration may rapidly occur. The infant shows signs such as loss of skin turgor, sunken eyes and fontanelle, dry mouth and oliguria.

Treatment consists of isolation from non-infected infants and replacement of electrolytes and water. Antibiotics are of no value unless there is evidence of systemic bacterial infection.

Prevention of acquired infections

The procedures detailed below will help to reduce and control infections. The 'Matching Michigan' initiative to prevent central venous catheter blood stream infections is now followed in the majority of units in the UK (for more information go to www.patientsafetyfirst.nhs.uk/).

Labour ward

- Fastidious care in hand-washing.
- The use of gloves for vaginal examinations, insertion of scalp electrodes and instrumental deliveries.
- Identification of risk factors for group B streptococcus and commencement of intrapartum antibiotics where appropriate.

Nursery

- Careful hand-washing is the key to reducing nosocomial infection. On entry into a neonatal unit, all staff and visitors should wash their hands carefully. Hands should be washed or an alcohol hand rub should then be used every time before and after an infant or the surrounding work space is handled.
- Cleansing of incubators and equipment, and frequent changes of humidifier and incubator sterile water.
- Have one stethoscope per baby.
- Routine baths for babies using hygienic soap solutions.
- Aseptic surgical techniques for procedures such as intubation, umbilical catheterization, peripherally inserted central catheters, intravenous cannulation, intercostal catheters and lumbar punctures. Chlorhexidine has been shown to be twice as effective as iodine.
- Fungal prophylaxis with fluconazole or nystatin/mycostatin.
- Isolation techniques for infectious babies.
- Avoidance of overcrowding and restriction of nursery 'traffic' to a minimum.

Adjunctive therapy

Intravenous immunoglobulin therapy

Intravenous immunoglobulin (IVIG) infusion has been used for sepsis prophylaxis in preterm and low birthweight infants. The Cochrane Review found a reduction in sepsis but no difference in mortality or other clinically important outcomes. IVIG has also been used in infants with suspected or proven sepsis. While there appears to be a modest reduction in mortality compared with controls, the Cochrane Review concluded that there is insufficient evidence to support the routine use of IVIG in infants with suspected or proven infection.

G-CSF or GM-CSF treatment

Haemopoietic colony stimulating factors (CSFs) for granulocytes (G-CSF) or granulocyte-macrophages (GM-CSF) have been evaluated either for prophylaxis or in the management of septic infants in a number of studies. The Cochrane Review failed to establish a clear benefit and there is currently insufficient evidence to support the practice.

SUMMARY

Infection is a commonly encountered problem in neonatal medicine. It has significant morbidity and mortality. Signs and symptoms may be present at or shortly after birth or may occur at any time during admission. Staff looking after neonates must have a high suspicion of infection, as prompt treatment is required. A number of measures have been proven to decrease the risk of nosocomial infection with the most important being careful hand-washing.

 Now visit **www.essentialneonatalmed.com** to test yourself on this chapter.

CHAPTER 11

The extreme preterm infant

Key topics

Introduction

About 7–8% of all births are born preterm (<37 weeks' gestation). Preterm births account for the majority of work on most neonatal intensive care units (NICUs) and preventing preterm birth has become the foremost challenge for obstetric practice today. The burden to society of preterm births is enormous – because of the expensive and lengthy intensive care required and the potential for long-term neurodisability in survivors. However, expert and careful intervention to support these infants in the immediate neonatal period also offers the opportunity to generate a lifetime of good-quality survival from what initially may be a life-threatening situation.

Gestational age

Establishing the exact gestational age is sometimes difficult and so for many years, especially in the USA, classification and outcome studies have been based on birthweight, which is measureable. However, it is clear that survival and neurodevelopmental outcome are more strongly determined by the degree of prematurity than by birthweight. Most recent studies and treatment protocols therefore use gestational age. Degrees of prematurity are defined in Table 11.1.

Gestational age can now be accurately determined by a first-trimester ultrasound 'dating scan'. If there is a big discrepancy between this and the estimated date of delivery (EDD) calculated from the mother's last menstrual period (LMP), or if there is an unbooked or concealed pregnancy, the gestation can be estimated by performing an objective examination of the newborn baby. The new Ballard examination (based on the original Dubowitz examination) is recommended. This quantifies

Table 11.1 Gestational age bands and their incidence

Gestational age (weeks after LMP)	Terminology	Approximate incidence (as % singleton live births)[a]
>42 weeks	Post term	4
37–42 weeks	Term	90
<37 weeks	Preterm	6–8
34–36 weeks	Mildly preterm[b]	4.9
32–34 weeks	Moderately preterm[b]	0.8
28–32 weeks	Very preterm[b]	
<28 weeks	Extreme preterm	0.4
≤24 weeks	Threshold of viability	0.14

[a] The frequency of preterm birth is much higher in multiples (twins, triplets, etc.).
[b] The definitions of these gestation bands vary between different countries and authors.

six neurological and six physical parameters and should be performed with the baby fully exposed under a radiant heat warmer (see Fig. 11.1).

Causes and management of preterm labour

Risk factors for preterm labour

The risk factors for preterm labour are shown in Table 11.2. In some cases labour can be suppressed (see below), but in many preterm delivery becomes inevitable. The biggest global causes of prematurity are social deprivation and multiple pregnancy: 6% of singletons, 51% of twins and 91% of triplets are delivered preterm. Infection is strongly implicated in 25–40% of preterm labour – evidence of chorioamnionitis is found in more than 50% of deliveries at less than 25 weeks. In some cases the 'cause' of preterm labour cannot be established.

Predicting preterm delivery

Accurate prediction of imminent preterm delivery allows targeted intervention and transfer, but is not yet an exact science. The following may be useful:
• Ultrasound measurement of the length of the cervix – cervical shortening is associated with a high risk of delivery.
• Fetal fibronectin (a glycoprotein produced by the fetus and act as 'biological glue'); its presence in vaginal/cervical secretions in mid-trimester is highly predictive of preterm labour, but is not valid in the presence of ruptured membranes.
• Frequency and duration of regular contractions.

Clinical management of preterm labour

Although the high mortality and morbidity associated with preterm delivery have prompted a great deal of research into ways of predicting preterm birth, only limited benefits have resulted. Where possible, the woman in preterm labour at less than 32 weeks' gestation should be transferred to a perinatal unit where optimal delivery, stabilization and subsequent management of her infant can be carried out. *In utero* transfer should only be attempted when the preterm labour is not advanced or can be

(a)

									Maturity rating	
Skin	Sticky friable transparent	Gelatinous red, translucent	Smooth pink, visible veins	Superficial peeling &/or rash, few veins	Cracking pale areas, rare veins	Parching deep cracking no vessels	Leathery cracked		Score	Weeks
									−10	20
Lanugo	None	Sparse	Abundant	Thinning	Bald areas	Mostly bald			−5	22
Plantar surface	Heel–toe 40–50mm:−1 <40mm: −2	>50mm no crease	Faint red marks	Anterior transverse crease only	Creases ant. 2/3	Creases over entire sole			0	24
									5	26
Breast	Imperceptible	Barely perceptible	Flat areola no bud	Stippled areola 1–2 mm bud	Raised areola 3–4 mm bud	Full areola 5–10 mm bud			10	28
									15	30
Eye/ear	Lids fused loosely: −1 tightly:−2	Lids open pinna flat stays folded	Slightly curved pinna; soft; slow recoil	Well-curved pinna; soft but ready recoil	Formed & firm instant recoil	Thick cartilage ear stiff			20	32
									25	34
									30	36
Genitals male	Scrotum flat, smooth	Scrotum empty Faint rugae	Testes in upper canal Rare rugae	Testes descending Few rugae	Testes down Good rugae	Testes pendulous Deep rugae			35	38
									40	40
Genitals female	Clitoris prominent Labia flat	Prominent clitoris Small labia minora	Prominent clitoris Enlarging minora	Majora & minora equally prominent	Majora large Minora small	Majora cover clitoris & minora			45	42
									50	44

(b)

	−1	0	1	2	3	4	5		Maturity rating	
									Score	Weeks
Posture									−10	20
									−5	22
Square window (wrist)	>90°	90°	60°	45°	30°	0°			0	24
									5	26
									10	28
Arm recoil		180°	140°–180°	110°–140°	90°–110°	<90°			15	30
									20	32
Popliteal angle	180°	160°	140°	120°	100°	90°	<90°		25	34
									30	36
Scarf sign									35	38
									40	40
Heel to ear									45	42
									50	44

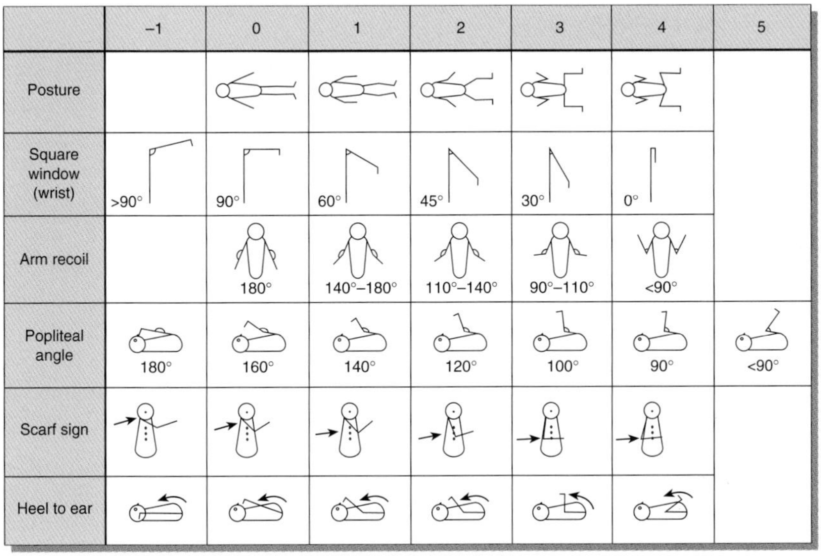

Figure 11.1 The expanded new Ballard score. Reproduced with permission from Ballard JL, Khoury JC, Wedig K, *et al.* New Ballard Score, expanded to include extremely premature infants. *J Pediatr* 1991;**119**:417–423.

Table 11.2 Risk factors for preterm labour and prematurity

Factor	Comment
Maternal age	Extremes of age (<18 yrs or >35 yrs) are associated with preterm labour
Maternal ethnicity	Afro-Caribbean mothers have a 15% incidence of preterm labour
Multiple pregnancy	The higher the multiple, the greater the chance of preterm delivery
Infection	Chorioamnionitis is strongly associated with extreme preterm labour
Hypertension, PET	Labour often induced early to maintain maternal health
Cervical weakening	Previous mid-trimester pregnancy loss or cervical surgery (e.g. cone biopsy)
Uterine malformation	Bicornuate uterus or massive fibroids
Antepartum haemorrhage	Abruption or placenta previa
Amniotic fluid volume	Polyhydramnios and oligohydramnios are both risk factors
Maternal substance abuse	Alcohol, cocaine and cigarette smoking all associated with preterm labour
Fetal abnormality	Congenital anomalies and trisomies associated with preterm delivery

Box 11.1 Approach to threatened preterm delivery

- Is the patient in active preterm labour?
- Is there an underlying cause for the onset of labour?
- Should steroids be given to the mother to enhance fetal lung maturity?
- Should drugs be used to reduce uterine activity?
- Are the mother and fetus at risk of infection?
- Where is the baby to be delivered?
- How is the baby to be delivered?
- Is a suitable neonatal intensive care cot available?

safely and effectively suppressed with tocolytic agents (see Chapter 25).

When a patient is admitted with a diagnosis of possible 'preterm labour', the management plan depends on the criteria listed in Box 11.1.

Obstetric management of preterm labour is rarely clear-cut and is a balanced decision between the relative risks to mother and fetus of continuing the pregnancy versus those of early delivery. Suppression of preterm labour is sometimes possible using tocolytic agents such as beta-adrenergic agonists (e.g. ritodrin), calcium channel blockers (e.g. nifedipine), oxytocin receptor antagonists (e.g. atosiban) or COX-2 cyclo-oxygenase inhibitors (e.g. indometacin). These can delay preterm delivery by 2–7 days but have not been shown to reduce neonatal mortality or morbidity. Magnesium sulphate does not delay delivery but reduces the risk of cerebral palsy in the preterm infant.

Temporary suppression of labour may 'buy time' for *in utero* transport to a perinatal centre or for the acceleration of fetal lung maturity with two doses of corticosteroids. Betamethasone has been shown to be associated with fewer adverse effects than dexamethasone. Meta-analyses have consistently shown that corticosteroids given for 48 h before delivery significantly reduce the incidence and severity of respiratory distress syndrome (RDS) and the incidence of intraventricular haemorrhage (IVH), and possibly improve neurodevelopmental outcome. Suppression of labour is **contraindicated** in the presence of intrauterine infection, congenital anomaly, signs of fetal compromise or significant antepartum haemorrhage.

Mode of delivery in preterm labour

Caesarean section or vaginal delivery

If delivery is inevitable then the best mode of delivery must be chosen. Where the mother's life is in danger (e.g. pre-eclampsia) urgent caesarean section is indicated. Where delivery is elective (e.g. for severe intrauterine growth retardation, IUGR) a balance must be struck between the risks to the fetus of labour and vaginal delivery and the risk to the mother from a caesarean section. In very early gestations (<26 weeks) a lower segment caesarean section (LSCS) may not be possible and a classical (vertical incision) caesarean is needed. This carries a greater risk of uterine rupture in future pregnancies.

Preterm breech presentation

Many extreme preterm babies are still in the breech position when the mother enters labour. The preferred mode of delivery for the preterm breech fetus has been the subject of considerable controversy. The hazards to the fetus of vaginal breech delivery include difficulty with delivery of the head and, rarely, entrapment of the aftercoming head. Although caesarean section in the preterm breech may be associated with some difficulties, it is probably the preferred method of delivery beyond 25 weeks' gestation.

Survival and outcome for the preterm infant

Decision-making in the management of the extremely preterm delivery is influenced by the improved short- and long-term outcomes observed with advances in perinatal care. Aggressive obstetric management and intervention for fetal reasons in late second-trimester deliveries is now practised in many tertiary perinatal centres, and these attitudes are partly responsible for the improved outcomes obtained. Units should develop their own guidelines for the management of extremely preterm labour.

Short-term survival and outcome

Published survival rates vary markedly from country to country and from centre to centre. Large geographically based population studies offer the least biased data. It is important to consider the following points:
• Are babies with lethal congenital abnormalities excluded?
• Is birthweight <500 g or gestation <24 weeks included or excluded?
• Are infants born alive but not resuscitated or not resuscitatable included?
• Is the denominator 'all live births' or 'all admissions to NICU' (the latter will have better outcomes)?
• Have late neonatal deaths (>28 days) been included?

Representative figures for survival after NICU admission are presented by birthweight and gestational age in Table 11.3. Figure 11.2 shows the risk of adverse outcome (death and severe neurodisability) for whole geographically defined populations of very immature babies born in Europe and Australia.

Table 11.3 Typical survival rates analysed by gestational age and birthweight for groups for Australian and New Zealand intensive care nurseries when baby is resuscitated and admitted for intensive care

Gestation at birth (weeks)	Survival (%)	Birthweight (g)	Survival (%)
≤22	<10	400–499	25
23	20	500–749	65
24	60	750–999	85
25	75	1000–1249	95
26	85	1250–1500	98
27	90	<1500	98
28–29	95		
30–32	99		

Source: Abeywardana, S. (2006). *Reports of the Australian and New Zealand Neonatal Network* 2004. ANZNN, Sydney.

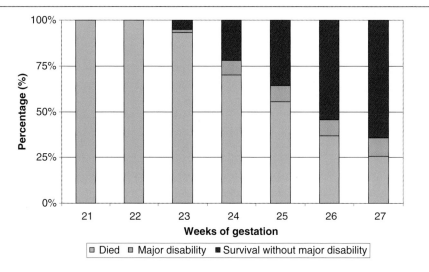

Figure 11.2 Death, severe disability and survival without major disability by gestational age, from five geographically based studies. Reproduced with permission from *Acta Paediatrica*.

Long-term outcomes

As more extreme preterm babies survive and are followed up into teenage and adult life it is clear that there is an additional hidden burden of subtle neurodisability occurring in the most preterm babies (<26 weeks). This can occur even in the absence of obvious central nervous system (CNS) damage or haemorrhage and may be related to subtle disruption of the neuronal pathways that are normally developing in the third trimester. There is a higher than expected incidence of attention deficit hyperactivity disorder (ADHD), autistic features and subtle learning difficulties than in term-born controls. Final stature, IQ and visual function may all be impaired, but often not to a degree that interferes with activities of daily living and not to a degree that is perceived as detrimental by the children themselves.

Preterm delivery at the margins of viability

Babies born at the margins of physiological viability (≤24 weeks) present particular challenges. These infants have a high chance of dying during labour, in the delivery suite or in the first few days after admission to the NICUs. Data from the EPICURE studies in the UK suggest the chances of survival

without disability are low at these extreme gestations (Table 11.4).

Practitioners will approach extreme preterm delivery differently depending on their experience, cultural and religious beliefs and the health care system they operate in. Extreme preterm babies less than 28 weeks are sadly not able to be treated in most developing countries where access to NICU is

Table 11.4 Survival without serious disability (Epicure 1,2)

	EPICURE 1 (1995)		EPICURE 2 (2006)[c]
	At birth[a]	After admission to NICU[b]	
22 weeks	1%	5%	–
23 weeks	3%	6%	11%
24 weeks	9%	12%	24%
25 weeks	20%	24%	40%

[a] Survival without serious disability.
[b] Survival without serious disability at 6 years of age.
[c] Estimated survival without disability at 6 years (outcomes of EPICURE1 applied to EPICURE 2 survival).

Box 11.2 Ethical decision making at extreme preterm gestations (<25 weeks)

- Discussions with parents should be undertaken by a senior, experienced neonatologist, in conjunction with the obstetrician
- Doctors must act with the best interests of the baby in mind.
- A management plan should ideally be agreed with both parents before delivery
- It is important to be sure about the gestation – on what basis has it been calculated? 23 weeks refers to 23^{+0} to 23^{+6} days.
- If in doubt, there should be a presumption of offering life support. A palliative care pathway may be chosen later if the progress is not favourable
- If a baby at these gestations has a low heart rate at birth then assessing the response to five inflation breaths via a mask is important. There is no evidence to support the use of adrenaline and CPR at these gestations

extremely limited. Even in developed countries attitudes vary widely. In the Netherlands infants <25 weeks are not routinely offered intensive life support. In most perinatal centres infants of 22 weeks are not offered intensive life support; at 23 weeks NICU care may be started if parents expressly want this and the baby is in good condition; and at 24 weeks most will offer intensive care, provided there are no other mitigating factors such as a severe congenital anomaly or perinatal asphyxia. In some countries national professional or ethical bodies have published guidelines to help doctors and parents make the right decisions. The important points outlined in Box 11.2 should be considered.

The ethical dilemmas posed by treating the most extreme preterm babies are discussed further in Chapter 28.

Stabilization at birth and management in the 'golden hour'

Experienced personnel should be present at delivery, preferably having had an opportunity to intro-

duce themselves to the parents and to have prepared equipment. They should be aware of any treatment plan agreed with the parents (see above) and be familiar with the obstetric history. Special considerations for extreme preterm births are listed in Table 11.5. In general it is best to think of the process as 'stabilization' rather than 'resuscitation'. These babies are fragile, and usually not severely asphyxiated. They benefit from a calm transition and avoidance of trauma or hyperoxygenation. Once in the NICU they should have vascular access secured and from then on have 'minimal handling' (see Chapter 24).

Transportation within and between hospitals

The baby must be transported from delivery suite to the neonatal intensive care unit (NICU) in a safe but efficient manner. A transport incubator that provides warmth and oxygen saturation monitoring is ideal. If the distance is very short the resuscitaire trolley may be used provided warmth and ventilation can be maintained. If the baby has been delivered in a low-intensity perinatal unit (and *in utero* transfer was not possible) then transfer to a regional NICU must be arranged urgently. This decision will be influenced by the expertise and facilities of the referring hospital, as well as the safety and availability of transportation. Increasingly, dedicated transport teams fulfil this role. Parents must be kept fully informed. Transport is discussed in detail in Chapter 25.

Link to *Nursing the Neonate*: Neonatal stabilization and transport, Chapter 13.

CLINICAL TIP: If the mother cannot be with the baby, either because she is ill or the baby has had to be transferred to another hospital, a photograph of the baby should be provided. Sometimes the mother will provide an item of clothing so that the baby can smell her. Achieving and maintaining breast milk expression is vitally important in this situation.

Table 11.5 Approach to stabilization of a preterm infant ≤28 weeks

Factor	Comment
Personnel	Experienced staff required – usually two neonatal doctors/practitioners and a neonatal nurse to attend
Thermoregulation	The room must be warm. An overhead heater should be turned on. Place the baby in a clear plastic bag/wrap immediately at delivery (without drying first) and place under the overhead heater (Fig. 11.3). Put a bonnet over the head. Monitoring of the heart rate can take place through the plastic bag. Do not remove until the baby is in a warm, humidified incubator. Hypothermia <36°C massively increases the mortality in preterm babies
Airway	As at term, keep the head in the neutral position. You will need a small face mask and should have a small laryngoscope and ET tubes (2.0, 2.5 and 3.0mm) available
Breathing	Use lower peak pressures (20–25cmH$_2$O) to prevent lung damage. PEEP (5–6cmH$_2$O) is very important and must be maintained throughout the stabilization. Use an air–oxygen mix and be prepared to increase the oxygen concentration. Avoid hyperoxia (see below). Give surfactant early, once the ET tube has been confirmed to be correctly located. If attempting CPAP (see below) then it is vital that PEEP is maintained throughout
Circulation	A rise in heart rate is a valuable sign of effective lung aeration, as chest movement is harder to see than at term. Saturation monitoring can measure the pulse and give valuable information about oxygenation
Drugs	These are rarely indicated. If there has been sufficient asphyxia that the heart rate does not respond to lung inflation then a senior doctor should consider whether it is in the best interests to continue aggressive resuscitation as the prognosis will be poor. A lower dose of prophylactic vitamin K is required than at term
Parents	Transfer the baby to NICU as soon as possible, but try to allow the mother to see her baby, even if only briefly, before you leave the room
Vascular access	Once the baby is in a warm, humidified incubator, a skilled operator should insert an umbilical venous and arterial line (see Chapter 29)

Common problems to be expected in the preterm infant

During the final 3 months of intrauterine life most organ systems undergo important structural and functional development. Premature birth requires rapid adaptation to extrauterine life before these organ systems are fully developed. The incidence and severity of all complications of prematurity are normally related to gestational age and birthweight. The main problems are shown in Table 11.6.

Supportive care on the NICU

Monitoring

Heart rate, respiratory rate, blood pressure and temperature must be monitored continuously, with appropriate alarm signals. An apnoea monitor is often used in the special care nursery.

Oxygen therapy

Many sick preterm infants require oxygen therapy to relieve hypoxia. Oxygen is a potentially toxic

Table 11.6 Common problems in the preterm infant

Problem	Impact
Perinatal asphyxia	Less able to tolerate asphyxial insult. Risk of periventricular leucomalacia (see Chapter 22)
Thermal instability	Hypothermia exacerbates RDS and increases mortality. If environmental temperature is too low the baby will expend energy keeping warm at the expense of growth
Lack of primitive survival reflexes	Immature or absent suck–swallow and gag reflex. Need NG feeding (see below)
Pulmonary disease	Apnoea, RDS, transient tachypnoea of the newborn, pneumothorax, pneumonia and chronic lung disease of prematurity (bronchopulmonary dysplasia)
Jaundice	High red cell mass and poor liver conjugation makes hyperbilirubinaemia almost inevitable. Acidosis and a poor blood–brain barrier increases the risk of kernicterus (see Chapter 19)
Metabolic disturbance	Hypoglycaemia, hypocalcaemia, hypomagnesaemia, hyponatraemia, hypernatraemia, hyperkalaemia are all common and must be anticipated
Patent ductus arteriosus (PDA)	Risk of congestive heart failure and risk factor for NEC and IVH
Fragile capillary network in the subependymal area	High risk of IVH, especially in response to swings in cerebral perfusion pressure and carbon dioxide level. Large IVH can cause venous infarction or hydrocephalus (see Chapter 22)
White matter injury	Periventricular white matter susceptible to ischaemic damage, especially if sensitized by fetal inflammation (infection). High risk of periventricular leukomalacia (PVL) – see Chapter 22)
Infection	Relative immunodeficiency and breech of natural barriers (e.g. by central venous lines) predispose to infection, which may be nosocomial or maternal in origin
Feed intolerance	Poor gut motility may cause feed intolerance. Prematurity is also the main risk factor for necrotizing enterocolitis (NEC) – see Chapter 17
Immature visual system	Risk of ROP (see Chapter 23) and myopia/strabismus
Surgical problems	Undescended testes, inguinal and umbilical hernias
Haematological disorders	Disseminated intravascular coagulation, vitamin K deficient bleeding and iatrogenic or iron-deficient anaemia are more common, but not inevitable
Renal immaturity	Inability to concentrate urine, and inability to excrete an acid load with a low renal bicarbonate threshold, resulting in late metabolic acidosis. Late metabolic acidosis may be associated with failure to gain weight satisfactorily. Treatment with sodium bicarbonate and feeding with breast milk or appropriate preterm formula feeds usually improves the acidosis

Box 11.3 Oxygen monitoring

- **Transcutaneous oxygen monitors** ($\pm$ transcutaneous carbon dioxide monitor). These devices utilize a small heating element to heat the skin to 43–44 °C and induce hyperaemia to arterialize the capillary blood and oxygen ($\pm CO_2$) diffusing through the skin, which is monitored continuously.
- **Pulse oximetry** utilizes analysis of red light transmitted through tissues to measure haemoglobin oxygen saturation in arterial blood. This provides continuous, non-invasive and well-tolerated monitoring. Research studies are currently underway to determine the optimum target O_2 saturation levels. Early results suggest the arterial oxygen tension should probably be maintained between 50 and 80 mmHg (6.2–10 kPa) and O_2 saturation at 90–95% (BOOST-2 and SUPPORT trials, 2011)
- Insertion of a catheter into an umbilical or peripheral artery (Chapter 29) provides a readily available site for sampling arterial blood for blood gases, electrolytes and blood glucose, and continuous BP monitoring. Intermittent arterial stabs are less reliable for monitoring P_aO_2, and capillary sampling is not reliable at all, although can be used to monitor pH and pCO_2 in the more stable infant

substance in the preterm infant, and may cause retinopathy of prematurity (ROP) and exacerbate lung inflammation. It must therefore be administered with the utmost care and the response continuously monitored with a pulse oximeter or transcutaneous monitor (Box 11.3). Regular measurements of P_aO_2 are made in premature infants requiring extra oxygen to minimize complications such as ROP and chronic lung disease. It is dangerous to treat ill premature infants without adequate blood-gas monitoring being available. Whether oxygen is administered directly into the incubator or via a headbox, nasal prongs, nasal continuous positive airway pressure (CPAP) prongs or through an endotracheal tube, its use must be monitored very carefully. Oxygen should be warmed to 35–37 °C, humidified to 28–38 mg H_2O/L, and the inspired concentration continuously recorded with high and low alarms set.

Respiratory distress syndrome

Even with the advent of suppression of preterm labour, antenatal corticosteroids and postnatal surfactant, which have radically reduced mortality and morbidity, RDS remains the major problem for the preterm baby in the first week of life. Surfactant-deficient RDS (hyaline membrane disease) is almost inevitable in babies born at less than 28 weeks' gestation. Those preterm infants who die usually have hyaline membranes in the lung at autopsy, but may also have evidence of IVH, patent ductus arteriosus, pneumothorax, necrotizing enterocolitis (NEC) and bronchopulmonary dysplasia. In this century the challenge has moved from preventing death from RDS to preventing chronic lung disease of prematurity. There has been a recent shift towards the use of early CPAP, even in the most extreme preterm infants, in the hope of avoiding mechanical ventilation. Up to 40–50% of even very preterm babies studied appear to manage without intubation or surfactant.

For infants of birthweight less than 800 g or less than 26 weeks' gestation it may be desirable to intubate and ventilate from birth to provide initial airway stabilization, with the aim of early extubation on to CPAP. For other infants at less than 32 weeks' gestation, airway stabilization at birth with CPAP is widely practised. If the baby is intubated, exogenous 'prophylactic' surfactant should be administered as soon after birth as possible. 'Rescue' surfactant treatment for those babies who do not cope on CPAP may be delivered by the 'InSurE' technique: <u>In</u>tubation, <u>Sur</u>factant, <u>E</u>xtubation.

Blood pressure

Arterial blood pressure (BP) is an important variable to measure. If an indwelling arterial catheter is in place, it can be attached to an electronic pressure transducer to measure BP. Alternatively, a mechanical oscillometric device can be used, attached to a BP cuff. Normal BP ranges are shown in Chapter

16. Blood pressure varies with gestational age and birthweight and normally increases over the first 24 h of life. Maintenance of an adequate and stable cerebral blood flow is important to avoid cerebral ischaemic and haemorrhagic injury. Management of hypotension is discussed in Chapter 16.

Thermoregulation

Body temperature must be maintained in the normal range by nursing the preterm infant in a closed, humidified incubator (see Chapter 24). Nursing on a servo-controlled heated platform is less desirable as humidity is not maintained, but may be required for some surgical conditions.

Feeding

Infants of less than 34 weeks' gestational age do not have a good suck or swallow reflex and should usually be fed via an orogastric or nasogastric tube. Premature infants with small gastric capacity require frequent feeding. Feeding the preterm infant is discussed in detail in Chapter 9. The ideal milk is mother's freshly expressed breast milk (EBM). This provides immunity, is easily absorbed and reduces the risk of NEC. If this is not available, stored (frozen) EBM or sometimes donor EBM may be used. Encouraging and supporting the mother to produce breast milk is vital. If formula is used it should be a specialized preterm formula (see Chapter 9).

Parenteral fluids

Sick babies and infants of less than 1500 g or 30 weeks' gestation may need intravenous fluids (10% dextrose and electrolyte solution) until feeding is established. Nutrition is vital and if feeds are going to be delayed or increased slowly, then parenteral nutrition (PN) should be administered early, even on the first day of life. PN is discussed fully in Chapter 9.

The fluid requirements of ill preterm infants depend on a variety of factors, including postnatal age, renal function and transepidermal water loss. Consequently, the fluid intake is adjusted (at least daily) on the basis of urine output, weight, serum electrolytes and urinary concentration. Water losses will be increased by multiple phototherapy and open radiant incubators (approximately an extra 20 mL/kg per day). Sick preterm infants, especially those with RDS and patent ductus arteriosus, should receive restricted fluid volumes until renal output is well established. Insensible losses can be reduced by environmental measures (see Chapter 24).

On the first day intravenous fluids should not contain sodium, but the sodium and electrolyte requirement for premature infants will increase as immature kidneys do not conserve sodium well. Close monitoring of serum electrolytes, including calcium, is necessary.

Jaundice

This is extremely common in the preterm infant and must be tracked with frequent bilirubin estimations. Jaundice of prematurity is a diagnosis of exclusion after other causes have been eliminated. Preterm infants are more prone to bilirubin encephalopathy than term infants, and factors that affect the entry of free bilirubin into the brain include low albumin levels, acidosis, hypoxia, hypoglycaemia, hypothermia, certain drugs and starvation. Jaundice is discussed thoroughly in Chapter 19.

Vitamins

A single intramuscular dose of 400 μg/kg of vitamin K is adequate unless the baby is receiving broad-spectrum antibiotics, when twice-weekly injections are necessary to compensate for loss of the endogenous vitamin K normally produced by bowel flora. Preterm infants who require PN receive supplemental vitamins. Preterm formulas are supplemented with vitamins. Preterm infants of less than 32 weeks' gestation should have human breast milk fortifier added to EBM. Once a preterm infant of less than 34 weeks' gestation is tolerating full feeds, most recommend a multivitamin preparation such as Pentavite or Abidec drops given daily and continued until the baby is fully weaned on to a mixed diet.

Anaemia

Some sick preterm infants will be anaemic at birth or develop anaemia as a result of frequent blood sampling and will require a transfusion with packed red blood cells. The venous haematocrit should be maintained at more than 0.35% (haemoglobin 12 g/dL) in all sick babies during the acute phase of RDS. However, during the physiological nadir of anaemia (at 5–7 weeks) preterm infants may tolerate a haemoglobin concentration of 7 g/dL (haematocrit 0.25%), especially if there is an adequate reticulocyte response (>5%). To prevent iron deficiency anaemia, preterm infants less than 2000 g birthweight or 34 weeks' gestation are usually prescribed supplemental iron (ferrous sulphate) from 2–6 weeks until fully weaned.

 Link to *Nursing the Neonate*: Haematology in the term and preterm neonate. Chapter 17.

Preparation for discharge home

The transition from hospital to home is a crucial step in the future well-being of the family. Once the requirements for intensive care are over, the baby will still need monitoring, incubator care and nasogastric feeding. This can be a very frustrating time for the parents, who have already been through a lot of stress. Early discharge for low-birthweight infants can be safely practised and may promote attachment. The baby may be discharged at 34–35 weeks provided feeding is progressing well, temperature control is good, weight gain is steady, the mother is handling her baby competently and the home situation is good. Some units promote short-term nasogastric feeding at home for selected, trained parents, with outreach nurse support, as a way of speeding the transition to full feeding. Other units will have a transitional care facility or invite the mothers in to be 'resident' on the neonatal unit for a few days before discharge to gain confidence in being the prime carer for their baby at last.

Community nursing support can be very helpful in allaying fears, monitoring well-being and preventing readmission to hospital. Outpatient follow-up should be arranged for all complex babies. Intermittent follow-up continuing to 2 years of age is desirable for all extreme preterm babies to allow data collection on outcomes which becomes part of the quality improvement audit cycle (see Chapter 26).

Link to *Nursing the Neonate*: Discharge planning and the community outreach service. Chapter 20.

SUMMARY

About 7% of all births occur preterm, but it is those at less than 32 weeks and especially less than 28 weeks that provide the greatest challenge. These births often occur unexpectedly and a skilled team must be mobilized. The use of antenatal corticosteroids has dramatically improved survival and every opportunity should be taken to administer these, even if labour needs to be delayed.

A philosophy of gentle 'stabilization' rather than aggressive resuscitation, with careful avoidance of extremes of temperature, BP, oxygen and carbon dioxide concentration will be beneficial in the longer term. In those babies born at the 'threshold of viability' good communication with the parents is essential. The right decisions need to be made in the best long-term interests of the baby, and they must be clinically, ethically and morally sound decisions that all can agree on.

The survival of extremely preterm infants is one of the successes of modern medicine. It is important that the long-term aim (survival with a good quality of life) is kept in mind and that these advances are also enabled in developing countries.

CHAPTER 12

The low-birthweight infant

Key topics

Introduction

Newborn infants can be classified according to birthweight, gestational age or size for gestational age (Table 12.1). Low birthweight is defined as less than 2500 g. However, a low birthweight (LBW) infant may be that size because they are either preterm or small for gestational age (SGA), or both. The problems these infants develop tend to be determined by whether the infants have been born too early or are born too small for the duration of gestation. The problems associated with LBW are described here. Those predominantly associated with prematurity are described in Chapter 11.

The infant who is small for gestational age

Although several synonyms have been used to describe the growth-restricted infant, including dysmaturity, light for dates, small for dates and intrauterine growth restriction, the preferred term is now SGA. There has been no such uniformity in the definition of SGA. From a statistical viewpoint, infants weighing more than two standard deviations below the mean can be defined as SGA, regardless of gestation. However, because they share common clinical problems, infants below the 10th centile for weight are often regarded as 'SGA'. It must be recognized that some of these will in fact be appropriately grown and are just smaller than average, for familial or racial reasons. Furthermore, many

Essential Neonatal Medicine, Fifth Edition. Sunil Sinha, Lawrence Miall, Luke Jardine.
© 2012 John Wiley & Sons, Ltd. Published 2012 by John Wiley & Sons, Ltd.

Table 12.1 Classification of newborn infants according to birthweight, gestational age or size for gestational age

Factor	Terminology	Incidence (%)
Birthweight		
<2500 g	Low birthweight (LBW)	6.5
<1500 g	Very low birthweight (VLBW)	1.3
<1000 g	Extremely low birthweight (ELBW)	0.6
Gestational age (completed weeks after last normal menstrual period)		
<37 weeks	Preterm	8.4
>41 weeks	Post-term	0.6
Size for gestational age		
Weight between 90th and 10th centiles for gestation	Appropriate for gestational age (AGA)	80
Weight <10th centile for gestation	Small for gestational age (SGA)	≈10
Weight >90th centile for gestation	Large for gestational age (LGA)	≈10

neonates with birthweight above the 10th centile will demonstrate evidence of acute or chronic weight loss, and should therefore fall into the spectrum of the growth-restricted infant. Variables such as sex, race and altitude should be considered when determining growth curves, because a birthweight below the 10th centile in one population may not fall below the 10th centile in another, even though both may be growth restricted. Table 12.2 lists important factors that predict birthweight of an individual fetus or neonate for a given population.

CLINICAL TIP: It is important that weight and length measurements are plotted on an appropriate growth chart. WHO have issued growth charts for preterm and term babies based on a breastfed population, which mean breastfed infants will no longer appear to be dropping centiles. Down's syndrome specific charts also exist. Growth-restricted infants should be plotted on a normal growth chart appropriate to their gestational age.

Link to *Nursing the Neonate*: The small baby. Chapter 5, pp. 65–70.

Classification of small for gestational age infants

Subdividing the heterogenous SGA population into subgroups offers the potential to better understand the underlying cause, and therefore allows a more accurate prognosis and appropriate postnatal management:
- SGA but appropriately grown (constitutionally small)
- SGA due to growth restriction (IUGR).

It is important to attempt to define the neonate 'starved' as a result of IUGR. These babies show greatest growth failure in terms of weight, then length; head circumference is the least affected. There is little subcutaneous fat, the skin may be loose and thin, muscle mass is decreased, especially the buttocks and thighs, and the infant often has a wide-eyed, anxious look. This pattern can be distinguished from the uniformly growth-restricted type, which implies either a fetal cause (e.g. chromosomal) or a very early insult.

Table 12.2 Determinants of birthweight	
Maternal factors before conception	Stature
	Weight
	Genotype
	Race
	Age
	Parity
	Socioeconomic status (occupation, education, income)
Factors at or around conception	Fetal genotype
	Singleton or multiple conception
	Fetal sex
	Genetic anomaly (chromosomal or major gene locus)
Factors between conception and birth	Altitude above sea level
	Fetal or maternal infection (rubella, malaria)
	Maternal work and ability to rest
	Maternal cigarette smoking
	Maternal diet
	Maternal alcohol, drugs, medications
	Placental dysfunction (e.g. PET)

Subcutaneous fat can be objectively assessed by measuring the circumference of the mid-upper arm or by measuring skinfold thickness with special calipers.

Causes of intrauterine growth restriction

The causes of IUGR can be classified according to whether they are fetal, placental or maternal (Table 12.4). The growth failure can be classified as 'intrinsic', which implies an abnormality at the time of conception or within the first trimester (fetal and some maternal causes), or 'extrinsic', implying a later onset of growth restriction (placental or maternal causes). See Table 12.3.

Intrinsic fetal growth restriction

Early-onset IUGR, which tends to give rise to an SGA infant who is proportionate, symmetrical and hypoplastic, is more likely to have an intrinsic cause of growth failure. During the first trimester, global

Table 12.3 Classification of the growth-restricted fetus and the SGA infant. Many growth-restricted infants exhibit a mixture of classifications

Proportionate (type I IUGR)		Disproportionate (type II IUGR)
Symmetrical	vs	Asymmetrical
Intrinsic cause	vs	Extrinsic cause
Hypoplastic	vs	Hypotrophic

insults include chromosomal anomalies (e.g. trisomy syndromes), perinatal infections (e.g. congenital viral infections (TORCH)), dwarfing syndromes (e.g. achondroplasia, chondrodystrophic dwarfism, Russell–Silver syndrome), maternal substance abuse (e.g. alcohol, opiates, cocaine) and exposure to teratogenic drugs and rarely, ionizing radiation.

These infants, sometimes referred to as having type I IUGR, show symmetrical growth restriction, with similar growth reductions in weight, length

Table 12.4 Cause of intrauterine growth restriction

Fetal	Placental	Maternal
Chromosomal abnormalities	Toxaemia of pregnancy	Maternal disease
Prenatal viral infection	Multiple pregnancy	Alcohol
Dysmorphic syndromes	Small placental size	Smoking
X-rays	Site of implantation	Malnutrition
	Vascular transfusion in monochorial twin placentas	Altitude

and head circumference see Table 12.3. They do not exhibit a head-sparing effect and, because of a decreased number of cells, as well as decreased cell size, do not have the potential for normal growth. This group comprises only about 10–30% of all SGA babies in modern Western societies. There is potential for miscalculation of gestational age if this is based on biparietal measurement at a late scan.

Extrinsic fetal growth restriction

Later-onset fetal growth restriction results from disorders of the placenta or from maternal problems. These are associated with impaired delivery of oxygen and nutrients from the placenta. These factors may become operative at different times during pregnancy, resulting in less predictable effects on fetal growth. Maternal factors include hypertension `(e.g. essential, pregnancy-induced, pre-eclampsia), diabetes mellitus with vascular complications, renal disease, cardiac disease, sickle cell disease and collagen disorders. Maternal smoking, alcohol and narcotic abuse and maternal hypoxia (e.g. cardiac disease, pulmonary disease, migration to high altitude) may also cause extrinsic IUGR.

Placental factors

These all have the common feature of diminished placental blood flow, which can become more severe later in pregnancy. Twins show a normal rate of intrauterine growth until the demands of the two fetuses outstrip the placental blood supply. This usually occurs at about 32 weeks' gestation, and fetal growth rates fall off from this time. SGA infants occur in 24–40% of twin pregnancies. Placental disorders associated with IUGR include chronic villitis, haemorrhagic endovasculitis, chorioangioma, chronic abruptio placentae, hydatidiform degeneration, single umbilical artery and twin–twin transfusion syndrome.

> CLINICAL TIP: Very disproportionate growth-restricted babies with large heads and small bodies were once a common site on special care baby units. This picture is now unusual as obstetricians usually make a decision to deliver the baby earlier, on the basis of serial ultrasound scans and Doppler measurements. They are still occasionally seen in the context of unbooked pregnancy or when one of twins or triplets is very growth restricted.

Problems to be expected in the growth-restricted fetus and small for gestational age infant

When IUGR results from a restricted nutrient supply, the fetus adapts to maximize the prospect of good outcome by redistributing blood to the brain, accelerating pulmonary maturity and increasing the red cell mass (polycythaemia). These features may initially represent useful adaptation, but they later become pathological when deprivation is more extreme and fetal distress supervenes. Table 12.5 summarizes the problems that these babies may face.

Table 12.5 Anticipated problems in the fetus/neonate who is small for gestational age (SGA)

Fetus	Neonate	Subsequent outcome
Congenital malformation		Dependent on malformation
Stillbirth		
Fetal distress or cord compression	Asphyxia	Intellectual deficit, poor growth
Meconium aspiration	Meconium aspiration syndrome	Cerebral palsy (due to asphyxia)
Oligohydramnios with possible deformation	Polycythaemia	Hyperviscosity, risk of thrombosis, NEC
Less subcutaneous fat	Hypothermia	Poor growth
Less glycogen stored	Hypoglycaemia	Intellectual deficit
Chronic asphyxia	Hypocalcaemia	Fits
Chronic ischaemia to organs (brain sparing)	Liver and renal impairment	Coagulopathy or oliguria
Premature rupture of membranes	Infection (impaired immune system)	
Preterm delivery	Pulmonary haemorrhage	Severe RDS Chronic lung disease of prematurity
Poor fetal growth	Poor growth	Short stature

Problems manifesting in the neonatal period

Perinatal asphyxia

Fetuses with chronic distress do not tolerate the additional hypoxic stress of delivery, and they readily develop hypoxia and acidosis.

Congenital malformations

There is a 20-fold increased incidence of congenital malformation in SGA babies compared with their normal birthweight peers. Cause and effect needs to be established.

Infection

There is a ninefold increased incidence of infection. This is partly explained by the association with TORCH infections, but also by a greater incidence of acquired infection.

Hypoglycaemia

SGA infants have insufficient hepatic and cardiac muscle glycogen stores and a limited capacity for gluconeogenesis. Hypoglycaemia is often asymptomatic.

Hypocalcaemia

The increased incidence of hypocalcaemia relates to perinatal asphyxia and not to SGA infants *per se*.

Polycythaemia

This is a common problem, when prolonged intrauterine hypoxia results in elevated levels of erythropoietin. Thrombocytopenia may also coexist.

Thermal instability

Maintenance of body temperature is a problem for the SGA infant, but less so than for the preterm infant. This relates to the large surface area to body weight ratio and reduction in subcutaneous fat.

Respiratory distress

Respiratory distress in the SGA infant may be due to meconium aspiration, polycythaemia, massive pulmonary haemorrhage or pneumonia, but is not usually due to RDS as fetal 'stress' leads to increased cortisol release and surfactant production. Growth restriction in extremely preterm infants, however, does not protect them against RDS to the same degree.

Problems manifesting in infancy and childhood

Growth

In the neonatal period the infant loses little weight and begins to gain weight rapidly after birth. This growth spurt is often not maintained and a permanent deficit in somatic growth may persist into childhood.

Full-term IUGR infants stand a good chance of catching up, particularly if growth restriction is due to maternal factors. Infants who are both severely preterm and growth restricted are much less likely to reach average size than infants of the same degree of prematurity but who are normally grown. If catch-up growth is going to occur, it usually does so by 6 months. Infants with intrinsic causes of fetal growth restriction exhibit minimal catch-up growth and remain lighter, shorter and with smaller head circumference at 3 years of age.

The Barker hypothesis (fetal programming)

A large number of epidemiology studies have shown a relationship between small birth size and the subsequent risk of type 2 diabetes, insulin resistance, hypertension, cardiovascular disease and stroke. This is thought to be mediated through insulin-like growth factor 2 (IGF-2) and is referred to as the Barker hypothesis after David Barker, who first made these observations. This programming is thought to be due to an evolutionary adaptation whereby the IUGR fetus alters its physiology in expectation of a 'thrifty' postnatal environment, which is an advantage in a hostile environment where food is not plentiful. In a modern society where food is plentiful and where small infants are often encouraged to gain weight rapidly, this phenotype predisposes to atherogenesis and cardiovascular disease in later life. For this reason, infants with severe IUGR should have their weight gain targeted to their birth centile, not the 50th centile.

Development

The ultimate developmental outcome relates to the cause of the IUGR, timing and duration of the insult, severity of growth restriction, degree of asphyxia, the postnatal course and the socioeconomic status of the infant's family.

A number of follow-up studies have shown that SGA infants born at term are prone to more developmental, behavioural and learning problems than infants of the equivalent weight due to prematurity. Males are more vulnerable than females. A baby who is both SGA and premature is predisposed to a greater risk of serious neurological abnormalities than if he/she were only premature or only SGA. Catch-up in head circumference (which reflects brain growth) is a good prognostic sign for cognitive development.

Management of the low birthweight infant

Perinatal management

Antenatal identification that a fetus is SGA will greatly influence management. If IUGR is suspected, careful monitoring of fetal and uteroplacental function will be necessary, with serial ultrasound scans, Doppler assessment of blood flow and biophysical monitoring (see Chapter 1).

A decision regarding the best method and timing of delivery needs to be made. If vaginal delivery is planned then continuous intrapartum fetal heart rate monitoring should be undertaken. A practitioner skilled in resuscitation should be present at delivery.

If severely IUGR, the baby should be transferred to a special care nursery or transitional care facility for close observation, monitoring for hypoglycaemia and temperature instability. Incubator care may be necessary.

Investigations for IUGR

Investigations as to the aetiology are only required if the cause is not obvious. Investigations to identify complications depend on the individual symptoms. Relevant investigations are listed in Table 12.6.

Feeding

If catch-up growth is to occur and the child is to reach his/her full growth and intellectual potential, adequate early nutrition is essential. The SGA infant should commence feeds soon after birth, and ini-tially feeding should be frequent with colostrum or high-energy formula. Estimates of blood glucose should be made before feeds. The infant should receive at least 60 mL/kg on day 1, and increase up to 180 mL/kg/day. In preterm IUGR infants enteral feeding should progress cautiously because of the increased risk of necrotising enterocolitis (NEC) from fetal redistribution of blood away from the gut. A feeding regime is helpful (see Chapter 9). Aggressive over-feeding to a calculated expected weight (e.g. the 50th centile) is no longer recommended because of the long-term risks of type 2 diabetes and cardiovascular disease.

CLINICAL TIP: In the preterm baby with severe IUGR or abnormal antenatal Doppler studies, rapid escalation of milk feeds, especially if not breast milk, may increase the risk of NEC. Feeds should be increased slowly, using a structured feeding protocol.

Table 12.6 Approach to the investigation of IUGR	
Investigation	**Comment**
Placental histology	May identify evidence of infarction or TORCH infection
FBC	If petechiae (low platelets) or plethora or hypoglycaemia (polycythaemia)
Glucose	To ensure normoglycaemia
Chest radiograph	Only if respiratory symptoms or very dysmorphic
Abdominal radiograph	If any concern about NEC
TORCH infection screen (IgG, IgM)	If hepatosplenomegaly, petechiae, cataracts or microcephaly present
CMV PCR (urine)	This is the most sensitive test for congenital CMV
Chromosomal analysis (karyotype)	If dysmorphic features present in addition to IUGR
Renal and brain USS, echocardiogram	Only if dysmorphic
LFT, clotting screen	Only if evidence of chronic fetal hypoxic–ischaemic injury

CMV, cytomegalovirus; FBC, full blood count; LFT, liver function test; NEC, necrotising enterocolitis; PCR, polymerase chain reaction; USS, ultrasound scan.

Supportive care

If the infant develops hypoglycaemia despite early feeding, 10% dextrose intravenous infusion may be required, in addition to milk. A capillary haematocrit should be performed. If it is greater than 70%, a venous haematocrit is indicated. If the venous haematocrit is greater than 70–75%, or the baby has symptomatic polycythaemia, a dilutional exchange transfusion with normal saline (30 mL/kg) is indicated.

A careful examination for congenital malformations should always be made. The most common anomaly is a single umbilical artery. Look for features suggestive of intrauterine infection, such as hepatosplenomegaly, petechiae, cataracts and microcephaly.

SUMMARY

When a baby is born with low birthweight it is important to know the gestation. If the baby is SGA then consider whether this is constitutional (familial) or whether there is growth restriction. If there is evidence of IUGR decide whether this is intrinsic or extrinsic and investigate appropriately. Early nutrition is important but beware of over aggressive feeding because of the short-term risk of NEC and the longer-term risk of cardiovascular disease. Severe IUGR may have lifelong consequences including short stature, metabolic disease and reduced cognitive ability.

 Now visit **www.essentialneonatalmed.com** to test yourself on this chapter.

CHAPTER 13
Respiratory disorders

Key topics

Introduction

At birth, major cardiorespiratory changes take place in order to prepare the baby for extrauterine existence. This includes replacement of fetal lung fluid by air and establishment of regular spontaneous breathing. Associated with lung inflation and increased oxygenation there is a marked decrease in the pulmonary vascular resistance with consequent increased pulmonary blood flow and closure of the ductus arteriosus, foramen ovale and ductus venosus. As a result, the lungs take over the respiratory function previously carried out by the placenta. Many pathological processes can interfere with this normal sequence of events and cause respiratory disorders. Their clinical presentation varies according to the severity of the illness and depends on which part of the respiratory apparatus is primarily involved such as:
- respiratory distress (due to primary lung disease)
- apnoea and bradycardia (due to immaturity or dysfunction of respiratory centres in brain)
- stridor (due to upper airway obstruction)
- chronic respiratory insufficiency (due to fatigue or weakness of muscles of breathing such as in neuromuscular diseases, see Chapter 22).

Essential Neonatal Medicine, Fifth Edition. Sunil Sinha, Lawrence Miall, Luke Jardine.
© 2012 John Wiley & Sons, Ltd. Published 2012 by John Wiley & Sons, Ltd.

Respiratory distress

Respiratory distress is a general term used to describe respiratory symptoms and is not synonymous with respiratory distress syndrome (RDS). Signs of respiratory distress include:

• tachypnoea – a respiratory rate greater than 60/min
• expiratory grunt – breathing against a closed glottis
• chest retraction or recession
• flaring of the ala nasae
• cyanosis or low arterial oxygen saturation in air.

Diagnosis

The presence of two or more of the above signs persisting for 4 h or more suggests respiratory distress. There are many causes of respiratory distress in the newborn (Table 13.1).

Diagnosis will be made by a full clinical history, physical examination and appropriate investigation, including a chest radiograph (Box 13.1). Perinatal history should include gestational age, the presence of polyhydramnios or oligohydramnios, anomalies on ultrasound, risk factors for sepsis, the passage of meconium, poor condition at birth and duration of amniotic membrane rupture. Physical examination includes observation of vital signs and auscultation of the lungs for symmetry of air entry, and heart sounds.

Treatment of respiratory distress

Supportive care

The supportive care of the infant with respiratory distress is similar regardless of aetiology. Infants with respiratory distress require frequent or continuous observations of respiratory and heart rates, temperature, blood pressure and signs of respiratory distress. Accurate fluid balance charts are essential. Adequate temperature control and provision of nutrition essential part of respiratory care in newborns.

Table 13.1 Common causes of respiratory distress in newborns

Primary respiratory causes	Secondary to extrapulmonary pathology
TTN (or retained fetal lung fluid)	Following birth asphyxia: surgical conditions, e.g. choanal atresia, Pierre Robin sequence, diaphragmatic hernia, lobar emphysema, oesophageal atresia with TOF
RDS due to surfactant deficiency	Persistence of fetal circulation (or PPHN)
Pneumonia	Congenital heart disease
Pneumothorax; pneumomediastinum; pulmonary interstitial emphysema	Anaemia
Aspiration syndromes, e.g. meconium, milk, blood	Polycythaemia
Pulmonary hypoplasia, e.g. associated with oligohydramnios	Infection
Pulmonary haemorrhage	Metabolic disease
Chronic neonatal lung disease, e.g. BPD	

BPD, bronchopulmonary dysplasia; PPHN, persistent pulmonary hypertension of newborn; RDS, respiratory distress syndrome; TOF, tracheo-oesophageal fistula; TTN, transient tachypnoea of the newborn.

Oxygen

Oxygen is a useful and life-saving therapeutic agent, but is also potentially dangerous, particularly in the preterm baby, as it may damage the eyes (retinopathy of prematurity) and the lungs (bronchopulmo-

Box 13.1 Investigations for respiratory distress

- Chest radiograph
- Bacteriological cultures on blood, urine and cerebrospinal fluid (CSF)
- Viral cultures and rapid-yield immunodiagnostic tests
- Haematocrit and full blood count
- Chest transillumination if pneumothorax suspected
- Passage of nasogastric catheters if choanal and oesophageal atresias suspected
- Hyperoxia test to differentiate between cardiac and respiratory disease
- Echocardiography

nary dysplasia). When administered, it should be warmed to 34–37°C and humidified. Oxygen therapy is discussed in Chapter 15.

Fluids

Infants with acute moderate to severe respiratory distress should not be enterally fed. With mild respiratory distress nasogastric feeding may be adequate, but with severe respiratory distress, intravenous fluids will be required. Usually a 10% dextrose saline solution or total parenteral nutrition (TPN) is used.

Monitoring of blood gases and acid–base status

With moderate or severe respiratory distress, assessment of the arterial acid–base status, with samples from an intra-arterial catheter or capillary blood gases may be necessary. Continuous transcutaneous monitoring of PO_2 and PCO_2 decreases the requirement for blood sampling and enables rapid detection of fluctuations in clinical status. If respiratory acidosis is severe (pH <7.20 with PCO_2 >60 mmHg, 8 kPa), assisted ventilation may be necessary. For a

severe metabolic acidosis (base deficit more than −8), an infusion of sodium bicarbonate may be indicated but one should always try to treat the underlying cause first. Arterial catheterization is indicated when there is a need for frequent sampling for gas analysis, and is used for direct aortic blood pressure monitoring.

Artificial respiratory support

In more severe cases artificial respiratory support may be necessary. This may be in the form of non-invasive respiratory support such as continuous positive airway pressure (CPAP) which can be escalated to bilevel positive airway pressure (BiPAP) or non-invasive positive-pressure ventilation (NIPPV) if needed. Yet, in a proportion of cases, such treatment may fail and hence the necessity to switch to mechanical ventilation. This is described in Chapter 15.

Transient tachypnoea of the newborn

Transient tachypnoea of the newborn (TTN) occurs in approximately 1–2% of all newborn infants and is due to respiratory maladaptation at birth causing retention of fluids in the lungs (which are normally replaced by air by this time). Tachypnoea is generally the outstanding feature. TTN is usually benign and self-limiting, with symptoms rarely persisting beyond 48 h.

Pathogenesis

Most of the fetal lung fluid is squeezed out during descent through the birth canal or within the first few breaths after birth, but some is reabsorbed into the pulmonary capillaries and lymphatics. Occasionally, there is an excess of fluid or the clearance mechanisms are inefficient. In these cases retained fluid causes respiratory distress by making the lungs stiff.

Predisposing factors for TTN are late preterm delivery (34–36 weeks), heavy maternal analgesia, birth asphyxia, prelabour caesarean section, breech presentation, hypoproteinaemia and excessive fluid administration to the mother in labour. Polycythaemia may produce a similar clinical picture resulting from hyperviscosity with resultant pulmonary plethora. Maternal asthma is said to be associated with TTN.

Diagnosis

The diagnosis of TTN is confirmed by chest radiograph and the clinical course. Resolution of the respiratory distress within 48 h confirms the clinical diagnosis retrospectively. Chest radiograph shows streakiness caused by interstitial fluid, fluid in the lung fissures and perihilar cuffing. Pleural effusions and cardiomegaly may also sometimes be seen.

Treatment

TTN does not usually require respiratory support, other than extra inspired oxygen. Regular blood-gas measurements should be performed in the early stages of the illness. In more severe cases CPAP may aid resolution. If the blood gases deteriorate, the diagnosis should be reconsidered or complications such as pulmonary hypertension or pneumothorax may have developed. Sometimes the typical picture of TTN evolves over several days into one of RDS.

Respiratory distress syndrome

RDS is a specific clinical entity occurring predominantly but not exclusively in preterm infants owing to a lack of surfactant (a surface tension-lowering agent) in the alveoli. It has a characteristic clinical course and specific radiographic changes.

Incidence

Incidence of RDS is related to the degree of prematurity and is unusual in full-term infants (Fig. 13.1). Some predisposing factors are listed in Box 13.2.

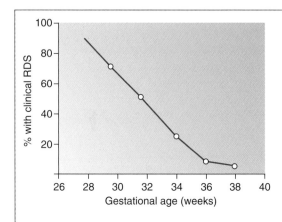

Figure 13.1 Incidence of RDS related to gestational age.

Box 13.2 Predisposing factors to RDS

- Prematurity
- Infant of a diabetic mother
- Antepartum haemorrhage
- Second twin
- Hypoxia, acidosis, shock
- Male sex
- Prelabour caesarean section (many factors involved)

Aetiology and pathogenesis

The major hallmark of RDS is a deficiency of surfactant which leads to higher surface tension at the alveolar surface and interferes with the normal exchange of respiratory gases. The higher surface tension requires greater distending pressure to inflate the alveoli, according to the Laplace law:

$$P = \frac{2\sigma}{r} \tag{13.1}$$

where P is the pressure required to inflate a sphere, σ the surface tension and r the radius.

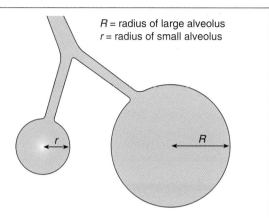

R = radius of large alveolus
r = radius of small alveolus

Figure 13.2 Schematic representations of two alveoli demonstrating the Laplace law (see text for details).

As the radius of the alveolus decreases (atelectasis) and as surface tension increases, the amount of pressure required to overcome these forces increases. The Laplace equation explains why, in the presence of high surface tension, large alveoli tend to become larger and small ones remain collapsed. Assuming that both small and large alveoli receive equal perfusion with blood, there will be a ventilation/perfusion (V/Q) imbalance. This results in severe biochemical disturbances, with hypoxia and acidosis, which give rise to a deterioration in pulmonary perfusion, thus causing further deterioration in V/Q. This may become progressively more severe and lead to persistent pulmonary hypertension (see Chapter 16).

Clinical features

The signs of RDS start immediately after birth or become obvious in the first 6 h of life. In the absence of surfactant each breath the infant takes is like the first breath in an effort to expand the alveoli. Fatigue contributes to the respiratory failure. The clinical course is usually associated with worsening of the symptoms, with a peak severity at 48–72 h, although occasionally maximum severity may occur in infants less than 12 h old. As the disease progresses the infant shows a need for increasing oxygen, the

expiratory grunt may diminish and prolonged apnoea may occur. Without intervention, recurrent and worsening apnoea superimposed on tachypnoea would indicate impending respiratory failure and the need for mechanical ventilation. The breath sounds are decreased and there may be a fall in blood pressure. The infant is oliguric initially and has evidence of increasing peripheral oedema due to fluid retention. At about 48 h a diuresis often occurs, with a concomitant clinical improvement in less severely affected infants.

It should, however, be realized that presentation of RDS in babies born at extreme preterm gestations, such as those born at 23 and 24 weeks' gestation, may have an entirely different pattern of clinical presentation and course of illness. Such babies may not show signs of respiratory distress. Their clinical condition appears quite stable with a normal chest radiograph. This, however, lasts for a short period of 2–3 days when their respiratory problem starts and they run into problems with prolonged ventilatory dependency and chronic lung disease. This may be because such infants are born with lungs in very early stages of development (see Chapter 15) which are more susceptible to lung injury particularly if requiring ventilation and oxygen treatment (pulmonary injury sequence).

Radiology

The radiograph is characteristic, showing under-aeration and a fine reticular or granuloreticular pattern, often referred to as 'ground glass'. In addition, air bronchograms are seen in the lung fields (Fig. 13.3). Severe cases with near-total atelectasis may show complete opacification of the lung fields ('white out'). The appearance of the chest radiograph may not correlate well with the clinical severity of RDS. Extremely preterm infants, in whom lungs are not fully developed, may actually have normal lung fields.

Laboratory abnormalities

Arterial oxygen tension is usually decreased. Arterial carbon dioxide tension may initially be normal (when breathing faster to compensate for

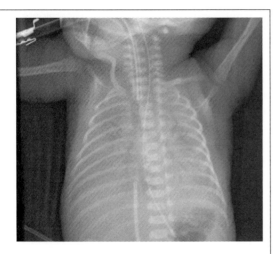

Figure 13.3 Chest radiograph showing the characteristic 'ground glass' appearance of RDS.

Establishment of adequate gas exchange

Oxygen

The aim of treatment is to maintain the P_aO_2 within the normal range. This is done in very mild cases by increasing the inspired oxygen concentration (F_iO_2). In more severe cases respiratory support may be necessary, but the further management depends on the size of the infant and degree of gaseous exchange abnormality.

Although CPAP may be administered shortly after birth, smaller infants are more likely to require mechanical ventilation. Indications for mechanical ventilation are listed in Box 13.3.

Supportive treatment

Chest physiotherapy

Infants receive regular position changes and airway suctioning to reduce the risk of mucus retention, airway plugging and pulmonary collapse. Routine chest physiotherapy is of no proven value in management of RDS.

Antibiotics

Broad-spectrum antibiotics are usually administered to all babies with RDS after suitable cultures have been taken. This is because sepsis/pneumonia, especially group B streptococcal infection, can produce a nearly identical picture. Antibiotics should be stopped once cultures, blood count and ancillary investigations for sepsis are reported as negative. The choice of antibiotics depends on the local preference keeping in mind the prevalence of local bacteriological spectrum.

Appropriate fluid balance

See Chapter 9.

respiratory difficulty), but is usually increased. Blood pH may reflect respiratory acidosis (from hypercarbia), metabolic acidosis (from tissue hypoxia) or mixed acidosis.

Treatment

Surfactant replacement therapy

The development and use of surfactant replacement therapy has revolutionized the treatment of RDS. Numerous preparations, including animal-derived surfactants and equally effective newer synthetic surfactants, have been developed and tested in numerous randomized controlled trials, all of which confirm the efficacy of surfactant in improving survival and reducing complications such as pneumothorax.

Surfactants can be used either 'prophylactically' in at risk infants (such as those born less than 27 weeks' gestation) or as a 'rescue' treatment whenever babies develop respiratory distress. Different surfactant preparations have different composition and dosing schedule but they are all effective. Normally one or two doses of surfactant should be sufficient and there is no evidence that further doses provide any real benefit.

Box 13.4 Common complications associated with RDS and its treatment

- Pneumothorax
- Patent ductus arteriosus (PDA)
- Necrotising enterocolitis (NEC)
- Subglottic stenosis (causing stridor)
- Chronic lung disease (CLD) and bronchpulmonary dysplasia (BPD)
- Intraventricular-periventricular haemorrhage (PVH-IVH)
- Periventricular leukomalacia (PVL)
- Retinopathy of prematurity (ROP)

Table 13.2 Typical incidence and survival rates for infants of different birthweight groups with a diagnosis of RDS

	Birthweight categories (g)	Incidence (%)	Survival (%)
	<500	100	10
	500–999	80	80
	1000–1499	55	95
	>1499	20	100
Total	500–5000	N/A	94

Blood pressure monitoring

See Chapter 16.

Minimal handling and nursing in a neutral environmental temperature

See Chapter 24.

Complications

In general, the risk of complications is related to the severity of the underlying RDS and its treatment. Box 13.4 lists the common complications. These complications in turn can lead to long-term morbidities such as cerebral palsy, and bronchpulmonary dysplasia (BPD).

Prognosis

Most infants who die do so not as a direct result of RDS but rather of a related complication (intraventricular haemorrhage, infection, chronic lung disease). Those weighing 1000 g or below are most at risk. More mature infants, even with severe RDS, survive but may require respiratory support for prolonged period. Survival figures by birthweight are shown in Table 13.2.

Pneumonia

Pneumonia in the newborn infant is relatively common especially among those who require ventilation or have undergone other invasive procedures as a part of their treatment or monitoring. The infecting agent may be viral, bacterial or fungal. Pneumonia may be contracted *in utero* and be present at birth (congenital) or acquired after birth (nosocomial). Congenital pneumonia may be due to ascending infection with prolonged rupture of membranes, or less frequently due to a transplacental infection (see Chapter 4). The diagnosis is suspected on maternal history, clinical examination and chest radiograph, and confirmed by bacteriological cultures from blood and tracheal aspirate. However, blood cultures may not be positive in all cases of pneumonia and its absence does not exclude the diagnosis. Indirect parameters such as WBC and CRP (C-reactive protein; a form of acute phase reactants) may help in diagnosing sepsis in a baby.

Aetiology

Pneumonia in the newborn is usually bacterial, and the most frequent bacterial pathogens causing congenital and acquired pneumonias are the Gram-negative bacilli (*Escherichia coli,* klebsiella, pseudomonas, serratia), group B streptococcus and staphylococcus.

Less common bacterial infections include *Listeria monocytogenes* and anaerobic bacilli. Occasionally, pneumonia is due to *Chlamydia trachomatis, Mycoplasma pneumoniae* or opportunistic pathogens such as *Candida albicans.* Viral pneumonitis is rare but occurs with cytomegalovirus (CMV), Coxsackie virus, respiratory syncytial virus (RSV) and human metapneumovirus (hMPV).

Clinical features

The early clinical signs and symptoms are non-specific and may include lethargy, apnoea, bradycardia, temperature instability and intolerance of feeds. At birth it may be difficult to distinguish pneumonia from other lung disease causing respiratory distress. The maternal and birth histories may reveal predisposing factors for neonatal infection.

Radiology

The appearances are non-specific and pneumonia may be difficult to distinguish radiologically from aspiration syndromes and even TTN. There are usually patchy opacities or more confluent areas of radiodensity through the lung. Lobar pneumonia is rarely seen in the newborn.

Treatment

Antibiotics

Broad-spectrum antibiotics should be administered after suitable cultures have been taken. Choice of antibiotics depends on the predominant pathogen causing sepsis and the antibiotic sensitivity pattern for the microorganisms causing early-onset sepsis in a given region (or hospital). Empirical therapy must cover both Gram-positive and Gram-negative organisms. The most frequently used combination is penicillin or ampicillin (or amoxicillin) and an aminoglycoside (frequently gentamicin). After an organism has been identified, the antibiotic therapy may be tailored according to the sensitivities.

Respiratory support

This is given according to the severity of signs and symptoms (see above as in RDS).

Pulmonary air leaks

This term refers to a collection of gas outside the pulmonary compartment, and a variety of disorders are included in this category (see Table 13.3).

The pathophysiology of these conditions is similar in that the alveoli become hyperinflated and rupture. Air then escapes into the lung interstitium

Table 13.3 Disorders categorized as pulmonary air leaks

Pneumothorax	Air in the pleural space (Fig. 13.4)
Pneumomediastinum	Air in the anterior mediastinum (Fig. 13.5)
Pneumopericardium	Air in the pericardial sac;
Pulmonary interstitial emphysema (PIE)	Air in interstitial lung spaces (Fig. 13.6)
Pneumoperitoneum	Air in the peritoneal cavity
Air embolus	Air dissecting into pulmonary veins

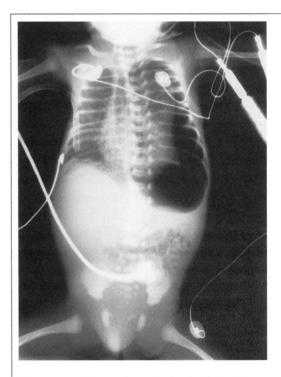

Figure 13.4 Chest radiograph showing left-sided tension pneumothorax.

(PIE) and tracks along the perivascular spaces into the mediastinum (pneumomediastinum) through the visceral pleura (pneumothorax), or rarely into the pericardium (pneumopericardium).

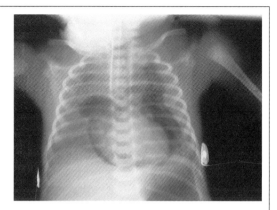

Figure 13.5 Chest radiograph showing pneumomediastinum. The heart and thymus are outlined by gas.

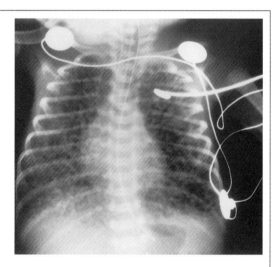

Figure 13.6 Chest radiograph showing extensive PIE. Note the overinflated chest with flattened diaphragm.

Spontaneous pneumothorax occurs in approximately 1% of vaginal deliveries and 1.5% of caesarean sections. Many of these have only minor symptoms, are discovered unexpectedly on a chest radiograph and may not require intervention. Resuscitation with positive-pressure ventilation is a recognized risk factor for development of pneumothorax. Antenatal steroids and surfactant therapy have markedly reduced the incidence of pulmonary air leaks in ventilated infants.

Pneumothoraces commonly occur in the following conditions or situations:
- stiff lungs, e.g. RDS
- hyperinflated lungs, e.g. in meconium aspiration syndrome
- hypoplastic lungs, e.g. Potter's syndrome, diaphragmatic hernia
- any form of intermittent positive pressure ventilation or continuous distending pressure such as CPAP. Prolonged inspiratory time and high end-expiratory pressures are particularly likely to cause pneumothorax in ventilated infants. Active expiration against a ventilator 'breath' (asynchrony between mechanical and spontaneous breaths) is also an important cause (see Chapter 15).

Clinical features

Infants with a tension pneumothorax exhibit signs of severe respiratory distress. Frequently a pulmonary air leak occurs in a baby who already has respiratory distress and there may be sudden deterioration, with cyanosis, poor peripheral perfusion and bradycardia. Specific signs of a tension pneumothorax are a shift of the mediastinum (apex beat) to the opposite side, asymmetrical chest expansion, asymmetrical air entry and weak peripheral pulses. A prominent sternum may suggest a pneumomediastinum.

Occasionally, unilateral PIE develops as a result of a ball-valve effect in a main bronchus. The emphysematous lung may cause compression of the more normal lung, thereby further embarrassing ventilation (Fig. 13.7).

Diagnosis

The definitive diagnosis is made by an anteroposterior chest radiograph. A lateral film may be necessary to diagnose air in the anterior mediastinum. When a pneumomediastinum is present, the chest radiograph may reveal the 'sail' or 'spinnaker' sign (air around the thymus). In the critically ill infant who has a tension pneumothorax, chest transillumination may be used to make the diagnosis. Occasionally, the insertion of a 21G butterfly needle with

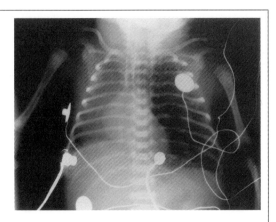

Figure 13.7 Chest radiograph showing left-sided PIE. The mediastinum and right lung are compressed by the overinflated left lung.

jet ventilation is a successful means of ventilation for infants with PIE (see Chapter 15). Localized PIE may resolve spontaneously or may persist for several weeks, and may or may not cause any further deterioration in the baby. Effort should be made to avoid any form of PPV or continuous distending pressure unless really needed.

Pneumomediastinum is often of little clinical importance and usually does not need to be drained. Pneumopericardium can cause life-threatening cardiac tamponade (compression), which requires pericardiocentesis (needle aspiration via the subxiphoid route). The procedure can be facilitated by transillumination guidance. Pericardial tube placement and drainage (like a chest tube for pneumothorax) may be necessary if the pericardial air reaccumulates.

three-way tap and syringe may be life-saving in suspected tension pneumothoraces. This is an emergency diagnostic and therapeutic procedure undertaken when there may be delay in obtaining an radiograph in a critically ill infant. Blind needling of the chest may create a pneumothorax and should not be attempted except in an emergency.

Management

A tension pneumothorax will need to be released immediately by inserting a chest drain into the intercostal space, connected to underwater seal drainage or a Heimlich one-way flutter valve (see Chapter 29). Occasionally, evacuation of the pneumothorax will be incomplete with this catheter, and an additional catheter will be necessary. For non-tension pneumothoraces in full-term infants, nursing in 100% oxygen for up to 12 h may accelerate reabsorption of the pneumothorax. The rare pleural effusion or chylous effusion in the newborn may require thoracocentesis.

Generalized management of PIE is focused on reducing or preventing further barotraumas to the lung by decreasing peak inspiratory pressure (PIP) to the minimum required attaining acceptable arterial blood gases. Reduction in positive end-expiratory pressure (PEEP) may also help in decreasing the PIE. High-frequency oscillatory or

Meconium aspiration syndrome

Meconium aspiration syndrome (MAS) is a serious and potentially preventable cause of respiratory distress in the newborn. It is not synonymous with MSAF (meconium staining of the amniotic fluid) which occurs in about 13% of all deliveries, whereas, MAS occurs only in 4–5% of newborns born through MSAF. The passage of meconium often indicates fetal distress, but in the breech presentation may be normal. Aspiration most commonly occurs *in utero* and less so after birth. The response of the infant to intrapartum asphyxia is to gasp, and if meconium is present it will be aspirated deep into the bronchi. Once respiration begins, distal migration of the meconium into small airways occurs.

Clinical features

There is a wide spectrum of presentations of MAS, ranging from severe birth asphyxia requiring active resuscitation through early onset of respiratory distress to a vigorous baby with no major problems. Typically the infant is born covered in meconium-stained liquor and has meconium staining of the umbilical cord, skin and nails. The chest appears to be hyperinflated and there may be a prominent sternum. Respiratory distress may be mild initially, becoming rapidly more severe after several hours. If asphyxia has occurred, the baby may also show signs of early-onset encephalopathy (see Chapter 22).

Pathogenesis and aetiology

Meconium causes a number of anatomical and physiological problems that make lung function worse:
• Plugging of the airways, with consequent atelectasis. It also causes a 'ball-valve' obstruction with hyperinflation of the lungs and a high risk of pulmonary air leaks.
• Irritation of the airways, causing a chemical pneumonitis.
• Antagonism of surfactant production.
• Possible secondary bacterial infection.
• In a proportion of babies with severe MAS, there is development of marked ventilation/perfusion inequality and right-to-left shunt due to persistent pulmonary hypertension (PPHN, see Chapter 16).

Radiology

Chest radiographs show hyperinflation (flat diaphragms, widening of rib spaces) with diffuse patchy opacities throughout both lung fields (Fig. 13.8). Pneumothorax or pneumomediastinum may also be seen.

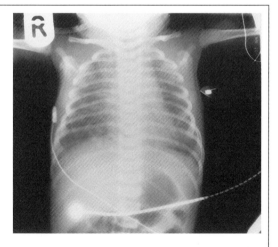

Figure 13.8 Chest radiograph showing meconium aspiration syndrome. There is extensive discrete shadowing throughout both lung fields.

Prophylactic management

Morbidity and mortality from MAS can be prevented or minimized by optimal perinatal management. There is controversy as to whether a neonatal paediatrician should attend every delivery where there is meconium staining of the liquor. It is important, however, that an experienced neonatal paediatrician be present for the delivery if thick meconium is present, especially if there are signs of intrapartum fetal distress.

Various therapeutic interventions have been used. Results of large controlled trials and systematic reviews suggest that
• Amnioinfusion therapy for thick-consistency MSAF does not reduce the risk of MAS.
• Intrapartum naso- and oropharyngeal suctioning does not reduce the incidence of MAS and hence is not recommended.
• Routine endotracheal intubation and suctioning is of no benefit in vigorous infants born through MSAF of any consistency. This should, however, be performed in infants born through MSAF if they are depressed, if they need PPV, or if they are vigorous initially but develop respiratory distress within the first few minutes of life.
• In such cases, the baby is intubated with a wide-bore suction catheter or endotracheal tube and the trachea is suctioned clear. Suctioning is facilitated by the use of a meconium aspirator. Further suction is applied directly to the endotracheal tube as it is being removed. If a large quantity of meconium is present in the endotracheal tube after extubation, the baby should be reintubated and further tracheal suction applied. The stomach should be aspirated following intubation. All depressed babies who are born through thick MSAF should be carefully assessed and regularly monitored for signs of MAS.

Treatment of established meconium aspiration syndrome

The treatment will be the same as for respiratory distress (see above). Particular emphasis or consideration should be given to the following points:
• Humidification of inspired oxygen.
• Postural drainage positioning, suctioning of airways and chest percussion are of unproven benefit.

• Antibiotics are usually given, although the efficacy has not been established.

• Both conventional and high-frequency ventilation can be used with multiple strategies to achieve normal gaseous exchange and prevent complications such as air trapping and air leaks, which are common in such infants.

• Exogenous surfactant has been used with success in some studies. In some centres lavage with surfactant is practised but its efficacy is not fully established.

• Inhaled nitric oxide (iNO) therapy should be considered in infants with concomitant PPHN who are not responding to conventional treatment. Other agents used in such condition are prostacyclin and sildenafil.

• Extracorporeal membrane oxygenation (ECMO) is considered as a rescue treatment when predicted mortality is running high. Overall success rate of ECMO in babies with MAS is over 80%.

Pulmonary hypoplasia

For adequate fetal lung development the fetus must be able to make breathing movements and move a column of amniotic and lung fluid up and down the trachea and main bronchi. Hypoplasia may therefore be due to

• failure of fetal breathing (neuromuscular disorders)

• inability to expand the lungs (diaphragmatic hernia, pleural effusions)

• lack of liquor (oligohydramnios) due to renal or urethral abnormalities or prolonged preterm rupture of the membranes causing leakage of amniotic fluid.

Clinical features

The infant develops severe respiratory distress from birth, with marked hypoxia, hypercapnia and metabolic acidosis. Pneumothorax is a common complication. The lungs are very stiff and there is little chest movement with mechanical ventilation. It may be difficult to diagnose lung hypoplasia on chest radiograph. Severe lung hypoplasia is incompatible with life, and less severe forms contribute towards chronic ventilator dependency and bronchopulmonary dysplasia.

Management and prognosis

Management of lung hypoplasia starts antenatally if diagnosed earlier and includes counselling by the obstetrician, neonatologist, clinical geneticist and surgeon (if appropriate). Pulmonary hypoplasia results from a large number of different conditions and hence the prognosis is governed mainly by the aetiology and associated anomalies. Lung biopsy may be difficult to perform safely while the infant is alive and hence postmortem studies should be made where possible. Where permission for a full autopsy is not granted, an open or needle biopsy of the lung obtained soon after death may provide a tissue diagnosis.

Pulmonary haemorrhage

Pulmonary haemorrhage has a characteristic clinical presentation in newborn infants, with cardiovascular collapse associated with an outpouring of blood-stained fluid from the trachea and mouth. The condition is often fatal and occurs in about 1/1000 births. Among survivors, there is a high incidence of chronic lung disease.

Pathogenesis

The underlying mechanism for pulmonary haemorrhage can be classified as:

• **haemodynamic:** a manifestation of an exaggerated haemorrhagic pulmonary oedema brought about by an acute increase in pulmonary blood flow as in large PDA

• **haematological:** due to associated coagulation abnormalities such as in disseminated intravascular coagulation (DIC) associated with sepsis or other coagulopathy.

Pulmonary haemorrhage is often associated with bleeding in other organs such as brain or gut.

Risk factors

The incidence of pulmonary haemorrhage is inversely related to the gestational age of the babies. Prematurity, RDS and exogenous surfactant therapy (in combination) are the three most important risk factors. Other antecedent risk factors include severe birth asphyxia, hypothermia, small for gestational age (SGA) infants, coagulation disturbances and congenital heart disease.

The severity and magnitude of clinical signs depend upon the magnitude of haemorrhage and the severity of the underlying condition leading to the episode. The clinical manifestations result from several interrelated pathophysiological consequences of blood loss and haemorrhage into the lung parenchyma and airways.

Treatment

The treatment will be that of respiratory distress as described earlier, but particular emphasis must be given to the following:
• Resuscitation of cardiovascular collapse with volume expanders such intravenous infusion of plasma protein fraction, blood or normal saline.
• Treatment of pulmonary oedema with furosemide and perhaps morphine.
• Correction of coagulation disturbances; fresh frozen plasma and/or recombinant factor VIIa (rFVIIa).
• If mechanical ventilation is required, high PEEP may help to decrease bleeding.
• Exogenous surfactant seem to improve the respiratory status in infants with pulmonary haemorrhage.

Congenital diaphragmatic hernia

Congenital diaphragmatic hernia (CDH) is a failure of normal development of the diaphragm during the first trimester. The hernia is usually a posterolateral (Bochdalek) type; 80% occur on the left side. This occurs through a defect in the diaphragm as a result of a persistent pleuroperitoneal canal caused by failure of the muscular components to develop. The defect in the diaphragm permits herniation of the abdominal contents into the thorax. Consequently, there is hypoplasia or compression of the lung on the side of the hernia, with displacement of mediastinum to the contralateral side. Sometimes there is hypoplasia of the contralateral lung. Babies with a large diaphragmatic hernia have rapidly progressive respiratory failure after birth, with persistent cyanosis. A less acute diaphragmatic hernia may

present in the nursery, with respiratory distress, or occasionally on routine examination a 'dextrocardia' or scaphoid abdomen will be found. On auscultation of the lungs, bowel sounds may be heard on the side of the lesion if gas has entered the gastrointestinal tract. The lungs will not inflate adequately with normal pressure.

Diagnosis

Most cases of CDH are now diagnosed *in utero* by routine obstetric ultrasound at 18–20 weeks' gestation or following investigation of polyhydramnios. The diagnosis of a diaphragmatic hernia is confirmed by chest radiograph, which shows bowel loops in the thorax (Fig. 13.9). If the radiograph is taken shortly after birth, there may be some difficulty in determining whether the bowel is in the chest, especially if there is little air in the gastrointestinal tract. Similarly, diagnosis may be delayed when the liver is in the chest, in cases of right-sided diapharagmatic hernia. The radiograph should include the abdomen, to show a paucity of abdominal gas pattern. A rarer form of diaphragmatic hernia is through an anteromedial defect beneath the sternum (Morgagni type). This typically contains part of the colon. It is usually symptomless

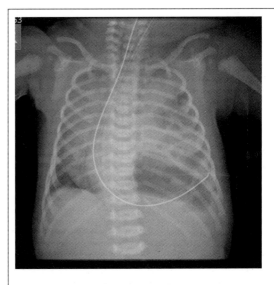

Figure 13.9 Chest radiograph showing a left-sided diaphragmatic hernia.

and often detected on a lateral chest radiograph. Eventration, which results from a failure of muscle development in the primitive diaphragm, is not a true hernia. CDH can be a part of a syndrome or associated with a chromosomal abnormality.

Treatment

If CDH is suspected, an orogastric tube should be inserted and the abdominal contents in the chest aspirated. If the baby requires assisted ventilation, it should be performed via an endotracheal tube and never by bag and mask, in order to prevent increasing gaseous distension of the bowel within the chest. Care must be taken to prevent rupture of the contralateral lung, as the baby is almost exclusively dependent on this lung for ventilation. Following initial diagnosis the baby should be stabilized and referred to a paediatric surgeon for operative treatment. Surgery for the more severe cases is often delayed for a few days to enable maximum stabilization, often with high-frequency oscillation ventilation. Surgery consists of reduction of the abdominal contents, closure of the diaphragmatic defect and correction of any bowel malrotation.

PPHN is a common complication of severe diaphragmatic hernia. Adequate ventilatory support, through either conventional or high-frequency ventilation, is required in all cases. Inhaled nitric oxide empirically would appear to be the drug of choice, but data in relation to CDH suggest that it its use is unhelpful. ECMO has been used to provide stability and for associated PPHN; however, it is of no clear benefit in terms of long-term outcome. The role of fetal surgery is being reinvestigated with procedures to plug the trachea at around 23 weeks' gestation, but the results do not show convincing benefit. Moreover, it can produce secondary problems such as hydrops.

Prognosis

The prognosis depends on the degree of pulmonary hypoplasia and the age at presentation. Infants with respiratory distress in the first 6 h have a high mortality (about 70%), whereas those presenting between 6 and 24 h have a much better prognosis (mortality rates 10–15%). Later presentation is not likely to be associated with pulmonary hypoplasia and the prognosis is very good.

Oesophageal atresia and tracheo-oesophageal fistula

Oesophageal atresia is a congenital anomaly in which there is usually complete interruption of the lumen of the oesophagus, in the form of a blind upper pouch. This is commonly associated with a tracheo-oesophageal fistula (TOF). The commonest variety of this condition is a blind-ending upper oesophageal pouch, with the lower oesophagus arising from the trachea above the carina (Fig. 13.10c). A variety of other patterns occur much less commonly (Fig. 13.10).

Clinical features

Maternal polyhydramnios occurs in 60% of cases and is largely responsible for the high frequency of

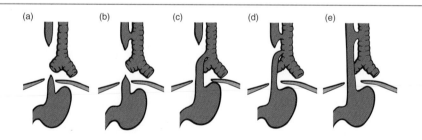

Figure 13.10 Variants of tracheo-oesphageal fistula with or without oesophageal atresia. Type c accounts for 85% of cases, the others being equally uncommon.

premature births. The oesophageal atresia is associated with excessive saliva and mucus production, with a high incidence of aspiration pneumonia. Abdominal distension is due to air passing down the fistula into the stomach, and may develop rapidly and irreversibly. Coexistent congenital anomalies may be present and may be either major or minor (e.g. VACTERL association – vertebral anomalies, anal atresia, cardiovascular anomalies, tracheoesophageal fistula, oesophageal atresia, renal anomalies, limb defects).

The most important aspect of oesophageal atresia is that it should be recognized as soon as possible after birth, preferably prior to the first feed, so that pulmonary complications (due to aspiration) are less likely to occur. All babies with suspected oesophageal atresia should have a size 5 nasogastric tube passed down each nostril in turn and into the stomach shortly after birth, preferably before the first feed. If this is not done, oesophageal atresia is generally diagnosed by excessive secretions or cyanosis and coughing with feeds. The definitive diagnosis is made by the inability to pass a firm radio-opaque no. 10 catheter or a replogle tube into the stomach, as it arrests about 10 cm from the lips. Once the catheter has been passed as far as possible, an radiograph of the neck and upper chest should be taken to confirm that it has become obstructed at this level. The abdominal radiograph should be inspected for gas in the stomach and the chest radiograph assessed for areas of collapse. Air is a useful contrast medium in the upper pouch. It is not usually necessary to put radio-opaque contrast medium into the upper pouch to confirm the diagnosis, but if this is done a non-irritant substance should be used. For an H-type fistula, which presents with recurrent aspiration or infections, radiological diagnosis may be difficult. A cine contrast swallow will usually confirm the diagnosis.

Treatment

A baby with oesophageal atresia and TOF should be nursed supine and propped head-up at 60° to avoid gastric contents spilling into the lung through the fistula. A replogle tube should be placed in the oesophagus and put on suction. Surgery should be performed by a paediatric surgeon as soon as the baby has been adequately resuscitated and stabilized. Surgery consists of division of the TOF and anastomosis of the two segments of the oesophagus if possible. Occasionally, the atretic segment is too long to enable primary anastomosis, and exteriorization of the cervical oesophagus as an oesophagostomy and the stomach as a gastrostomy will be necessary. A definitive operation can be delayed to a later date.

With a cervical oesophagostomy the baby should be encouraged to practise sucking on a dummy during gastrostomy feedings ('sham feeding'). Complications and sequelae from surgery are frequent and include a brassy cough, associated with coexistent tracheomalacia, oesophageal stricture, breakdown of the anastomosis with mediastinitis, recurrence of the TOF and gastro-oesophageal reflux.

Lobar emphysema

Congenital lobar emphysema is a rare anomaly due to a cartilaginous deficiency of the lobar bronchus, most commonly involving the left upper lobe (50%), the right middle lobe (24%) or the right upper lobe (18%), and frequently associated with congenital heart disease (30%), such as tetralogy of Fallot, ventricular septal disease (VSD) or total anomalous pulmonary venous drainage (TAPVD). The onset of respiratory distress is frequently insidious, usually taking 2–3 weeks to develop, and is caused by lung collapse around the hyperinflated lobe. The mediastinum becomes displaced and the chest wall is prominent over the affected area. Breath sounds are diminished and the percussion note is hyper-resonant. Once a definitive diagnosis is made, a lobectomy is generally required. Acquired lobar emphysema may be secondary to an extrinsic or intrinsic bronchial obstruction, such as a mucous plug. This type should be treated conservatively but may require bronchoscopy.

Congenital cystic adenomatous malformation

Congenital cystic adenomatous malformation (CCAM) is a rare cystic lesion found more often in males than females, and often diagnosed on antenatal ultrasound. This emphysematous lesion may be associated with polyhydramnios, hydrops fetalis, prematurity and stillbirth. There are three distinct types: type I CAM (70%) presents as single or multiple large cyst(s) confined to one lobe; type II (18%) is composed of multiple medium-sized cysts and 50% have other anomalies; type III (10%) is a large bulky lesion with evenly distributed small cysts. Asymptomatic lesions may not require removal. This is one of the few conditions that is successfully treatable by fetal surgery in selected cases.

Chronic lung disease and bronchopulmonary dysplasia

The term chronic lung disease (CLD) is a non-specific term, commonly used to describe a group of heterogeneous condition characterized by signs of chronic respiratory sign and symptoms. It should not be used interchangeably with diagnosis of BPD, which is a specific condition that develops in newborns who are born preterm. It is usually defined as the presence of chronic respiratory signs, a persistent oxygen requirement or dependence on any form of respiratory support, and an abnormal chest radiograph persisting at 36 weeks corrected age. Other causes of CLD are shown in Box 13.5.

Although surfactant treatment has improved overall survival of premature infants, the incidence of BPD remains approximately 30–40% in very preterm babies. With the use of standardized oxygen saturation monitoring as required in the new physiological definition of BPD, the incidence may further decrease by as much as 10%.

BPD is usually associated with severe RDS, but occasionally complicates meconium aspiration, pulmonary haemorrhage and severe neonatal pneumonia. This was first described by Northway *et al.* (1967), but since then the characteristics of the disease have changed and it is now essentially a condition seen mostly in babies who are born very premature and require mechanical ventilation. The incidence of BPD varies according to the definition used, and recently a physiological definition of BPD has been introduced. The latter facilitates the meas-

> ### Box 13.5 Conditions causing chronic lung disease
>
> - Bronchopulmonary dysplasia
> - Recurrent aspiration:
>   Pharyngeal incoordination
>   Gastro-oesopheageal reflux
>   Tracheo-oesophageal fistula
> - Interstitial pneumonitis:
>   Cytomegalovirus
>   *Candida albicans*
>   Chlamydia
>   *Pneumocystis jirovecii*
>   *Ureaplasma urealyticum*
> - Chronic pulmonary oedema (due to left to right shunt as in PDA)
> - Rickets of prematurity
> - Neuromuscular diseases affecting intercostal muscles and diaphragm (spinal muscular atrophy, myotonic dystrophy and mysthenia gravis)

urement of BPD as an outcome in clinical trials and comparisons between and within centres over time.

Aetiology

BPD is multifactorial in origin and results from a sequence of events occurring in a preterm infant which increases the infant's dependency on ventilation and oxygen (known as the 'pulmonary injury sequence'). The incidence relates to the severity of RDS and the degree of prematurity. It has only been described in infants who have received PPV, and probably relates to barotrauma or more importantly volutrauma (alveolar overdistension due to excessive tidal volume delivery). Oxygen therapy for prolonged periods of time also appears to be linked with its development.

Clinical features

Infants who develop BPD have signs of persistent chest retractions, crepitations and rhonchi on chest auscultation, gross hyperinflation of the lungs and an increased anteroposterior chest diameter. Most of these infants also have a patent ductus arteriosus, and after a period of time may develop right heart failure (cor pulmonale). There is often associated developmental delay in such children, requiring input from multiple agencies.

Radiology

The original description of BPD by Northway *et al.* (1967) staged the radiological appearances in four grades. The first two are indistinguishable from RDS and are not helpful for descriptive purposes. In the most severe form there is an irregular honey-comb appearance to the lung, with overinflated lung fields, extensive fibrosis and multiple cysts of irregular size (Fig. 13.11). The majority of infants with BPD now do not develop these gross radiological signs but exhibit a finer, more homogeneous pattern of abnormality.

Management

The prevention of BPD requires careful management of infants who are receiving mechanical ventilation. Pulmonary interstitial emphysema, pulmonary oedema, PDA and sepsis appear to increase the risk of BPD developing. The following therapies have been used to treat BPD with varying effects but they are not supported by any robust scientific evidence.

• **Dexamethasone**. Studies have shown that dexamethasone reduces the ventilatory dependency and should be considered after the first 2 weeks of life in infants with severe lung injury who remain ventilator-dependent. The dose and duration of treatment must be kept to the minimum necessary to achieve the desired effects, as indiscriminate use of postnatal dexamethasone has been linked with excessive prevalence of cerebral palsy..

• **Diuretics**. Diuretic therapy reduces interstitial lung fluid and has been used for acute deterioration associated with pulmonary oedema. However, routine prolonged use is not recommended because of lack of evidence that it improves the incidence or severity of BPD and concern over side effects.

• **Therapy directed at reducing oxygen toxicity**. Antioxidants such as vitamin E and superoxide dismutase appear to be of no benefit, but vitamin A has been shown to reduce BPD and death in very low birthweight (VLBW) infants.

• **Adequate oxygenation** throughout all daily activities (O_2 saturation 92–96%) minimizes progressive pulmonary vascular disease.

• **Nutritional supplementation** is necessary to obtain optimal growth in the presence of high energy consumption due to the work of breathing. Adequate nutrition is a key aspect of care for the infants with CLD.

Prognosis

Children with BPD have been shown to have increased airway resistance and are more likely to wheeze. They also have increased airway reactivity and viral-induced wheeze. Episodic wheezing is commonly seen in infants and children who have had BPD in the newborn period.

Lower airway infection in the first year of life is a particular risk to children who have had CLD in the neonatal period. Pneumococcal vaccine is now in routine use. Such children appear to be particularly likely to develop RSV-positive bronchiolitis,

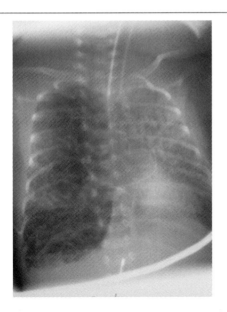

Figure 13.11 Chest radiograph showing severe bronchopulmonary dysplasia.

which may cause very severe respiratory failure. Monoclonal RSV antibody (palivizumab) is used for prophylaxis during the RSV season. Advice must be given to the parents to avoid exposing the baby to the risk of viral infection in the first year or two of life.

SUMMARY

Respiratory disorders are the commonest cause of illness in newborns. Their severity varies according to the underlying pathology.

Respiratory distress is a non-specific term used to describe a combination of symptoms which indicate involvement of respiratory system including lungs, airways, thoracic cage and breathing centre in the brain.

RDS is a specific diagnosis related to surfactant deficiency due to immaturity of lungs in preterm babies. In severe cases it can lead to severe respiratory failure and death.

Other causes of respiratory distress include congenital and acquired pneumonia, cardiorespiratory maladaptation at birth (see Chapter 16), aspiration syndromes and congenital abnormalities of lungs.

Treatment of respiratory disorders ranges from simple supportive measures such as ambient oxygen and artificial respiratory support to intensive cardiorespiratory support including mechanical ventilation and other strategies (see Chapter 15).

 Now visit **www.essentialneonatalmed.com** to test yourself on this chapter.

CHAPTER 14

Apnoea, bradycardia and upper airway obstruction

Key topics

Introduction

Normal respiratory function is essential for successful transition to the extrauterine environment. The control of breathing is complex and is not fully developed at birth, particularly if the infant is preterm. Apnoea is one of the commonly encountered problems in the neonatal intensive care unit (NICU), and considerable time and effort goes into monitoring, preventing and treating babies with apnoea. The aetiology, investigation and management of apnoea is therefore discussed in detail in this chapter. Acute life-threatening events (ALTE) and sudden infant death syndrome (SIDS) are uncommon but serious events which are more commonly encountered in graduates of the intensive care nursery. Obstruction to gas flow in the upper airway can present in babies as apnoea, respiratory distress, coughing, a hoarse cry, or stridor. Common causes of airway obstruction and their management will be discussed.

Physiology

The onset of breathing begins early in fetal life. It is initially intermittent, irregular and occurs only during periods of active rapid eye movement (REM) sleep. The function of fetal breathing is not fully understood but, along with adequate amniotic fluid

Essential Neonatal Medicine, Fifth Edition. Sunil Sinha, Lawrence Miall, Luke Jardine.
© 2012 John Wiley & Sons, Ltd. Published 2012 by John Wiley & Sons, Ltd.

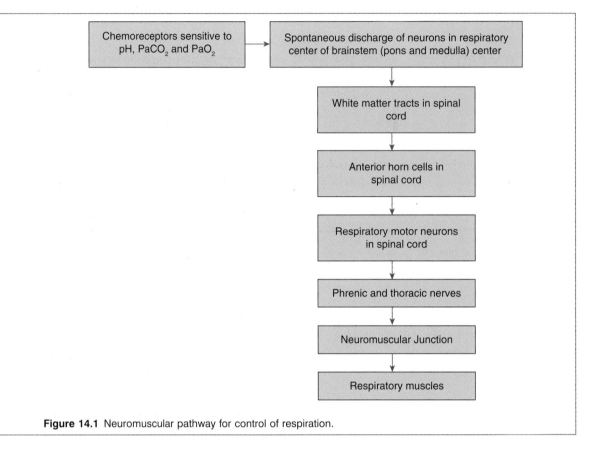

Figure 14.1 Neuromuscular pathway for control of respiration.

volume, it probably has an essential role in lung growth. Fetuses that do not breathe (due to either neurological or muscular disorders) are at significant risk of lung hypoplasia (see Chapter 13).

Successful transition to the extrauterine environment requires a marked change from the intermittent breathing of a fetus to the continuous breathing of a newborn baby. The control of breathing is complex (see Fig. 14.1), but we know that respiration is initiated in the respiratory nuclei found in the brainstem (pons and medulla). Hypercapnia increases respiratory activity and hypoxia causes an initial increase in respiratory activity lasting several minutes, followed by a decrease in ventilatory frequency. Preterm infants have less well-developed chemoreceptor responses to hypoxia and hypercapnia.

Breathing patterns in the newborn can be divided into four different types:

- **Regular:** there are nearly equal breath-to-breath intervals; this is infrequent
- **Irregular:** unequal breath-to-breath intervals; this is particularly common in preterm infants
- **Periodic breathing:** cycles of hyperventilation alternating with periods of hypoventilation and pauses in breathing lasting about 3 s
- **Apnoea** (see below).

With advancing gestation to term, the proportion of time the infant is breathing regularly increases, and phases of irregular, periodic and apnoeic periods decline. Further maturation occurs in the months after birth.

Apnoea

Clinically significant apnoea is defined as a cessation of breathing (absence of respiratory airflow) lasting for 20 s or more. Apnoea lasting for 10 s or more is also significant if accompanied by a desaturation (cyanosis or decreased SpO_2), or bradycardia of less than 100 beats/min.

Apnoea is most common in preterm babies, particularly those born at less than 34 weeks' gestation. It is seen in 25% of infants of birthweight less than 2500 g, and in over 80% of infants with birthweight below 1000 g. It is uncommon in the first 24 h of life, increasing towards the end of the first week of life, and then tends to become less frequent as the baby matures.

Types of apnoea

Central apnoea

Central apnoea accounts for 25% of all cases of neonatal apnoea. It is due to factors affecting the respiratory centre in the brainstem or the higher centres in the cerebral cortex.

Obstructive apnoea

Complete obstruction of the airways will cause obstructive apnoea. Nasal obstruction (by bone/mucus/milk) will cause obstructive apnoea in babies as they are obligatory nose breathers. Obstructive apnoea is characterized initially by increased respiratory effort (baby attempts to overcome the obstruction) before the cessation of breathing. Obstructive apnoea accounts for 15% of cases and occurs with congenital malformations, such as choanal atresia and the Pierre Robin sequence. Preterm infants with small upper airways may have apnoea when in the supine position, especially during active (REM) sleep. Apnoea of this type may be minimized by nursing the infant in the prone position. Presence of milk, mucus or meconium in the upper airway is likely to provoke severe episodes of obstructive apnoea.

Mixed apnoea

Mixed apnoea accounts for the majority (approximately 60%) of cases particularly in preterm infants, but may be difficult to diagnose clinically. Superficially it resembles central apnoea initially, with cessation of respiration, but then the baby makes intermittent respiratory efforts without achieving gas exchange.

Reflex apnoea

Babies may develop reflex apnoea or vagally mediated apnoea due to vigorous suction of the pharynx, passage of a nasogastric tube, physiotherapy or sometimes even in response to defecation. Apnoea associated with gastro-oesophageal reflux may be reflex and/or obstructive.

Aetiology of apnoea

A number of factors can increase the frequency of apnoea. Common causes are listed in Box 14.1. In the term infant the aetiology is usually identified. In the preterm infant, 'apnoea of prematurity' is the primary cause, but should be considered a diagnosis of exclusion. Apnoea of prematurity is predominantly a mixed apnoea.

Investigation of apnoea

Investigations are carried out to determine treatable causes of apnoea and will depend on the prevailing clinical condition. Investigations are listed in Box 14.2.

Box 14.1 Causes of apnoea

- Apnoea of prematurity
- Lung disease (e.g. RDS, pneumothorax)
- Infection
- Airway obstruction (e.g. secretions, micrognathia, choanal atresia)
- Hypoxia
- Intracranial haemorrhage
- Metabolic causes (acidosis, hypoglycaemia, hypocalcaemia, hypomagnesaemia)
- Drugs (e.g. maternal narcotics, trishydroxyaminonethane (THAM), prostin (PGE1), magnesium sulphate)
- Gastro-esophageal reflux
- Seizures
- NEC
- Patent ductus arteriosus
- Temperature instability
- Polycythaemia with hyperviscosity syndrome
- CNS abnormalities (including Ondine's curse – see Clinical Tip)

Box 14.2 Useful investigations in determining the underlying cause of apnoea

- Full blood count
- Blood culture
- Other cultures as indicated (urine, CSF, tracheal aspirate, nasal/pharyngeal, surface swabs, etc.)
- Chest radiograph
- Blood glucose
- Serum electrolytes, including calcium, magnesium and sodium
- Blood gas (arterial, venous or capillary)
- Continuous monitoring of oxygen saturation
- Ultrasound examination of the brain
- (In special circumstances) further neurological investigations, i.e. electroencephalogram (EEG), polygraphic sleep studies; PCR for the *PHOX2B* gene may identify cases of PAHS

CLINICAL TIP: New onset or increasing frequency of apnoea in a premature baby is of great clinical concern. It should not be presumed to be secondary to apnoea of prematurity. The baby should be carefully examined for the other possible causes. A septic work-up and commencement of intravenous antibiotics should be seriously considered if no obvious cause is found. Apnoea in a term infant is always abnormal and a cause must be sort.

Apnoea monitoring

A variety of respiratory monitors are available, including a pressure-sensitive pad on which the infant lies, an air-filled plastic blister attached to the abdomen (SIMS Graseby Medical Ltd, Watford, UK) and impedance monitors using electrodes attached to the chest wall. None of these will detect obstructive apnoea until the infant stops fighting for breath. The use of an oxygen saturation monitor or an ECG monitor together with an apnoea monitor is recommended in high-risk infants in order to recognize bradycardia occurring with an obstructed airway.

Treatment of apnoea

General management

Any obvious cause of apnoea (see Box 14.1) should be treated. Apnoeic episodes should be prevented whenever possible. This involves careful handling of low birthweight infants and attention to feeding techniques, with avoidance of stomach distension and rapid feeding. The infant's temperature needs to be maintained in the thermoneutral range. Careful suctioning of the airway and positioning of the infant should minimize obstruction.

Management of acute apnoea

A suggested approach to managing an acute episode of apnoea on the NICU is shown in Fig. 14.2.

Management of recurrent apnoea

This usually occurs in preterm infants and may be very difficult to manage. There are clinical concerns that these episodes might be harmful to the developing brain or cause dysfunction to the gut and developing organs.

The following techniques are employed in the management of recurrent apnoea:
- Nurse in the prone position with careful attention to maintenance of the airway.
- Stimulation (see below).
- Consider altering the feeding regimen, i.e. very occasionally, a continuous milk infusion may be better tolerated than intermittent feeds.
- If anaemia is thought to be a contributing factor, then it should be treated by blood transfusion, but the lowest acceptable level of haemoglobin may be difficult to determine (see Chapter 20).
- Increasing the inspired oxygen will decrease the incidence of apnoea. Oxygen saturations should be targeted at 91–95% in preterm infants and oxygen concentrations should be decreased if saturations are above 95%.
- Specific treatment includes drugs, continuous positive airway pressure (CPAP), non-invasive posi-

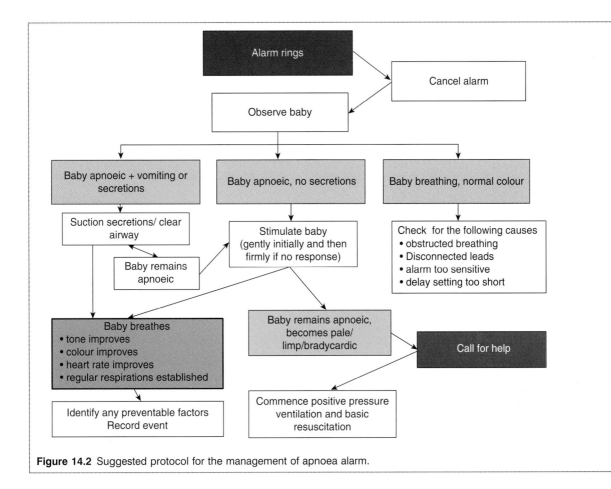

Figure 14.2 Suggested protocol for the management of apnoea alarm.

tive pressure ventilation (NIPPV) and mechanical ventilation (see below).

Stimulation

Tactile stimulation by regular stroking of the infant has been shown to reduce the number of apnoeic episodes, but this is not a feasible method for routine use. In the past, a variety of rocking mattresses that gently rock or undulate the baby have been used; although these appeared to reduce the frequency of apnoea, they have been largely replaced.

Drug treatment

This is only indicated when specific causes of apnoea have been treated. They are frequently prescribed in extremely preterm infants prior to extubation. Drugs for apnoea are usually continued until the baby is 32–34 weeks of gestational age.

Caffeine citrate is now the drug of choice for apnoea of prematurity. Its mechanism of action is not certain. Possibilities include increased chemoreceptor responsiveness, enhanced respiratory muscle performance and generalized central nervous system excitation. The main mechanism of action appears to occur centrally as a respiratory stimulant. An initial loading dose (given intravenously or orally) is followed by a daily dose. Serum levels of caffeine do not need to be routinely monitored but can be considered if there are any side effects. While caffeine does reduce the rate of apnoea, the major benefit is that it improves the rate of survival without neurodevelopmental disability at 18–21 months in infants with VLBW.

Older methylxanthines such as theophylline and aminophylline are still used in some centres. Tachycardia and irritability are the first signs of overdosage. Doxapram has been used only in selected infants in whom recurrent apnoea cannot be controlled by methylxanthines. Extreme jitteriness is a well-recognized side effect.

Ventilatory support

CPAP is effective in treating or preventing apnoea. The major benefit is that it holds the airway open and prevents collapse during expiration. It is probably most useful in treating the obstructive component of apnoea but may also have an effect on central apnoea by stimulating respiration via the Hering–Breuer reflex. The administration of CPAP is described in Chapter 15. In infants who are resistant to CPAP and respiratory stimulants, and who continue to have frequent or severe episodes, an attempt at NIPPV may be worth while (see Chapter 15). Occasionally, intubation and mechanical ventilation are required to avoid major physiological changes associated with the apnoeic episodes. Only minimal pressures and rates are usually required.

Prognosis

With respect to prognosis it is important to distinguish the cause of the apnoea from its effect. There is an association between recurrent apnoea and later cerebral palsy, but this may reflect the common origin of the brain lesion that causes the movement disorder, the prematurity and the resultant apnoea. In general, outcome is related to the underlying cause, and when correction is made for confounding factors, apnoea *per se* has no additional deleterious effect on outcome.

Recurrent apnoea of prematurity has usually resolved by 37 weeks' gestational age, but in some infants apnoea may persist beyond the expected date of delivery and no cause can be found. In rare cases discharge home on caffeine may be required, and home apnoea monitors may be of benefit.

> **CLINICAL TIP:** Ondine's curse (also known as primary alveolar hypoventilation syndrome or congenital central hypoventilation syndrome) is a very rare syndrome where infants have life-threatening apnoea while sleeping. It is fatal if left untreated. A mutation in the *PHOX2B* gene is found in the majority of cases.

Acute life-threatening events

ALTEs are sudden unexpected episodes of colour change with limpness, collapse or apnoea in an otherwise apparently well baby. These are very worrying episodes, both for the parents and for clinical staff. Appropriate investigations must be performed to elucidate a cause, but if no cause is found then anxiety may persist about the risk of a similar event occurring again once the baby has gone home.

Research has confirmed that there is an association between ALTE and SIDS cases, but when multivariate regression analysis is performed these studies show that the risk is not increased if the data are adjusted for factors such as maternal age, education, smoking, alcohol consumption, social deprivation, tog value of the bedding, co-sleeping with a parent and the baby being placed to sleep prone. Consequently it is believed by some authorities that ALTEs do not predict an increased risk of SIDS when the child goes home.

Sudden infant death syndrome or sudden unexpected death in infancy

SIDS (also known as sudden unexpected death in infancy, SUDI) is the unexpected death of an infant between 1 month and 1 year of age that remains unexplained despite extensive review of the medical records, a postmortem examination and a death scene investigation. To date no exact cause for SIDS has been identified, and it appears likely that it represents a final common pathway for a number of unrelated clinical phenomena.

Neonatologists must be aware of the risk of SIDS in survivors of neonatal care and give appropriate advice to reduce the risk once the baby has gone home. There are a number of risk factors for SIDS. These include

- maternal smoking or drug abuse
- prematurity
- low birthweight
- multiple births
- infant–parent co-sleeping

The introduction of risk reduction procedures has decreased the incidence of SIDS by up to 75%. These are listed in Box 14.3.

Additional factors that may be important include early advice about minor illnesses, using a new mattress and discouraging co-sleeping. Co-sleeping is completely contraindicated if either parent is taking drugs or sedative medications. It is important for staff on neonatal units to recognize those babies at high risk and to discuss risk reduction procedures with the parents. Instruction on resuscitation (showing the parents an appropriate video followed by a question and answer session) should be provided.

CLINICAL TIP: The parents of premature babies may request apnoea monitors for use at home. There is no evidence that home monitors reduce the risk of a major life-threatening event occurring out of hospital, nor do they prevent death: babies have died despite being monitored. Each case should be considered individually and the parents carefully counselled. In any case, before giving the parents an apnoea monitor for home use it is essential to show them how to apply basic resuscitation skills in case the baby is found apnoeic or collapsed at home.

Upper airway obstruction

The normal anatomy of the upper airway is shown in Fig. 14.3. Upper airway obstruction frequently presents in the delivery room or nursery as a result

Box 14.3 Measures to reduce risk of SIDS

- Put babies to sleep on their backs with no soft toys or cushions in the cot
- Avoid exposing babies to tobacco smoke
- Avoid overwrapping babies and prevent overheating
- Breastfeed

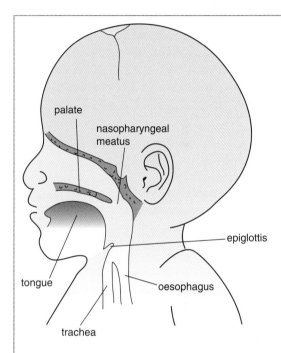

Figure 14.3 A normal upper airway. Reproduced with permission from South M, Isaacs D (eds) *Practical Paediatrics*, 7th edition. Elsevier Health Sciences, London.

of foreign material in the airway, and can readily be relieved by suction. Upper airway obstruction not relieved by suction is unusual and may be mild, occurring only when the infant is distressed, crying or during feeds. Severe airway obstruction at birth due to anatomical abnormalities may be life threatening.

A spectrum of pathological conditions can affect the neonatal upper airway, and these can be

conveniently divided into the following groups according to the site of the lesions:
• **nasal and nasopharyngeal lesions:** choanal atresia, intranasal tumours, nasolacrimal duct cysts
• **oral and oropharyngeal lesions:** micrognathia, large tongue, lymphatic malformation at base of tongue, tongue cysts
• **laryngeal lesions:** laryngomalacia, bifid or absent epiglottis, vocal cord paralysis, laryngeal web, subglottic stenosis, laryngeal cleft, subglottic haemangioma, intubation trauma
• **tracheal lesions:** tracheomalacia, tracheal stenosis, haemangioma.

Clinical features

Despite the varied pathophysiology, the clinical presentations of these disorders can be remarkably similar and may include any of the following;
• **Stridor:** this is the most common symptom. It is mostly inspiratory but there may be an expiratory component if the obstruction is below the glottis (intrathoracic).
• **Suprasternal and sternal retractions:** although chest retractions may be evident, the most marked retractions will be suprasternal.
• **Croupy cough.**
• **Hoarse cry.**
• **Difficulty in feeding.**

With increasing upper airway obstruction the baby may develop cyanosis followed by apnoea and bradycardia. Besides looking for the cause of the upper airway obstruction, it is of primary importance to determine the degree of emergency and decide whether the infant needs an artificial airway (nasopharyngeal, oropharyngeal, endotracheal or tracheostomy). This decision can be made mostly on clinical evaluation.

Causes of persistent stridor are shown in Box 14.4.

Laryngomalacia (infantile larynx)

The larynx in children with this condition is unusually floppy and narrows on inspiration, with resultant stridor. The stridor is often only present on crying. In most cases, it is a benign condition that improves with age, but the stridor may not disappear until 6–9 months from birth. Diagnosis is

---

Box 14.4 Causes of persistent stridor

• supraglottic – 62% (mostly laryngomalacia, rarely lingual cysts)
• vocal cord – 15% (nerve palsies, webs, papilloma, foreign body)
• subglottic stenosis – 14%
• tracheomalacia – 9%

---

made by seeking a paediatric ear, nose and throat (ENT) opinion and having laryngoscopy performed. In mild cases the parents should be reassured that the condition is self-limiting. In more severe cases, endoscopic laser aryepiglottic fold excision can provide symptomatic relief. Rarely, for cases of laryngomalacia resulting in significant airway obstruction, tracheostomy may be required.

CLINICAL TIP: Tracheostomy is the creation of an artificial airway through the trachea for the purposes of establishing either airway patency below an obstruction or an airway for prolonged ventilatory support. It is used either as an emergency procedure in cases of acute upper airway obstruction (rarely) or as an elective procedure, as in chronic lung disease or neuromuscular diseases, where the infant requires prolonged ventilatory support. Caregivers require training on how to replace the tube if it becomes dislodged or blocked. The tracheostomy can be closed when the underlying pathology improves.

Choanal atresia

This is a developmental anomaly of the nasal airways and can present as an acute emergency at birth. The condition is suspected by the finding of apnoea when the baby stops crying and confirmed by an inability to pass a catheter through the nasal passage. It is caused by a bony or membranous obstruction, of the nasopharyngeal meatus, which is usually unilateral and rarely bilateral. Bilateral obstruction can be temporarily managed by the insertion of an oral airway but will require surgical correction, with stents left in the posterior nares for up to 6 weeks to prevent the bone overgrowing and closing the posterior nares again. Unilateral atresia rarely requires surgical intervention during infancy. Associated anomalies occur in 20–50% of infants with choanal atresia, such as the CHARGE association, which includes coloboma or other ophthalmic abnormality, heart disease, choanal atresia, developmental delay, genital hypoplasia, and ear abnormality with hearing loss.

Pharyngeal obstruction

Micrognathia (e.g. Pierre Robin sequence) causes a backward displacement of the tongue which obstructs the pharynx. Severe macroglossia (sometimes seen in trisomy 21 or Beckwith–Wiedemann syndrome) can also cause pharyngeal obstruction. Pharyngeal obstruction can be temporarily managed by the insertion of a nasopharyngeal airway (see Fig. 14.4).

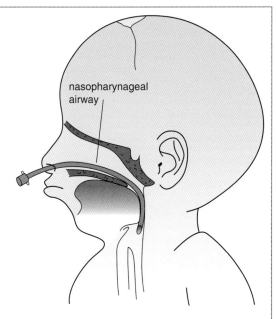

nasopharynageal airway

Figure 14.4 Nasopharyngeal tube used for micrognathia. Reproduced with permission from South M, Isaacs D (eds) *Practical Paediatrics*, 7th edition. Elsevier Health Sciences, London.

Subglottic stenosis

This is most commonly an acquired condition, and in the rarer congenital cases the baby often presents early with stridor. Acquired subglottic stenosis is usually related to trauma of the glottic structures by vigorous suction or intubation. More commonly it is related to prolonged intermittent positive pressure ventilation (IPPV) through an endotracheal tube. With modern endotracheal tubes the incidence of this condition has fallen, and it now occurs in only 1% of ventilated infants.

The mechanisms by which stenosis develops are multifactorial, but physical ulceration from the tube, together with the piston action of the ventilator, is a very important causative factor. In addition, poor humidification of inspired gases and local infection may be contributory. The duration of intubation is important, but stenosis has been reported not uncommonly in infants intubated for only a few days.

Most infants with stridor following extubation have some subglottic oedema. If subglottic stenosis is suspected, direct laryngoscopy by an experienced ENT surgeon must be urgently arranged before extubating the baby if possible. Those with mild stenosis usually do not present until after discharge, when an intercurrent upper respiratory tract infection precipitates serious upper airway obstruction. Tracheostomy should be avoided wherever possible as, in many of these children, later closure of the tracheostomy is difficult. Surgical procedures such as repeated dilatation, or cryo- or laser surgery to split the cricoid cartilage anteriorly, may be successful in managing the condition.

Tracheal obstruction

Tracheal obstruction may be caused by a number of factors including mucus, blood, haemangiomas or tumours (either in the airway itself or externally causing compression). Congenital airway haemangiomas respond very rapidly to treatment with propanolol. Tracheomalacia or bronchomalacia is a condition where the airway cartilage is incompletely formed, allowing the airway to fold in on itself during inspiration. In the majority of cases it is self-limiting.

CLINICAL TIP: Bronchoscopy is another useful procedure for evaluating upper airway problems. A flexible 2.2 mm or 2.7 mm bronchoscope should be able to pass through a 2.5 mm or 3.0 mm endotracheal tube and visualize the upper airway structures. Common neonatal diagnoses that may be made by bronchoscopy include laryngomalacia, subglottic stenosis, laryngeal oedema and/or inflammation, laryngeal haemangioma, and broncho-tracheomalacia.

SUMMARY

Successful transition to the extrauterine environment requires the establishment of continuous breathing. Apnoea is very common in preterm infants (<35 weeks) and is called apnoea of prematurity if no other cause can be identified. It is always abnormal in a term infant and specific causes should be sort. CPAP and caffeine are the mainstays of treatment for apnoea of prematurity.

SIDS or SUDI is the unexpected death of an infant aged between 1 month and 1 year. A number of important preventative measures can be undertaken to reduce the risk of SIDS, including avoidance of cigarette smoke, safe sleeping position and prevention of overheating. Upper airway obstruction has a number of causes and babies will often present in the delivery room with respiratory distress or apnoea.

 Now visit **www.essentialneonatalmed.com** to test yourself on this chapter.

CHAPTER 15
Respiratory physiology and respiratory support

Key topics

Introduction

Prenatal development of the respiratory system is not complete until sufficient gas exchange surface has formed to support normal breathing at birth. Therefore, prenatal development of the lungs occurs in stages and may not be complete until after birth. Structural maturity of the airways and chest wall is a part of lung development. Fundamental processes that impact on respiratory function include ventilation and distribution of gas volumes, gas exchange and transport, and pulmonary circulation. There is an unique interaction between lungs and brain, and hence maturation of the respiratory centres in the brain is also integral to normal respiratory function.

Fetal lung development

An insight into lung development is important to understand the diseases of the lungs and lung function in newborns. Fetal lung development takes place in several phases (Fig. 15.1). Demarcations are not exact, with transition and progression occurring between each. The lungs of premature babies born at around 24–25 weeks' gestation and onward are in the canalicular or saccular stages. The saccule or terminal sac is the distal airway structure which

Essential Neonatal Medicine, Fifth Edition. Sunil Sinha, Lawrence Miall, Luke Jardine.
© 2012 John Wiley & Sons, Ltd. Published 2012 by John Wiley & Sons, Ltd.

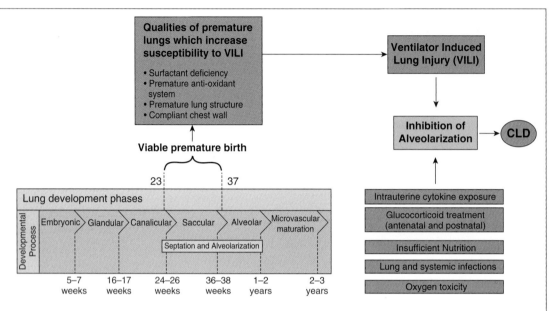

Figure 15.1 Stages of fetal lung development. From Attar MA, Donn SM. Mechanism of ventilator-induced lung injury in premature infants. *Semin Neonatol* 2002;7:353–360. With permission from Elsevier.

further branches into respiratory bronchioles by about 32 weeks' gestation. Alveolization starts from about 32 weeks and continues until 2 years of age. The large increase in lung surface areas does not occur until after the saccular lung begins to alveolize.

Physical factors such as fetal breathing and movements play a crucial role in structural development and may influence the size and capacity of the lungs. Hormonal factors also influence alveolization and can be either stimulatory (vitamin A, retinoids) or inhibitory (antenatal and postnatal glucocorticoids). Congenital infection (chorioamnionitis), inflammation and mechanical ventilation also inhibit lung development through arrest of alveolarization.

Pulmonary surfactants

Pulmonary surfactant, a multicomponent complex of several phospholipids, neutral lipids and specific proteins, is synthesized and secreted into alveolar spaces by type II epithelial cells. Pulmonary surfactant reduces the collapsing forces in the alveoli, conserves mechanical stability of the alveoli, and

maintains the alveolar surface relatively free of liquid. Preterm infants are deficient in endogenous surfactant and administration of exogenous surfactant in such cases reduces the pressure required to open the lung, increases the maximum lung volume, and prevents lung collapse (atelectasis) at low pressure. Surfactant is primarily composed of phospholipids (85%) and proteins (10%). Dipalmitoyl phosphatidylcholine (DPPC) is the predominant phospholipid in surfactants. The structure of DPPC is suited to form a stable monolayer generating the low surface tension required to prevent alveolar collapse at end expiration.

However, phospholipids alone do not make up for all the biophysical properties of pulmonary surfactant. The contribution of surfactant proteins, especially the low molecular weight components SP-B and SP-C, is essential for structural organization and functional durability of surfactants. They both promote the rapid dispersion of phospholipids at the air–liquid interface and account for the sustained low surface tension activity after dynamic compression. However, in several laboratory investigations, SP-B has been found to reduce surface tension to a greater extent than SP-C. SP-B also participates in intracellular and extracellular regulation of surfactant structure and function, and without SP-B, SP-C is not expressed properly. Congenital absence of SP-B is lethal, with respiratory failure occurring soon after birth. In contrast, SP-C deficiency is not associated with respiratory failure at birth, but may lead to interstitial lung disease in later childhood. The structure and function of the SP-B and SP-C proteins, including the effect of their mutations on lung function, have been the subject of recent reviews, which show a clear difference between the structures of SP-B and SP-C, thus predicting differing functions. There are two other surfactant proteins, SP-A and SP-D, which are only marginally involved in the surface tension-lowering ability of pulmonary surfactant but play an important role in the innate lung defence barrier against pathogenic organisms.

Respiratory physiology

Oxygen transport

Oxygen is essential for the production of adenosine triphosphate (ATP), a molecule that stores and releases energy. Severe hypoxaemia greatly reduces the production of ATP and the resultant anaerobic metabolism produces lactic acid. Lactic acid accumulation significantly contributes to the development of metabolic acidosis.

Oxygen diffuses across the alveolar membrane from a higher to a lower concentration. It is carried in the blood attached to haemoglobin, or to a lesser degree dissolved in plasma. The partial pressure of oxygen (PO_2) refers to the amount dissolved in plasma. Delivery of oxygen to the tissues depends on oxygen concentration and tissue perfusion. Oxygen combines with haemoglobin to be transported as oxyhaemoglobin. The saturation of the haemoglobin refers to the percentage of it that carries oxygen. The relationship between oxygen saturation and PO_2 is not constant, so that at a relatively low tissue PO_2 larger amounts of oxygen are released than when the PO_2 is higher. The P_{50} is the P_aO_2 (partial pressure in artery) at which the haemoglobin is half saturated with O_2; the higher the P_{50}, the lower the affinity of haemoglobin for oxygen. The

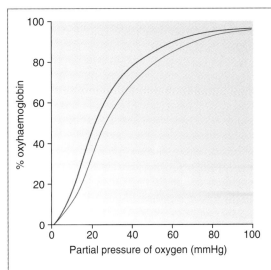

Figure 15.2 Oxygen dissociation curve for fetal haemoglobin (upper red line) and adult **haemoglobin** (lower blue line).

Table 15.1 Factors that influence the oxygen dissociation curve

Factors producing (L) shift	Factors producing (R) shift
↓ Temperature	↑ Temperature
↓ Basal metabolic rate	↑ Basal metabolic rate
↓ P_aCO_2	↑ P_aCO_2
↑ pH	↓ pH
↓ 2,3-DPG	↑ 2,3-DPG
↑ Fetal haemoglobin	↓ Fetal haemoglobin

2,3-DPG, 2,3-diphosphoglycerate.

oxygen dissociation curve for fetal haemoglobin (HbF) is different than that for adult haemoglobin (HbA) in that it is shifted to the left (Fig. 15.2). The fetus lives in a relatively hypoxic environment and the oxyhaemoglobin saturation is greater at lower partial oxygen pressures. This is of benefit to the fetus but is disadvantageous to the newborn infant, who at any given PO_2 level gives up less oxygen to the tissues than older children with HbA. Table 15.1

lists the factors responsible for a shift in the oxygen dissociation curve. A right shift of the curve means a higher P_{50} (i.e. a higher P_aO_2 is required for haemoglobin to bind a given amount of O_2).

Carbon dioxide transport

Carbon dioxide may be transported dissolved in the blood, but is mainly present as bicarbonate ions (HCO_3^-). Carbon dioxide is produced as a byproduct of cellular respiration and is liberated into the blood. It diffuses through the alveoli to be excreted in the expired air. The CO_2 content of the blood is referred to as the partial pressure of CO_2, or PCO_2.

Acid–base balance

In the presence of the enzyme carbonic anhydrase (CA), carbon dioxide dissolved in plasma forms carbonic acid, which in turn dissociates to H+ and HCO_3^- ions.

$$H_2O + CO_2 \xrightleftharpoons{CA} H_2CO_3 \rightleftharpoons HCO_3^- + H^+$$

As a result of this dissociation carbonic acid can be indirectly excreted through the lungs. Lactic acid must be excreted through the kidneys, and this occurs more slowly.

Buffer systems exist in the body to prevent rapid pH changes. The HCO_3^-/CO_2 relationship is an important buffer system; other buffers include haemoglobin and, to a lesser extent, plasma proteins. Disturbance of the acid–base balance can produce either acidosis or alkalosis, which may be due to either metabolic or respiratory causes.

During aerobic metabolism CO_2 is produced, and in the presence of respiratory disease is less effectively excreted, causing the P_aCO_2 to rise. As a result the infant becomes acidotic – respiratory acidosis. If the infant with relatively normal lungs breathes or is ventilated rapidly, more CO_2 is excreted and the reaction moves in the other direction to produce a respiratory alkalosis.

Lactic acid, the product of anaerobic metabolism, can only be excreted by the kidneys and, if in excess, the H^+ ions are buffered by haemoglobin,

proteins and H_2CO_3. The HCO_3^- cannot be excreted through the lungs to compensate, thereby leaving an excess of H^+ causing a metabolic acidosis. Persistent vomiting causes loss of H^+, resulting in an excess of HCO_3^- with consequent metabolic alkalosis.

In practice a simple respiratory acidosis rarely occurs, and in neonatal lung disease there is likely to be impairment of CO_2 excretion, together with production of lactic acid as a result of anaerobic metabolism, leading to a mixed respiratory and metabolic acidosis.

The base excess is derived from the relationship between pH and PCO_2 using the Siggaard Anderson nomogram. It is the amount of buffer base added to blood, assuming that PCO_2 is <5.5 kPa (40 mmHg), to correct the pH to 7.40. Thus, it is a direct measurement of the metabolic component of acidosis or alkalosis. Positive values represent excess of base and negative values excess of acid. The base excess is therefore valuable in assigning a predominant metabolic or respiratory component to acidosis or alkalosis.

The acid–base status of the infant can be derived from the blood gases. Normal biochemical ranges for arterial blood in term and preterm infants are shown in Table 15.2.

Specific treatments for various abnormalities of acid–base balance are described below.

Table 15.2 Normal biochemical range for arterial blood in term and preterm infants

Parameter	Term	Preterm
P_aO_2 mmHg (kPa)	60–90 (8–12)	50–80 (6.7–10.7)
PCO_2 mmHg (kPa)	35–42 (4.7–5.6)	30–40 (4–5.3)
pH	7.35–7.42	7.32–7.40
Base excess (BE) (mmol/L)	–2–0	–4–0
Bicarbonate (mmol/L)	22–26	19–24

Metabolic acidosis

Metabolic acidosis arises when there is tissue hypoxia (inadequate perfusion, hypoxaemia), excessive acid intake (total parenteral nutrition (TPN)), the production of excessive or abnormal acids (inborn errors of metabolism) or renal inability to excrete the acid load (tubular acidosis). In the presence of normal lungs the pH may be normal but the PCO_2 is low, and the base excess may be -8 mmol/L or more. Treatment is directed at the underlying problem.

In addition, metabolic acidosis may be treated by infusion of a molar (8.4%) solution of sodium bicarbonate. A solution containing 8.4% $NaHCO_3$ has 1 mmol of $NaHCO_3$ in 1 mL of solution and is usually infused slowly as a half-strength solution (4.2%). The dose (for a full correction) is calculated as follows:

$$\text{volume of } 8.4\% \text{ NaHCO}_3 \text{ (mL)}$$
$$= \text{base excess} \times \text{weight in kg} \times 0.6$$

The factor 0.6 represents the proportion of extracellular fluid to body weight in infants. Many people will initially give a half correction first.

Sodium bicarbonate combines with excess hydrogen ions to produce unstable carbonic acid, which in turn is hydrolysed to CO_2 and H_2O. The CO_2 is excreted by the lungs. For this reason, bicarbonate should not be given in the presence of high P_aCO_2. Under these circumstances, trishydroxyaminomethane (THAM) is preferable to bicarbonate, and this is described in the section on respiratory acidosis.

Metabolic alkalosis

This metabolic derangement usually occurs following excessive vomiting or the overuse of sodium bicarbonate. The pH may be normal or high. The P_aCO_2 is usually raised and the base excess is positive. Treatment is by infusion of normal saline.

Respiratory acidosis

This is due to lung disease and is usually aggravated by a metabolic acidosis as a result of anaerobic metabolism and poor tissue perfusion. If there is a mixed acidosis the pH is low, P_aCO_2 high and base excess strongly negative. Treatment depends on the severity of the lung disease, but if the pH is below 7.25 the infant will usually require mechanical ventilation. Sodium bicarbonate should not be given if the P_aCO_2 is more than 6 kPa. (45 mmHg)

If the base excess is more than -10 mmol/L and the P_aCO_2 exceeds 6 kPa (45 mmHg), then THAM can be used. THAM buffers H^+ and binds CO_2, thus lowering the P_aCO_2. It may cause apnoea and should only be used in infants being mechanically ventilated.

Respiratory alkalosis

This is due to overventilation and if it occurs while an infant is receiving mechanical ventilation it is simply treated by reducing the ventilator rate or inspiratory pressure/volume.

Typical examples of acid–base derangements in the newborn, with interpretation and possible causes, are shown in Table 15.3.

Assessment of respiratory function

This should be done on a composite of information obtained from:

- clinical observation
- blood gas measurements
- chest radiograph
- pulmonary function tests
- echocardiography.

Information obtained from these observations provide useful assessment of the underlying respiratory status and their progression but may have poor specificity when used individually

Clinical assessment

Five common physical signs associated with respiratory disorders are respiratory rate, chest wall retraction, nasal flaring, grunting and cyanosis.

Blood gas measurements

See Table 15.3.

Table 15.3 Examples of abnormal arterial blood gas results and their interpretation

F_iO_2	P_aO_2 mmHg (kPa)	pH	P_aCO_2 mmHg (kPa)	BE	Bicarbonate (mmol/L)	Interpretation	Possible cause
0.21	75 (10)	7.13	60 (8)	−10	13	Mixed acidosis	Severe birth asphyxia
0.65	53 (7)	7.18	60 (8)	−8	15	Mixed acidosis Hypoxia	Acute RDS
0.35	53 (7)	7.33	68 (9)	8	34	Chronic respiratory acidosis with renal compensation	Bronchopulmonary dysplasia
0.21	83 (11)	7.53	53 (7)	15	44	Metabolic alkalosis with mild respiratory compensation	Vomiting Pyloric stenosis

Radiographic evaluation

Radiography of the chest is an integral part of the diagnostic evaluation of respiratory disorders and remains the introductory and primary imaging examination for evaluation of the neonatal chest. Other modalities, including CT and MRI, are valuable only in certain selected cases.

Pulmonary function tests

These tests provide information about pulmonary mechanics and lung volumes. These are now available as bedside measurements and can be used for newborns.

Pulmonary mechanics

Pulmonary mechanics data is about the force (**pressure**) required to drive an amount of gas (**volume**), and provide information as to how this gas is flowing in and out of the lungs (**airflow**). This can be presented either in scalar form or as loops showing relationship between two variables such as pressure/volume and flow/volume loops (see Figs. 15.3 and 15.4). These data then automatically calculate compliance, resistance and time constant.

Compliance

The compliance is a measure of elasticity or distensibility of the lungs (Fig. 15.3) and is calculated by the formula

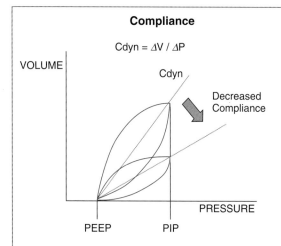

Compliance

$Cdyn = \Delta V / \Delta P$

Figure 15.3 Pressure-volume loop showing compliance of the lung.

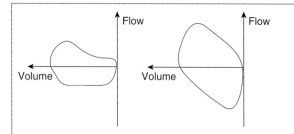

Figure 15.4 Flow volume loop showing resistance to airflow. The loop on the left shows increased resistance causing impedance to airflow, which has improved after treatment as shown in the loop on the right.

compliance = change in lung volume/

change in intrathoracic

pressure

A typical value for lung compliance in a young healthy newborn is $1.5–2.0\,mL\,cmH_2O^{-1}\,kg^{-1}$. Compliance in infants with RDS is lower and often ranges from 0.1 to $1\,mL\,cmH_2O^{-1}\,kg^{-1}$.

Resistance

Pulmonary resistance is a measure of the friction encountered by the gas flowing through the airways. By definition, resistance to airflow is equal to the resistive component of the driving pressure divided by the resulting airflow (V); thus

resistance = pressure/flow

Nearly 80% of the total resistance to airflow occurs in large airways and since the newborn airway lumen is approximately half the adult size, the neonatal airway resistance is considerably higher than that of an adult. Normal airway resistance in a term newborn is approximately $20–40\,cmH_2O/L/s$ which is about 16 times the value observed in adults ($1–2\,cmH_2O/L/s$).

Time constant

The time constant is the time (expressed in seconds) necessary for the alveolar pressure (or volume) to reach 63% of a change in airway pressure (or volume). Duration of inspiration or expiration equivalent to $3–5 \times$ time constant is required for relatively complete inspiration or expiration. It is calculated as

time constant = compliance $\times$ resistance

These days it is possible to assess this by using flow-volume loops on a pulmonary graphics machine, which provide information as to how the gas is moving in and out of the lung as well as giving an estimate of the work of breathing done by the patient.

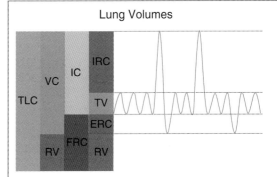

Figure 15.5 Lung volumes. TLC – total lung capacity, VC – vital capacity, RV – residual volume, IC – inspiratory capacity, FRC – functional residual capacity, IRC – inspiratory respiratory capacity. ERC – expiratory respiratory capacity, TV – tidal volume, RV – residual volume.

Lung function testing

Bedside pulmonary mechanics testing requires calibration and careful interpretation, but the information obtained is useful, particularly in babies requiring assisted ventilation for respiratory failure.

Lung function tests include assessment and measurement of total volume of gas in the lungs and its different components (Fig. 15.5). Helium dilution and nitrogen washout techniques have been adapted to measure **functional residual capacity** (FRC) in infants. FRC is the volume of gas in the lung that is in direct communication with the airways at the end of expiration. The volume of gas in the FRC serves as an oxygen storage compartment in the body and a buffer so that large changes in alveolar gas tension are reduced.

Cardiac assessment

The respiratory system has an unique relationship with the cardiovascular system, and hence assessment of respiratory function is not complete without the evaluation of cardiac status (cardiorespiratory assessment). This requires bedside echocardiography (ultrasound Doppler studies) which provides important information regarding the systemic and pulmonary circulation and is increasingly being used in many neonatal intensive care units as a routine investigation, particularly in babies with refractory respiratory failure.

Respiratory failure

Respiratory failure is present when there is a major abnormality of gas exchange resulting in hypoxaemia, hypercarbia and acidosis. Hypoxaemia may be due to either respiratory or cardiac abnormalities and, as an isolated factor, is not of great value in predicting the need for respiratory support. Hypercarbia is a much better indicator of respiratory failure. A rising P_aCO_2, particularly in the presence of a falling pH (respiratory acidosis), is an ominous sign. A value for P_aCO_2 of above 60 mmHg (8 kPa), with a respiratory acidosis (pH <7.25), indicates the need for mechanical ventilation. Some infants, particularly if very small, may require ventilation before these criteria are met. Hypercarbia and acidosis are strongly associated with the development of intraventricular haemorrhage in premature infants (see Chapter 22). The causes of respiratory failure are listed in Table 15.4.

Treatment of respiratory failure

Babies with signs of respiratory failure require artificial respiratory support, which can be given as follows:
- oxygen therapy
- continuous positive airway pressure (CPAP)
- non-invasive forms of mechanical respiratory support
- assisted ventilation through mechanical ventilators.

Oxygen therapy

Oxygen is the most commonly used therapy in neonatal intensive care units. The ultimate aim of oxygen therapy is to achieve adequate tissue oxygenation without creating oxygen toxicity and harmful oxidative stress. Tissue oxygenation in turn depends on a number of factors (see Box 15.1).

Commonly used indices of oxygenation are:
- alveolar-arterial oxygen pressure difference (P(A-a)O_2)

Table 15.4 Causes of respiratory failure in the neonate

Poor respiratory effort	Extreme immaturity, CNS depression, postoperative infections, metabolic, neuromuscular disease
Abnormal lungs	Surfactant deficiency – RDS Retained fetal lung fluid –TTN Pulmonary oedema – hydrops, CCF
Abnormal airways	Infections – pneumonia Obstructed airways – meconium, pneumothorax
Hypoplastic lungs	Obstructive uropathy Very early PROM Diaphragmatic hernia
Small thoracic volume	Bowel obstruction, exomphalos/gastroschisis repair, ascites, chondrodystrophic dwarfism

CCF, congestive cardiac failure; PROM, premature rupture of membranes; RDS, respiratory distress syndrome; TTN, transient tachypnoea of the newborn.

Box 15.1 Factors affecting tissue oxygenation

- Inspired oxygen (ambient oxygen)
- Adequacy of gas exchange in lungs (ventilation/ perfusion balance)
- Oxygen carrying capacity of the blood
- Cardiac output and right to left shunt
- Local tissue oedema or ischaemia
- Altitude

- oxygenation index (OI) OI = Mean Airway Pressure × FiO_2(%)/P_aO_2 (mmHg), multiply by 100
- arterial to alveolar oxygen tension ratio (a/A ratio)

An OI greater than 25 is indicative of severe ventilation/perfusion imbalance and values reaching 40 are associated with very poor prognosis. Although OI is the commonly used index, both for clinical and research studies, none of the above indices has a clear advantage over the others, and any of them can be used to assess the severity or progression of the respiratory illness requiring change in treatment.

Blood oxygen monitoring

Oxygen therapy is associated with toxicity and hence should be monitored closely. This can be done either by continuous non-invasive monitoring using pulse oxygen saturation (pulse oximetry) or transcutaneous oxygen levels ($TCPO_2$). However, where possible, arterial blood sampling for both PaO_2 and other blood gas indices remains the 'gold standard'. Although pulse oximetry is simple and easy to use, it is important to know the limitation of any device used. For example, a pulse oximeter showing a saturation above 95% may be associated with PaO_2 ranging anywhere from 10 to 16 kPa (80–120 mmHg) which is recognized to cause damage to the eyes (retinopathy of prematurity, ROP). Current saturation target is 91–95%, based on the results of a recent trial in which there was increased mortality if babies were nursed at 85–89% saturation. However, the higher range increases the risk of ROP and visual deficit.

Continuous positive airway pressure

CPAP is a form of positive pressure applied to the airways of a spontaneously breathing baby throughout the respiratory cycle. A similar positive pressure when applied through an endotracheal tube in a ventilated infant is called **positive end-expiratory pressure** (PEEP). CPAP and PEEP do not provide ventilation and hence should not be given if the baby is not breathing adequately. The rationale for using CPAP and PEEP is to maintain patency of the airways and avoid alveolar collapse on expiration and thus maintain FRC. Application of CPAP to preterm infants also helps to stabilize the chest wall and prevents collapse of upper airways. CPAP/PEEP improves lung compliance and decreases airway resistance. This allows a greater tidal volume for a given negative pressure,

with subsequent reduction in the work of breathing. CPAP improves oxygenation but has a variable effect on $PaCO_2$.

Indications for CPAP

CPAP is indicated:
- as a primary mode of support for respiratory distress at or soon after birth
- to facilitate extubation of a ventilated infant
- for the treatment of apnoea.

Applying CPAP

The optimal pressure is difficult to predict. Generally CPAP of 4–6 cmH$_2$O is appropriate, but some infants benefit from higher pressures. The lowest pressure that produces the best arterial oxygenation is the optimal CPAP pressure. Regular evaluation of P_aCO_2 and arterial pH is necessary to assess the infant's response to CPAP, and mechanical ventilation may be necessary if deterioration occurs.

CPAP can be administered in a variety of ways:
- **Nasal mask:** this can be effective but is difficult to attach and get a good seal without undue pressure.
- **Endotracheal tube:** this should only be used for a short period in a ventilated infant who is ready for extubation.
- **Nasal prongs:** this seems to be the most satisfactory (or least unsatisfactory) method of delivering CPAP. It can be accomplished by inserting nasopharyngeal tubes, but short nasal prongs are more suitable as this causes the least resistance. Binasal (double) short prongs are more effective than a single long prong.

Contraindications for CPAP

CPAP should not be used in the following situations:
- severe acute episode(s) of complete apnoea
- inability to maintain normal oxygenation with an FiO_2 >0.6, especially if the CO$_2$ is rising above 8 kPa (60 mmHg) or the pH is falling below 7.25
- upper airway abnormality (cleft palate, choanal atresia, tracheo-oesophageal fistula)
- severe cardiovascular instability
- unstable respiratory drive with frequent apnoeas and or bradycardia
- severe gaseous distension of the bowel (e.g. ileus, NEC)

Complications of CPAP

The possible complications are:
- pneumothorax or pulmonary interstitial emphysema due to overdistension of alveoli
- gastric distension and vomiting with face mask and nasal prongs
- hypercapnia
- nasal septum injury due to pressure necrosis
- nasal secretion, mucus plugs
- loss of pressure through an open mouth.

Other forms of non-invasive respiratory support

High-flow nasal cannulae (HFNC)

These have recently been introduced to the neonatal unit and seem to provide similar benefit to CPAP, but there is not yet enough data to support their full efficacy and safety.

Bilevel pressure support

This describes the delivery of two different pressure levels during the respiratory cycle. A baseline continuous airway distending pressure is provided which is then augmented by intermittent pressure rises. These pressure rises can be large, similar to those delivered via an endotracheal tube during invasive ventilation, or small (2–3 cmH$_2$O), and can be synchronized or non-synchronized. **Synchronized** pressure rises are triggered by the baby's own respiratory effort: every time the baby starts to breathe in, the pressure will rise to a set peak pressure. **Non-synchronized** pressure rises occur intermittently at regular intervals which can be set by the clinician. As with invasive ventilation, the duration of these pressure rises can also be set by the clinician.

Non-invasive/nasal intermittent positive pressure ventilation (NIPPV)

This describes the use of a conventional ventilator to provide bilevel support with large pressure rises, which are non-synchronized. Ventilation is delivered through a nasal patient interface (nasal prongs or mask) instead of an endotracheal tube. Bilevel pressure support with small pressure rises can be delivered by specialized devices which offer both synchronized and non-synchronized options.

Mechanical ventilation

Despite the successes of CPAP and NIPPV, a significant proportion of babies, particularly those born too prematurely (<27–28 weeks' gestation), require mechanical ventilators through an endotracheal tube. Indications for mechanical ventilation are summarized in Box 15.2 and its aims in Box 15.3.

Basic principles of mechanical ventilation

The ventilatory need of a patient depends largely on the mechanical properties of the respiratory system (compliance, resistance and time constant), and the type of abnormality in gas exchange (level of pO$_2$ and pCO$_2$). The ventilatory parameters which

> ### Box 15.2 Indications for mechanical ventilation
>
> - Failure to initiate or establish spontaneous breathing
> - Worsening apnoeas and bradycardias
> - Major respiratory or cardiac collapse
> - Surfactant administration
> - Need to maintain airway patency
> - Impaired pulmonary gas exchange

> ### Box 15.3 Goals of mechanical ventilation
>
> These should be considered no matter what ventilatory device, mode or modality is chosen.
>
> - Achieve adequate pulmonary gas exchange
> - Decrease patient's work of breathing
> - Overcome alveolar atelectasis
> - Avoid ventilator-induced lung injury
> - Maximize patient comfort

Box 15.4 Factors affecting Po_2 and Pco_2

Determinants of oxygenation

- Fraction of inspired oxygen (FiO_2)
- Mean airway pressure, which is determined by
  Positive end-expiratory pressure (PEEP)
  Peak inspiratory pressure (PIP)
  Inspiratory time
  Gas flow rate
  Respiratory rate (sometimes)

Determinants of CO_2

- Minute volume = frequency × tidal volume
  (tidal volume is dependent on distending pressure
  ΔP (=difference between PIP and baseline PEEP)

control oxygenation and CO_2 removal are shown in Box 15.4.

Classification of mechanical ventilators

Over the past decade, a number of newer techniques of ventilation have evolved with different terminology and nomenclatures. This often causes confusion and can be better understood by using a simple classification using a hierarchal system of control mechanism.

Control variables (ventilatory modalities)

At any one time, a ventilator can only be operated using one of the following controls:
- pressure control
- volume control
- flow control (same as volume control, as flow is the integral of volume)
- time control (e.g. high-frequency ventilators).

Phase variables (ventilatory modes)

These variables determine the type of the delivered breath and are interchangeable:
- trigger (what starts inspiration)
- limit (what sustains inspiration)
- cycle (what ends inspiration and starts expiration).

Various types of ventilatory modes and modalities

Pressure-controlled ventilation

Pressure-targeted modalities limit the amount of pressure that can be delivered during inspiration. The operator sets the maximum pressure and the ventilator does not exceed this level. Although pressure is fixed, the volume of gas delivered to the lungs varies according to lung compliance. If compliance is low (stiff lungs), less volume is delivered than if compliance is high.

Volume-controlled ventilation

In volume-controlled modalities, a set tidal volume is delivered irrespective of lung compliance or the pressure required to deliver it. As it is now increasingly recognized that it is the volume rather than the pressure which is more useful in terms of efficacy and safety of mechanical ventilation, volume-targeted modes of ventilation are becoming more popular. They include:
- volume-controlled ventilation (VCV)
- volume-guarantee ventilation (VG) (also known as volume-guided ventilation)
- pressure-regulated volume-controlled ventilation (PRVC)
- volume-assured pressure support ventilation (VAPS).

The principal feature of VCV is that it delivers the set tidal volume regardless of the underlying lung compliance by automatically adjusting the peak inspiratory pressure (PIP). Another important feature of VCV that differentiates it from pressure-limited ventilation (PLV) is the way that gas is delivered to the lungs during the inspiratory phase. In traditional VCV, a square flow waveform is generated so that alveolar filling is complete only at the end of inspiration. VCV, like PLV, can be provided as intermittent mandatory ventilation (IMV), synchronized intermittent ventilation (SIMV), and assist control ventilation. It may also be combined with PSV during SIMV.

Volume-guarantee ventilation

VG is primarily a pressure form of ventilation but has inbuilt microprocessor technology (closed-loop ventilation) to adjust the pressure up or down, to maintain the tidal volume delivery in the desired range. VG can only be used in conjunction with patient-triggered modes, such as assist/control (see below), SIMV and PSV.

Pressure-regulated volume-control ventilation

PRVC is another modality of ventilation which combines the benefits of PLV and VCV. PRVC is also a form of closed-loop ventilation in which pressure is automatically adjusted.

Volume-assured pressure support ventilation

VAPS combines the advantage of both pressure and volume ventilation within a single breath and makes adjustments on a breath to breath basis, in contrast to VG and PRVC where adjustment takes place on an average of 4–6 breaths.

Intermittent mandatory ventilation

IMV delivers mechanical breaths at a rate set by the operator. Breaths are provided at regular intervals and baby may breathe spontaneously with, between or even against mechanical breaths. This can cause patient–ventilator asynchrony resulting in inconsistency in tidal volume delivery affecting gaseous exchange and cause complications such as air leaks and pneumothorax.

Synchronized intermittent mandatory ventilation

SIMV is a ventilatory mode in which mechanical breaths are synchronized to the onset of a spontaneous breath and delivered at a fixed rate set by the clinician. Between these set breaths, the patient breathes spontaneously, supported only by the machine's baseline pressure. Thus SIMV offers some improvement over IMV in that it provides synchrony during the inspiratory phase, but because the inspiratory time of the machine-delivered breath and the baby's spontaneous breaths are not the same, this mode provides only partial synchrony.

Assist/control ventilation

In assist/control mode – synchronized intermittent positive pressure ventilation (SIPPV), also called patient-triggered ventilation (PTV) – a synchronized mechanical breath is delivered each time the machine detects the patient's inspiratory effort (assist), but if the patient fails to breathe (becomes apnoeic) the machine will deliver the breaths at a 'back-up' rate as a safety net. Although the spontaneous and mechanical breaths are completely synchronized to the onset of inspiration, again the possibility exists (as with SIMV) that dyssynchrony will occur during the expiratory phase because of different inspiration time. This problem has been overcome by the introduction of a second signal detection system that determines when the patient's inspiratory effort is about to cease and then synchronizes the termination of the mechanical breath to this signal (assist/control, flow cycled).

Pressure support ventilation

PSV is also a patient-triggered (synchronized) mode of ventilation in which spontaneous breaths are fully or partially supported by an inspiratory pressure assist ('boost') above baseline pressure, thus decreasing any imposed work of breathing such as that created by the endotracheal tube. The amount of flow delivered to the patient during the inspiratory phase is variable and proportional to the patient effort in this mode. PSV is generally used during the weaning stages of ventilation. Thus PSV provides complete synchrony and resembles a normal breath.

Proportional assist ventilation

In proportional assist ventilation (PAV), the ventilator is continuously sensitive to the spontaneous respiratory efforts and adjusts the assist pressure in a proportionate and ongoing fashion. During episodes of apnoea or hypoventilation, PAV reverts to back-up conventional ventilation.

High-frequency ventilation

High-frequency ventilation (HFV) is conceptually different from conventional ventilation (CV). In HFV, gas exchange is achieved using a very high breathing rate but with much smaller tidal volumes and pressure amplitude than with CV, features that are thought to reduce ventilator-associated lung

Table 15.5 Comparison of basic parameters of high-frequency (HFV) ventilation and conventional ventilation (CV)

Parameter	HFV	CV
Rate (breaths/min)	180–1200	0–60
Vt (mL/kg)	0.1–5	4–20
Alveolar pressure (cmH$_2$O)	0.1–20	5–50
End-expiratory lung volume	High	Low
Minute ventilation	Rate$^{(0.5-1)}$ × Vt$^{(1.5-2)}$	Rate × Vt

Vt, tidal volume

injury. A comparison of the basic parameters of HFV and CV is given in Table 15.5.

HFV can be accomplished in various ways. The most commonly used method is high-frequency oscillatory ventilation (HFOV). Essentially this is a safer way of using 'super' PEEP. The lungs can be inflated to higher mean volumes without having to use high peak airway pressure to maintain ventilation (CO$_2$ removal). This produces more uniform lung inflation and reduces the risk of air leaks. Nonetheless, as with CV, there is the potential for gas trapping, which can cause overinflation of lungs with potential adverse consequences. Despite the putative advantages of HFOV in physiological terms, there is no scientific evidence of its superiority over CV when used as the primary mode of ventilation. However, when it is used as an early rescue treatment in specific situations such as severe RDS, air leak syndromes and pulmonary hypoplasia, the results are encouraging.

Another method of providing HFV is high-frequency jet ventilation, but this is not practised as widely as HFOV. It works by providing pulses of high-velocity gas (jet-stream) down the centre of the airway, penetrating through the dead space gas. The kinetic energy of the gas emerging from the jet nozzle at high velocity, rather than the pressure gradient, drives gas movement in large airways. Air leak syndrome has been the most commonly treated underlying disorder but jet ventilation has been successfully used in a variety of other respiratory conditions in newborns.

Alternative strategies for refractory respiratory failure

Despite the introduction of newer modes of ventilation and strategies such as HFV, a number of babies still fail treatment and require adjunctive treatment. Two such methods, inhaled nitric oxide (iNO) therapy and extracorporeal membrane oxygen (ECMO), are now considered to be a part of the armamentarium of various treatment strategies and have been proven to be of value in selected cases (Cochrane Review).

Inhaled nitric oxide therapy

This form of treatment of newborns with hypoxaemic respiratory failure and pulmonary hypertension has dramatically changed management strategies for this critically ill group of babies. In 'term' newborns it causes potent, selective and sustained pulmonary vasodilatation (without causing systemic hypotension), and improves oxygenation with dramatic results and a reduced need for ECMO. However, the potential role of iNO in 'preterm' newborns is currently controversial and remains under investigation. The recommended starting dose for iNO in term newborns is 20 ppm, and the typical duration of therapy is less than 5 days, which parallels the clinical resolution of persistent pulmonary hypertension. Babies undergoing iNO therapy require monitoring of NO$_2$ and methaemoglobin. A combination of iNO and HFOV seems to provide good results in babies with persistent pulmonary hypertension of the newborn (PPHN).

Extracorporeal membrane oxygenation

In ECMO an artificial lung circuit is used to provide 'lung rest' in babies (usually term) with reversible lung disease. Such a period of rest may allow lung recovery and help survival of the infant who has intractable respiratory failure not responding to conventional methods of respiratory support. ECMO circuits are of two types: venovenous (VV), which increases oxygen content; and venoarterial (VA), which also increase cardiac output (pump flow).

For VA bypass, the right internal jugular vein and common carotid artery are used as access points and are often ligated as a part of the bypass procedure. Venous blood is passively drained via the right atrium and passed via a roller pump to a venous capacitance reservoir (bladder box), membrane lung, heat exchanger and arterial perfusion cannula.

For VV bypass, a double-lumen cannula is used to remove and return the blood to the right atrium; the rest of the circuit is the same as in VA ECMO. To prevent thrombotic complications while on ECMO, the infant is treated with systemic heparinization.

A randomized controlled trial of ECMO versus CV in term infants with severe respiratory failure showed that ECMO was very effective in reducing mortality compared with conventional respiratory management. The developmental outcome in babies treated with ECMO was also very good.

General management of ventilated infants

The following aspects are of fundamental importance when managing ventilated infants:
• Regular arterial blood gas assessment, initially 4 hourly and less frequently as the infant stabilizes. Continuous monitoring of oxygenation with a transcutaneous PO_2 monitor and/or pulse oximetry and CO_2 with a transcutaneous PCO_2 monitor. Most of the newer ventilators now provide online continuous pulmonary graphics that can provide useful information regarding pulmonary mechanics. Avoidance of hypocapnia is important as this can impair cerebral perfusion, leading to cerebral palsy.
• Regular or continuous blood pressure monitoring with vigorous treatment of hypotension (see Chapter 16) by volume expansion with normal saline and inotropes such as dobutamine and/or dopamine.
• Regular bacteriological surveillance and appropriate use of antibiotics.
• Nutritional care through enteral feeding and/or parenteral nutrition (TPN).
• Adequate humidification of inspired gases.
• Nursing in a thermoneutral environment.

• Careful assessment of fluid balance.
• Provision of adequate analgesia and sedation.

Troubleshooting

If a sudden deterioration occurs during mechanical ventilation, then check ventilator failure, for example tube disconnection, tube blockage, accidental extubation into the oesophagus and tension pneumothorax.

When hypoxia or hypercapnia occur during ventilation it is essential to check whether a mechanical mishap or medical complication has occurred. If these factors are excluded, it may be appropriate to alter the ventilator settings.

Depending on the clinical circumstances, hypoxia would generally be defined as a PO_2 <50 mmHg (6.7 kPa); the clinical response would depend on circumstances and ventilator settings, but would include increasing F_iO_2, increasing PIP, increasing PEEP or lengthening inspiratory time.

The concept of permissive hypercapnia ($P_aCO_2 = 45–60$ mmHg) is widely accepted, but a P_aCO_2 greater than 60 mmHg would generally necessitate a change in ventilator settings, including increasing rate, increasing PIP, reducing PEEP and minimizing dead space if possible.

Analgesia and sedation

Mechanical ventilation in immature infants has been shown to be stressful, and many neonatologists sedate babies for at least some of the time that they are ventilated. An opiate (morphine or fentanyl) by continuous infusion is the most widely used sedative drug and also provides analgesia. If sedation without analgesia is required then midazolam or lorazepam is used, also by continuous infusion. These drugs may be required only for the first few days of mechanical ventilation and must be stopped before elective extubation for fear of causing respiratory depression. The use of morphine is currently the subject of some controversy, as one study (NEOPAIN study, Anand *et al.* 2004) showed an adverse neurodevelopmental outcome in those given morphine.

Some babies on CV breathe out of synchrony with the ventilator. This is often termed 'fighting the ventilator' and has been associated with the development of pneumothorax and intraventricular haemorrhage. If the baby 'fights' with vigorous out-of-phase spontaneous breaths, adequate sedation and occasionally muscle paralysis with atricurium is necessary. The newer techniques such as PTV and HFV are known to reduce this asynchrony between patient and ventilator.

Complications of mechanical ventilation

Ventilator-induced lung injury

Although life saving, the use of mechanical ventilation is associated with complications which are mostly iatrogenic and can be ameliorated by using appropriate ventilatory strategies to match the underlying pathophysiology. Various terms have been used to describe the individual components of ventilator-induced lung injury (VILI) but they are probably inter-related and likely act synergistically.

The mechanisms of VILI include:
- volutrauma (overstretching of lungs)
- atelectotrauma (incomplete expansion of lungs
- barotrauma (use of excessive inspiratory pressure)
- biotrauma (oxygen toxicity, inflammatory agents), and
- rheotrauma (turbulent and excessive gas flow)

Other complications

Other possible complications of mechanical ventilation include
- pneumothorax and pulmonary air leak
- intraventricular haemorrhage
- patent ductus arteriosus
- subglottic stenosis
- bronchopulmonary dysplasia.

SUMMARY

Respiratory disorders constitute the major workload in neonatal intensive care units. Although mostly related to prematurity, these can be associated with a variety of conditions and a significant proportion of affected babies develop respiratory failure requiring artificial respiratory support.

Moderate degrees of respiratory failure can be treated non-invasively by giving oxygen therapy and/or CPAP, which provides a continuous distending pressure and helps to improve lung volumes.

A smaller proportion of babies with severe respiratory failure require assisted mechanical ventilation, which can be given by using different ventilatory modalities. Although based on sound physiological principles, these modalities are relatively new and require further scientific validation through clinical trials.

Despite adequate ventilatory support through conventional methods, some babies may require alternative methods of treatment including high-frequency ventilation, inhaled nitric oxide therapy and extracorporeal membrane oxygenation.

Whatever method is used, one should always compare the risks and benefits in order to prevent iatrogenic complications such as VILI.

 Now visit **www.essentialneonatalmed.com** to test yourself on this chapter.

CHAPTER 16
Cardiovascular disorders

Key topics

Introduction

Congenital heart disease is one the most common significant abnormalities in the newborn and acquired cardiovascular problems are common in preterm or sick infants in the neonatal intensive care unit (NICU). A thorough understanding of the presentation and management of the common cardiovascular disorders is therefore important. This chapter focuses on the medical management of common disorders. Surgical management is not discussed as this generally takes place after the neonatal period. Nursing management is discussed thoroughly in *Nursing the Neonate*.

Link to *Nursing the Neonate*:
Nursing newborn babies with congenital heart disease.
Chapter 11.

Physiology of the cardiovascular system

The cardiovascular system undergoes major changes in the hours and days after birth. The transition of the circulation from fetal to neonatal is described in

Chapter 1. Failure of organ perfusion is a major component of many neonatal disorders, and an understanding of cardiovascular physiology is important in analysing the most appropriate management strategies.

Cardiac output

Cardiac output (CO) is the volume of blood ejected from the heart per minute. In the neonatal period pulmonary vascular resistance falls rapidly after birth, with a consequent reduction of right ventricular afterload, whereas systemic vascular resistance gradually increases, resulting in an increasing left ventricular afterload; this leads to a doubling of left ventricular stroke volume with no significant change in right ventricular stroke volume. This means cardiac output increases after birth with cardiac performance near the upper limit of its range. Cardiac output (mL/min) is defined as stroke volume (mL/beat) times heart rate (bpm):

$$CO = \text{stroke volume (SV)} \times \text{heart rate (HR)}$$

Cardiac output can only be measured directly using an invasive pulmonary artery catheter. Proxy measures use echocardiography to measure the velocity of flow through the aortic valve in conjunction with the diameter of the valve. Ultrasound cardiac output monitors are now becoming available.

Stroke volume

Stroke volume (volume ejected per heart beat) is a complicated function, dependent on the stretch undergone by individual heart myofibrils.

$$\text{stroke volume (SV)}$$
$$\sim \text{preload} + \text{afterload} + \text{contractility}$$

- **Preload.** This represents the passive stretching of the resting heart (end diastole), and is largely influenced by venous return and hence vascular volume. Starling's law states that stroke volume increases with increasing end-diastolic volume until a maximum myofibril stretch is reached. Underfilling

Table 16.1 Adrenergic receptors and effect of stimulation

Receptor	Effect
β_1	Increases myocardial contractility and heart rate
β_2	Increases pulmonary and systemic vasodilatation
α_1	Causes arteriolar constriction (vasoconstriction)
Dopaminergic	Vasodilatation in vascular beds such as the kidney, brain and gut

(reduced preload) or overfilling (increased preload) causes contraction to be less efficient.
- **Afterload.** This is the resistance to ventricular contraction distal to the ventricles. A variety of factors are involved, including peripheral vascular resistance and the viscosity of the blood.
- **Contractility.** This refers to the metabolic state of the heart muscle itself and is largely independent of both preload and afterload.

Cardiac output can be increased by increasing myocardial contractility (inotropy) or increasing the heart rate (chronotropy). These changes are mediated through α, β or dopaminergic adrenergic receptors. These effects are summarized in Table 16.1.

Blood pressure

Blood pressure (BP) is important to maintain organ perfusion. It is defined as the product of flow and resistance according to the formula:

$$BP = \text{blood flow} \times \text{peripheral resistance}$$

Normal range

Blood pressure (BP) normally varies with gestational age and postnatal age, and both need to be considered when deciding whether a baby needs treatment for low BP. The normal range against birthweight is shown in Fig. 16.1.

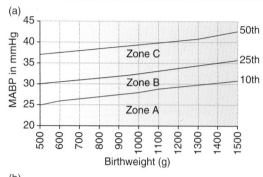

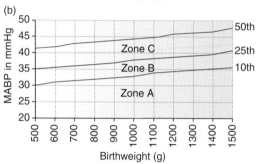

Figure 16.1 (a) Range of mean arterial blood pressure (MABP) measurements in very low birthweight infants less than 36 h of age and (b) more than 36 h old. Zone A: Hypotension requiring treatment (see Fig. 16.2). Zone B: Possible hypotension requiring clinical assessment. Zone C: BP unlikely to require treatment but clinical signs should be assessed.

Box 16.1 Consequences of failure of organ perfusion

- **Metabolic acidosis.** Tissue hypoxia leads to anaerobic metabolism and lactate production
- **Reduced urine output.** Failure to perfuse kidneys leads to oliguria or eventually anuria
- **Poor skin perfusion.** Capillary refill time (normally ≤2 s) is a good way to assess the circulation. Prolonged capillary refill may indicate shock. Mottling of the skin (cutis marmorata) occurs with prolonged underperfusion
- **Reduced conscious level.** With sever circulatory failure brain perfusion is diminished and the baby may become encephalopthic
- **Reduced gut perfusion.** The splanchnic blood vessels may vasoconstrict to maintain central BP. This relative gut ischaemia can predispose to NEC

Hypotension

Hypotension is a common and important complication of the sick newborn infant, but BP is not in itself the critical measure in which the clinician is interested. **Tissue perfusion** is essential, because once this falls below a critical limit, organ function will fail. The clinical measurement of blood flow and vascular resistance is not possible, and so BP is the physiological measurement that is used instead; see Box 16.1.

Management of hypotension

In general the mean arterial blood pressure (MABP) or the systolic BP is used to guide therapy. An open arterial duct (PDA) may cause a very low diastolic BP. A common rule of thumb is to maintain the minimum MABP above the infant's gestational age in weeks + postnatal age in days, up to 4 days of age (e.g. a 27 week infant on day 2 of life should have a MABP no lower than 29 mmHg).

The thresholds at which to consider treating hypotension by birthweight are shown in Fig 16.1.

- **Zone A.** Treatment mandatory because the BP is critically low.
- **Zone B.** Possible hypotension and potential uncertainty, as the patient may either cope without support or show signs of failing organ perfusion. If clinical signs are present, such as metabolic acidosis, decreasing peripheral perfusion, poor capillary return, poor colour and low peripheral temperature, then treatment should commence.
- **Zone C.** Satisfactory BP; treatment required only if there are obvious clinical signs of poor perfusion.

In addition to the BP measurement there are two important factors to consider:
- What is the **cause** of the hypotension? This must be identified and treated.

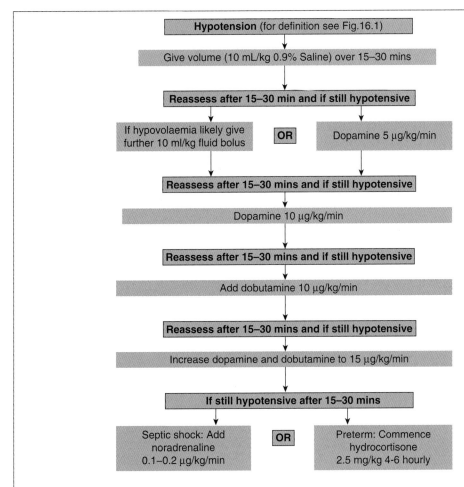

Figure 16.2 Flow diagram showing a suggested graded management response to neonatal hypotension.

• What is the **best therapeutic option** in restoring adequate BP?

In considering the first-line management of hypotension it is important to think through the possible physiological mechanisms:

- **Preload:** is the vascular compartment adequately filled? Is there volume depletion (e.g. blood loss)?
- **Afterload:** is this reduced (e.g. septic shock); should vascular resistance be increased?
- **Contractility:** is the myocardium working efficiently? Profound acidosis will affect muscle function.
- **Heart rate:** is it fast enough to maintain adequate cardiac output?

Figure 16.2 illustrates an approach to the incremental management of neonatal hypotension.

Volume replacement

Many sick premature infants are hypovolaemic. It is difficult to measure circulating blood volume, but serum electrolytes, urinary specific gravity (SG), capillary refill time and daily weight may be helpful in assessment of circulating volume. If the baby is thought to be hypotensive due to volume depletion, an infusion of either a crystalloid or colloid should be given (10 mL/kg, repeated once if necessary). There is considerable controversy as to what fluid should be used. Normal saline (0.9%) is the first-line volume expander. If the vasculature is 'leaky' both crystalloid and colloid will be rapidly lost into the tissues, causing a further osmotic loss of fluid from the vascular compartment.

Giving fluid to a baby who already has increased preload may further decompensate cardiac output. Repeated fluid boluses should not be given in the absence of hypovolaemia. Measuring central venous pressure (CVP) via a central line or assessing cardiac filling by echocardiogram can be helpful.

Inotropic agents

The action of **dopamine** depends on the dose. In low dose $(1–5\,\mu g\,kg^{-1}\,min^{-1})$ it primarily has dopaminergic actions and vasodilates the renal, coronary and possibly the cerebral circulation. In higher dose $(5–10\,\mu g\,kg^{-1}\,min^{-1})$ it stimulates β_1 receptors, enhances myocardial contractility and increases heart rate. At yet higher dosage $(10–20\,\mu g\,kg^{-1}\,min^{-1})$ the main effects are α-adrenergic, with an increase in peripheral vascular resistance and a reduction in renal blood flow (see Table 16.1)

Dobutamine $(5–20\,\mu g\,kg^{-1}\,min^{-1}$ by continuous infusion) has mainly β_2 effects, increasing BP by increasing myocardial contractility with some reduction in systemic resistance, thereby reducing afterload, which may be valuable in the failing heart. There is little effect on heart rate.

Noradrenaline (norepinephrine; $0.1–0.2\,\mu g\,kg^{-1}\,min^{-1}$ by continuous infusion) is sometimes used once dopamine and dobutamine have been given in maximum dosage. It has both α and β effects, causing an increase in contractility, tachycardia and vascular resistance. Peripheral perfusion may become compromised.

Hydrocortisone (2.5 mg/kg 4–6 hourly) can be used to treat intractable hypotension in extreme preterm infants, some of whom have adrenal dysfunction. It has a slow onset of action and is associated with small bowel perforation, but can be life-saving.

Hypertension

Neonatal hypertension is not uncommon in sick neonates. It is rarely due to essential hypertension and can be associated with congenital malformations

Table 16.2 Causes of neonatal hypertension

Vascular	Renal artery thrombosis Coarctation of the aorta
Renal	Renal vein thrombosis Renal dysplasia Obstructive uropathy Polycystic/multicystic disease
Drugs	Corticosteroids Methylxanthines
Endocrine	Congenital adrenal hyperplasia (rare forms) Phaeochromocytoma Neuroblastoma
Miscellaneous	Bronchopulmonary dysplasia Intracranial hypertension Convulsions Extracorporeal membrane oxygenation (ECMO) Essential

such as coarctation of the aorta, endocrine disorders, renal artery thrombosis, bronchopulmonary dysplasia (BPD) or steroid therapy. Table 16.2 lists the commoner causes of neonatal hypertension.

Management is directed at the underlying cause, and may sometimes include renal or aortic surgery. Thrombolysis for renal artery thrombosis remains controversial; the potential benefit (rescuing the kidney) has to be balanced against the risk of intracranial haemorrhage.

The threshold at which anti-hypertensives should be commenced is difficult to define. Empirically systolic BP >90 mmHg (diastolic >60 mmHg) in a term infant and systolic >80 mmHg (diastolic >50 mmHg) in a preterm infant should be treated. The BP should be reduced slowly. Antihypertensives used include angiotensin-converting enzyme (ACE) inhibitors (e.g. captopril), nifedipine, beta-blockers (e.g. propranolol) and hydralazine.

Congenital heart disease

Congenital heart disease (CHD) refers to abnormal structure or function of the heart from birth. Many

Table 16.3 Contribution of the commoner congenital heart malformations to neonatal congenital heart disease

Malformation	% of total
Ventricular septal defect	25
Patent ductus arteriosus	15
Atrial septal defect	15
Pulmonary stenosis	10
Aortic stenosis	5
Coarctation of the aorta	5
Transposition of the great arteries	5
Tetralogy of Fallot	5
Tricuspid atresia	1
Other individually rare conditions	14

Box 16.2 Cardiac disease in the newborn

This presents in the following ways:

- **Antenatally diagnosed:** expected complex CHD should be delivered in a cardiac centre
- **Murmur heard on routine examination** in hospital or by family doctor
- **Circulatory maladaptation at birth** (especially PPHN)
- **Cyanosis:** respiratory causes of cyanosis must be quickly excluded
- **Congestive cardiac failure:** usually left-to-right shunts (e.g. VSD, PDA) or obstructive lesions (e.g. CoA).
- **Dysrhythmias**
- **Low (postductal) oxygen saturation.**

abnormalities remain asymptomatic and undetected in the neonatal period, only to be diagnosed weeks or years later. The generally accepted incidence is approximately 8/1000 live births, and CHD is the commonest form of major congenital abnormality in developed countries. Table 16.3 lists the frequency of different congenital cardiac anomalies. With advances in second trimester ultrasound examination, 70% of major congenital heart lesions are diagnosed antenatally.

Aetiology

The aetiology of CHD is multifactorial and depends on the type of abnormality, but overall 75% have no identifiable cause. The main aetiological groups are shown in Table 16.4.

Mode of presentation

Between 25 and 60% of CHD is detected on the standard 'four-chamber' view during the 20 week anomaly scan. With specialist fetal echocardiography the detection rate can rise to 85–90%. Fetal echocardiography is not yet widely available but is recommended for those with an antenatally detected anomaly or abnormal function such as hydrops or

arrhythmia and for those with an increased nuchal translucency in the first trimester. After birth CHD is either detected by a murmur found on routine examination or by the baby developing symptoms of cyanosis or heart failure.

Heart murmur found on newborn examination

When a murmur is heard on routine examination in a healthy, asymptomatic infant, and no pathological features are present, then outpatient follow-up can be arranged. The parents will need reassurance. Most murmurs detected in the neonatal period will disappear in infancy, but if the murmur persists more than a few weeks or there are other abnormal signs then referral for echocardiography must be arranged.

Increasingly, the newborn examination includes a postductal saturation measurement, to detect duct-dependent lesions (see Chapter 6). Obstructive lesions will often present acutely as the duct closes within the first days of life. Heart failure due to left-to-right shunting presents later, at 3–6 weeks of age, as the pulmonary resistance falls. Dysrhythmias are relatively rare and may present antenatally (fetal tachycardia) or much later in childhood.

Table 16.4 Aetiological factors in congenital heart disease

Factor	Examples
Chromosomal disorders (5% of all children with CHD)	Trisomy 21: 30–40% have CHD – AVSD, VSD, ToF, ASD Trisomy 18: 90% have major cardiac defect, especially VSD Trisomy 13: 80% have major CHD – VSD Turner's syndrome: 10% have coarctation of aorta, also aortic or mitral stenosis
Single-gene defects (3% of CHD)	Noonan's syndrome: pulmonary valve stenosis Marfan's syndrome: aortic valve disease and aortic dissection Holt–Oram syndrome: VSD and ASD Williams' syndrome: supravalvular aortic stenosis DiGeorge syndrome (deletion 22q11): interrupted aortic arch, ToF Cornelia de Lange syndrome: VSD
Associations with other defects	Oesophageal atresia: VACTERL Pierre Robin: VSD CHARGE: ToF, AVSD, DORV, TGA
Polygenic	Sibling with CHD = 2–5% risk, parent with CHD = 5–10% risk
Infection	Maternal rubella infection: coarctation, VSD, PDA
Drugs and teratogens	Maternal lithium is associated with Ebstein's anomaly. Amphetamines, antimetabolites and anticonvulsants have been associated with CHD Alcohol: 30% of infants with fetal alcohol syndrome have CHD
Maternal conditions	Diabetes mellitus: VSD, TGA, hypertrophic cardiomyopathy SLE: congenital heart block

ASD, atrial septal defect; AVSD, atrioventricular septal defect; DORV, double outlet right ventricle; PDA, patent ductus arterioisus; ToF, tetralogy of Fallot; TGA, transposition of the great arteries; VSD, ventricular septal defect.

CLINICAL TIP: Saturation screening for CHD measures postductal saturations alone (<95% requires evaluation) or compares pre- and postductal SAO$_2$ (<3% drop expected). As well as detecting some duct-dependent defects, this can also pick up other sick newborns with sepsis or respiratory disorders. Remember preductal saturations must be measured on the **right** arm; see Chapter 6.

Investigations

Where there is no direct access to a paediatric cardiologist, it may be necessary to undertake basic investigations to decide which babies require referral for definitive echocardiography. These include chest radiograph, ECG and nitrogen washout test. Modern echocardiography has supplanted the need for many of these investigations but echocardiography requires considerable expertise, and is not available in all centres. Telemedicine is being used in some networks to prevent babies being transferred unnecessarily.

Chest radiograph

This is used to assess
• **Heart size.** This is assessed by measuring the cardiothoracic ratio. Cardiomegaly is seen in hypertrophy, congestive heart failure and cardiomyopathy.

• **Abnormal heart shape**, e.g. 'egg on side' for transposition of the great arteries (TGA), 'boot shaped' for tetralogy of Fallot.
• **Vascularity of lungs.** This may be difficult to interpret in the newborn, especially if taken on day 1 of life, due to residual fetal lung fluid. Increased vascularity (pulmonary plethora) suggests a left-to-right shunt, and reduced vascularity (oligaemia) suggests obstruction of right-sided flow to the lungs.
• **Position of heart.** Dextroposition is when the heart is further to the right than normal. Dextrocardia is when the apex of the heart points to the right. It may be associated with situs inversus (stomach gas bubble on the right).
• **Vertebral anomalies** that may suggest cardiac anomalies (e.g. VACTERL, Goldenhar syndrome).

Electrocardiograph (ECG)

This may be helpful in elucidating the nature of a cardiac abnormality prior to transfer to a cardiac centre for full assessment and is mandatory in the assessment of arrhythmias. In infants it is necessary to record from the V4R position (over the right nipple) as well as the traditional chest leads V1–V6. The parameters that must be assessed are listed in Box 16.3.

Nitrogen washout test

This may be helpful in distinguishing congenital cyanotic heart lesions from respiratory pathology. Arterial blood-gas estimations are performed before and after the infant has been breathing 100% oxygen (measured with an oximeter) for 10 min. In normal babies the PaO$_2$ should rise to 80 kPa

---

Box 16.3 Features to assess on the ECG

• **Heart rate.** The heart rate varies with gestational and postnatal age. Normal heart rates are 110–180 bpm in premature infants and 90–160 bpm at full-term.
• **QRS axis.** The QRS axis in neonates is further to the right than in older children, but moves to the left within the first month of life. The QRS vector is markedly abnormal in tricuspid atresia (left axis −45°). The axis is vertical (−90°) in endocardial cushion defects (AVSD).
• **P wave.** A tall P wave exceeding 3 mm in lead II indicates right atrial hypertrophy, and a broad P wave suggests left atrial hypertrophy but is rarely seen in the newborn.
• **P-R interval.** This measures the time from the onset of atrial contraction to the onset of ventricular contraction. A prolonged P-R interval indicates a degree of heart block. Normal PR interval is 0.08–0.14 s, typically 0.12 s (3 small squares). It can be shorter in preterm infants.
• **Right ventricular hypertrophy (RVH).** This is estimated from the right chest leads. The criteria for diagnosis of RVH are:
  1 upright T wave in V4R or V1 with dominant R after the first 5 days of life
  2 the voltage of R or S in V1 or V6 exceeds the normal range (approximately 10 mm)
  3 Q wave in V1
  4 right-axis deviation
• **Left ventricular hypertrophy (LVH).** This is diagnosed according to the following criteria:
  1 tall R waves in V6 (>12 mm) and deep S waves in V1 (>20 mm)
  2 a combined voltage of R in V5 or V6 and S in V1 exceeding 30 mm
  3 inverted T waves in the left chest leads – this suggests ischaemia, but digoxin may also cause this appearance
• **QT interval.** The time from the start of the q wave to the end of the T wave represents the time the ventricles take to depolarize and repolarize. It should be less than 0.44 s after correction for heart rate. In long-QT syndromes there is a risk of 'torsades de pointes' ventricular tachycardia. QT interval can be prolonged by certain drugs (e.g. erythromycin)

(600 mmHg). With intrinsic lung disease the PaO_2 increases to 20–53 kPa (150–400 mmHg), depending on the severity of disease. In the presence of cardiac abnormalities with a right-to-left intracardiac shunt there is little increase in PaO_2.

CLINICAL TIP: In centres with immediate access to a cardiologist or a neonatologist with skills in echocardiography the nitrogen washout test is no longer performed, as an echocardiogram will be a more accurate assessment of whether there is cyanotic CHD and avoids the potential danger of hyperoxia closing the arterial duct.

More specialized investigations

Echocardiography

The investigation of CHD has been revolutionized by the introduction of high-resolution, two-dimensional echocardiography. This allows the heart to be scanned in a number of standard planes, giving fine detail of anatomical structure:
- **Parasternal long-axis view** shows the left-sided structures, including left atrium, mitral valve, ventricles, septum, aortic valve and ascending aorta (Fig. 16.3a).
- **Parasternal short-axis view** shows the structure of the aortic and pulmonary valves and the main pulmonary artery (Fig. 16.3b).
- **Apical four-chamber view** shows all four chambers simultaneously – the atrioventricular (a-v) valves are particularly well seen (Fig. 16.3c).

Most abnormalities can be readily recognized by an experienced cardiologist. Cardiac Doppler with colour flow imaging is also very helpful in highlighting cardiac function and blood turbulence through small lesions. Blood flow velocity can be measured and if increased to more than 2 m/s suggests restrictive flow through a valve or vessel.

Cardiac catheterization

This is only undertaken in a specialist children's cardiac unit. Catheters are inserted via the femoral artery or vein or SVC and contrast injected under radiographic control to confirm anatomy (e.g. total anomalous pulmonary venous drainage, TAPVD). Interventional catheterization can be used to dilate stenosed valves or to insert coils to occlude a PDA. Transcatheter radioablation of an aberrant conduction pathway can be performed to prevent supraventricular tachycardia (SVT).

Cardiac catheterization in the newborn has a very low mortality rate but a significant morbidity rate, including infection and necrotising enterocolitis (NEC).

Cyanotic heart disease

Persistent central cyanosis in the newborn is usually due to respiratory or cardiac disease, but rarely may be due to persistent pulmonary hypertension, methaemoglobinaemia or shock. Central cyanosis occurs when there is more than 5 g/dL of deoxygenated haemoglobin in the blood. Apparent cyanosis can occur in the absence of hypoxia with severe polycythaemia (Hb >20 g/dL). Central cyanosis must be distinguished from peripheral cyanosis with a poor circulation due to cold, shock or hyperviscosity.

Most neonates presenting with CHD do not pose a diagnostic problem as they show central cyanosis with little or no respiratory distress. However, if there is difficulty distinguishing pulmonary disease from cyanotic CHD, a hyperoxia (nitrogen washout) test or echocardiogram should be performed.

The causes of cyanotic CHD are shown in Table 16.5. Most are due to right-to-left shunting (blood bypassing the lungs), abnormal connections (e.g. TGA or TAPVD) or 'common mixing' of oxygenated and deoxygenated blood (truncus arteriosus or a huge atrioventricular septal defect, AVSD).

Some causes of CHD rarely present in the neonatal period because the cyanosis does not develop for several months (see 'Tetralogy of Fallot' below).

An approach to the diagnosis of cyanotic CHD is shown in Fig. 16.4.

Transposition of the great arteries

TGA is the commonest heart defect presenting with cyanosis in the newborn (1 in 3500 births). The

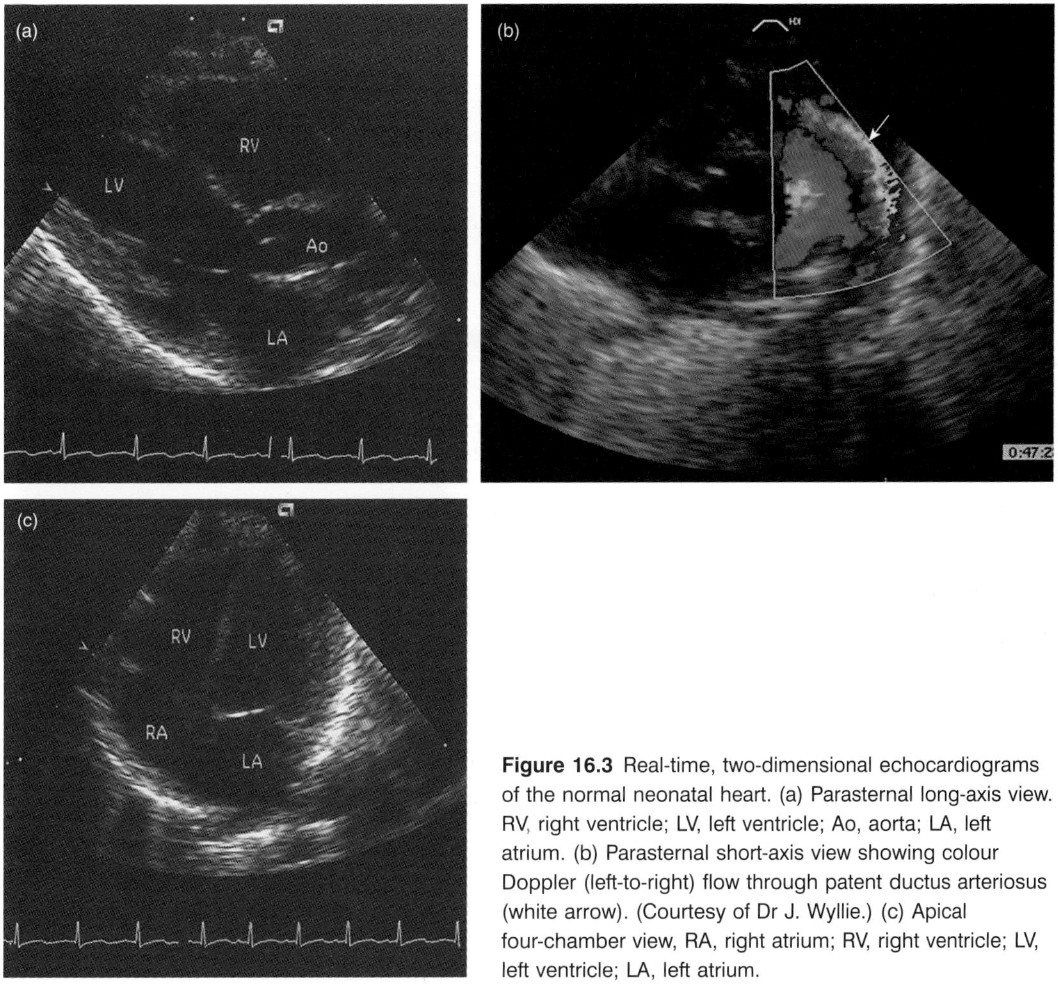

Figure 16.3 Real-time, two-dimensional echocardiograms of the normal neonatal heart. (a) Parasternal long-axis view. RV, right ventricle; LV, left ventricle; Ao, aorta; LA, left atrium. (b) Parasternal short-axis view showing colour Doppler (left-to-right) flow through patent ductus arteriosus (white arrow). (Courtesy of Dr J. Wyllie.) (c) Apical four-chamber view, RA, right atrium; RV, right ventricle; LV, left ventricle; LA, left atrium.

Table 16.5 Causes of cyanotic congenital heart disease

Restrictive pulmonary blood flow (right-to-left shunt)	Tricuspid atresia
	Pulmonary atresia or pulmonary stenosis
	Hypoplastic right heart syndrome
	ToF with severe pulmonary stenosis
	Ebstein's anomaly
Abnormal connections	TGA
	TAPVD
Common mixing	Truncus arteriosus
	Massive AVSD (usually presents with failure)

AVSD, atrioventricular septal defect; TAPVD, total anomalous pulmonary venous drainage; ToF, tetralogy of Fallot.

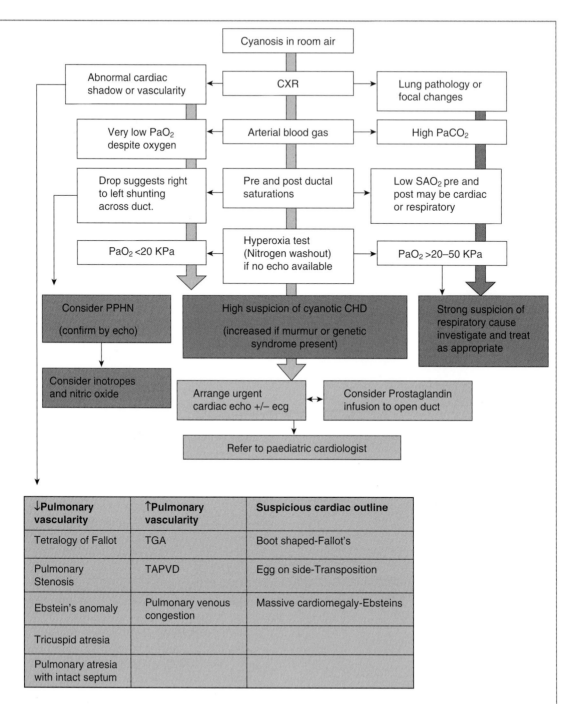

Figure 16.4 A diagnostic approach to cyanotic CHD.

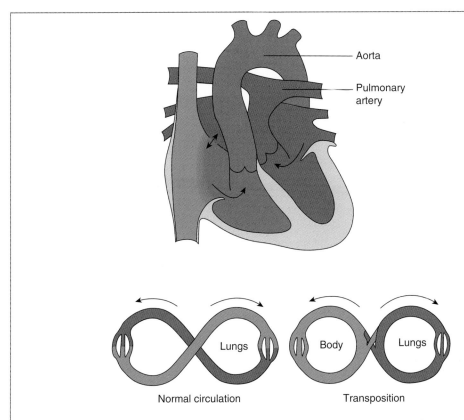

Figure 16.5 Schematic diagram of simple transposition of the great vessels without VSD.

aorta arises from the right ventricle and the pulmonary artery from the left, with the aorta lying in front of the pulmonary artery. The degree of cyanosis depends on the mixing of pulmonary and systemic blood. Without a large ventricular septal defect (VSD) or atrial septal defect (ASD) or an open duct the systemic and pulmonary circulations are totally separate and the baby will die. If a VSD is present a murmur may also be heard (see Fig. 16.5).

Investigations

There is a characteristic chest radiograph appearance with a narrow pedicle (an 'egg on its side'). The lung markings are often increased. The ECG shows right-axis deviation and right ventricular hypertrophy (RVH).

Treatment

Metabolic acidosis may be severe due to tissue hypoxaemia and should be corrected. Keeping the duct open with PGE_1 infusion is crucial. If oxygenation does not improve with prostaglandin therapy, the foramen ovale is enlarged by a balloon atrial septostomy (Rashkind procedure). Many cardiologists prefer to perform a balloon septostomy before the switch operation so that PGE_1 can be discontinued and surgery performed more electively. The treatment of choice for simple transposition is the arterial switch operation. In experienced hands this has a mortality of less than 5% and involves a full anatomical correction by switching the two major arteries and reconstructing the insertion of the coronary arteries. This is usually performed within the first 3 weeks of life. High-risk patients are those with additional cardiac lesions or low birthweight.

Tricuspid atresia

Tricuspid atresia (TA) affects 1 in 10,000 births. There is obstruction at the level of the right atrium to ventricle, often with hypoplasia of the right ventricle. It may be associated with pulmonary stenosis (PS) and a VSD. Pulmonary blood flow is often poor and the pulmonary arteries small. A systolic murmur is usually heard and the infant is severely cyanosed. Pulmonary blood flow is from the left ventricle via an open ductus arteriosus.

Investigations

On a chest radiograph there is pulmonary oligaemia but not cardiomegaly. The ECG shows left-axis deviation and left ventricular hypertrophy (LVH), and usually tall P waves in lead II. Echocardiography should confirm the diagnosis.

Treatment

Maintaining the ductus open with infusion of PGE_1 may keep the infant relatively pink so that growth can occur and a palliative shunt operation can be performed. When the child is older a further procedure will be necessary.

Pulmonary atresia or pulmonary stenosis

These conditions occur in 1 in 5000 births and involve a number of different anomalies of the pulmonary valve. TGA is present in 30% of cases of pulmonary atresia (PA). The symptoms depend on the associated cardiac abnormalities. More than 90% of babies with PA have an associated VSD. PA or stenosis with VSD is very similar to Fallot's tetralogy but usually presents earlier. Rarely the ventricular septum is intact: the right ventricle is then hypoplastic and the prognosis is very poor.

Investigations

The lung fields are oligaemic. There is right-axis deviation with right atrial and RVH on ECG if there is a coexistent VSD. LVH is seen in PA without VSD.

Treatment

PGE_1 infusion is useful to maintain the ductus open and allow pulmonary perfusion. Later the stenotic valve may be dilated or ablated by cardiac catheter or a shunt may needed to deliver blood from the right ventricle to the pulmonary artery.

Tetralogy of Fallot

Affecting 1 in 3600 births, this does not classically present with cyanosis in the newborn period, but a murmur may be detected early and on investigation some infants are found to be cyanosed. There is a combination of VSD, over-riding aorta, RVH and PS (Fig. 16.6). Treatment is ideally complete intracardiac repair in infancy, but occasionally a temporary Blalock–Taussig shunt is required as a temporary measure. The long-term prognosis following successful surgery is excellent.

Ebstein's anomaly

In this rare condition (1 in 25,000 births), there is downward displacement of the tricuspid valve into

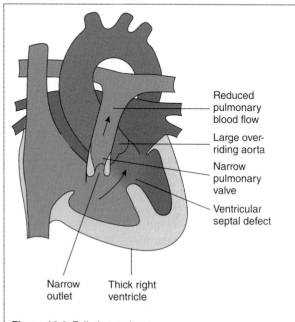

Reduced pulmonary blood flow

Large over-riding aorta

Narrow pulmonary valve

Ventricular septal defect

Narrow outlet

Thick right ventricle

Figure 16.6 Fallot's tetralogy.

the right ventricle with obstruction to pulmonary blood flow. In some it presents early with intense cyanosis and cardiac failure. The tricuspid valve is regurgitant, resulting in marked right atrial enlargement, cardiomegaly and congestive heart failure (often occurring *in utero*). Chest radiograph shows a very large heart ('wall to wall') with oligaemic lung fields. ECG is pathognomonic, with complete bundle branch block and right atrial hypertrophy (very tall P waves).

Medical management aims to support the baby through the transitional circulation by decreasing PVR with PGE$_1$ infusion, high FiO$_2$ and inhaled nitric oxide (iNO). Definitive surgical repair (valve repair and closure of ASD) follows as a multistage procedure. Further complications include *in utero* SVT and Wolff–Parkinson–White syndrome in 30%.

Total anomalous pulmonary venous drainage

In TAPVD, affecting 1 in 15,000 births, the pulmonary veins drain either directly or indirectly into the right atrium rather than the left atrium. If the drainage is obstructed, little oxygenated blood enters the right atrium and the infant is cyanosed. There is also pulmonary congestion, and sometimes cardiac failure with respiratory distress. It is one of very few CHD conditions that presents with both cyanosis and failure. It can be very difficult to distinguish from RDS and may require extensive investigation.

The anomalous pulmonary veins may be supracardiac (usually right-sided superior vena cava), cardiac (right atrium or coronary sinus), infracardiac (portal system) or mixed.

Chest radiograph shows a normal-sized heart with pulmonary oedema. Echocardiography may be diagnostic, but with severe obstruction pulmonary veins may be small and difficult to visualize even with colour flow Doppler. The diagnosis may require cardiac catheterization. Medical support with PGE$_1$, ventilation and extracorporeal membrane oxygenation (ECMO) is often necessary until neonatal surgical repair can be performed.

Prostaglandin treatment in congenital heart disease

Prostaglandin causes the ductus arteriosus to open and can be given as an emergency to any severely cyanosed infant in an attempt to improve pulmonary blood flow. There are two preparations: PGE$_1$ (alprostadil) and PGE$_2$ (dinoprostone). As the infusion starts the duct widens and if successful, the infant rapidly 'pinks up'. Doses of 10–50 ng kg^{-1} min^{-1} are given by infusion, preferably through a vein draining into the SVC. Oral therapy is usually problematic and if prolonged is associated with cortical bone proliferation. PGE$_1$ may also be life-saving in left-sided obstructive lesions, such as hypoplastic left heart and critical coarctation of the aorta, when systemic blood flow is achieved from the right ventricle through the duct.

Prostaglandins may cause pyrexia, jitteriness and apnoea in doses >15 ng kg^{-1} min^{-1}, requiring ventilation. Great care should be taken to avoid flushing the intravenous infusion, thereby giving a bolus of prostaglandin. Infants should not be transported between units on high-dose prostin without the facility to intubate and ventilate.

Congestive heart failure

Acute left ventricular failure rapidly progresses to congestive heart failure and occasionally to cardiovascular collapse. Table 16.6 lists causes of congestive cardiac failure in the neonatal period, which can be divided into left-to-right shunts, obstructive lesions or 'pump failure' (arrhythmias and cardiomyopathy).

Clinical features

Congestive heart failure causes respiratory compromise and presents with breathlessness, feeding difficulties and sometimes failure to thrive. On examination there is tachypnoea, tachycardia, recession and sometimes sweating. There is usually palpable hepatomegaly, a vigorous precordium and cardiomegaly (often only detected on chest radiograph). Other signs, such as oedema or excessive

Table 16.6 Causes of congestive heart failure in the neonatal period

Left-to-right shunts	PDA VSD AVSD Truncus arterisosus Peripheral AV malformation (e.g vein of Galen or haemangioma)
Obstructive lesions	Hypoplastic left heart syndrome Aortic stenosis Coarctation of the aorta Interrupted aortic arch Hypertrophic subaortic stenosis (especially in infant of diabetic mother)
Abnormal drainage	TAPVD
Pump failure	Transient myocardial ischaemia (with perinatal asphyxia) Viral myocarditis (especially Coxsackie, echovirus, rubella, CMV) Endocardial fibroelastosis Severe polycythaemia Hydrops fetalis (antenatal heart failure) Fluid overload Electrolyte imbalance: hypoglycaemia, hypocalcaemia Cardiomyopathy Arrhythmias

AVSD, atrioventricular septal defect; CMV, cytomegalovirus; PDA, patent ductus arteriosus; TAPVD, total anomalous pulmonary venous drainage; VSD, ventricular septal defect.

weight gain, triple or gallop rhythm, crepitations on chest auscultation, peripheral cyanosis and cardiovascular collapse, are variable. The position, quality and radiation of any murmurs may be useful in identifying the cardiac lesion.

Left-to-right shunts

Ventricular septal defect

VSD occurs as an isolated lesion in 1 in 280 live births, and accounts for 40% of all cardiac abnormalities. Lesions may vary in size, but only large defects cause symptoms in infancy. Cardiac failure due to VSD usually occurs at 4–6 weeks as the pulmonary vascular resistance naturally falls (Fig. 16.7). Usually the only sign in the first weeks of life is a murmur. About 70% will close spontaneously, especially apical muscular and small VSDs. Large defects in the membranous part of the ventricular septum will need surgical closure in early childhood, otherwise the persistently increased flow to the lungs will cause pulmonary hypertension.

Investigations

If there is a significant left-to-right shunt, the heart is enlarged on radiograph and pulmonary plethora may be seen. The ECG shows RVH and LVH. A VSD should be visible using echocardiography and flow through the defect can be measured to see whether it is 'restrictive' or not.

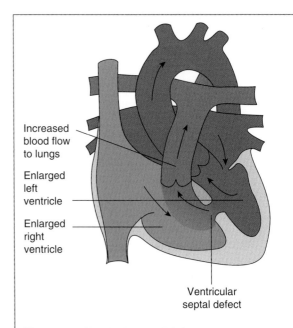

Increased blood flow to lungs

Enlarged left ventricle

Enlarged right ventricle

Ventricular septal defect

Figure 16.7 Ventricular septal defect.

Treatment

Diuretics are the first-line treatment for failure due to a VSD shunt. If growth can be achieved then a primary closure is preferable, but if there is intractable heart failure then banding of the pulmonary artery will protect the pulmonary circulation. Later surgery to patch the defect will be necessary, even after banding.

Patent ductus arteriosus

Normally the ductus arteriosus is functionally closed 10–15 h after birth and anatomically closed by 5–7 days of age. In preterm infants patency of the ductus arteriosus (PDA) is common. It is rare in term infants unless they are born at high altitude or have congenital rubella. A relatively high proportion of very preterm (<32 week) infants requiring mechanical ventilation develop delayed closure of the ductus. High fluid volumes are a major contributory factor. The incidence of PDA is commoner in those units that actively screen for it with early echocardiography.

Clinical features

Preterm infants with respiratory distress develop clinical features of a PDA within the first week or two of life, unlike term infants, who present at 4–6 weeks when the pulmonary vascular resistance has decreased.

The classic signs are bounding (collapsing) pulses, a wide pulse pressure (due to diastolic steal) and a hyperdynamic precordium with initially a systolic murmur at the upper left sternal edge. A diastolic component develops later, giving a 'machinery' murmur. If the duct is wide open there may be little audible murmur (the 'silent duct'), but the peripheral pulses are always abnormal.

Once cardiac decompensation occurs congestive heart failure develops, with tachycardia, tachypnoea, cardiomegaly, hepatomegaly, gallop rhythm and crepitations. Preterm infants with a PDA often develop increasing apnoea and ventilator and oxygen dependence and may be predisposed to NEC.

Investigations

Chest radiograph may show an enlarged heart and pulmonary oedema. The diagnosis is confirmed by echocardiography. The significance of a PDA shunt can be assessed by measuring the direction of Doppler flow, the diameter of the duct (>3 mm) (see Fig 16.3b) and the left atrial/aortic ratio (>1.3:1) (see Fig 16.3a).

Treatment

Careful fluid management with avoidance of fluid overload is essential in preventing this condition. Once evidence of a significant shunt exists, fluid restriction should be instituted. Diuretic therapy and correction of anaemia may be beneficial.

The duct can be successfully closed in about two-thirds of cases with a prostaglandin synthetase inhibitor (indometacin or ibuprofen) administered over 3–6 days. Medical closure is mostly likely to be successful within the first 2–3 weeks of life. Some units use indometacin prophylactically in the most extreme preterm infants. This has been shown to reduce the risk of significant intraventricular haemorrhage (IVH) but can have complications as indometacin has an effect on all vascular beds, reducing renal, gut and cerebral blood flow. Indometacin is contraindicated in NEC, thrombocytopenia, renal impairment, and severe unconjugated hyperbilirubinaemia. Ibuprofen has been shown to be as effective as indometacin in closing the duct, with fewer complications for the renal vascular bed.

If medical closure fails and the infant remains ventilator dependent owing to the large left-to-right shunt, then surgical ligation is necessary. This involves applying a clip across the PDA. In some cardiac centres this may be undertaken on the NICU to avoid moving an already unstable baby.

Obstructive lesions

Hypoplastic left heart

In this condition, affecting 1 in 5500 births, there is failure of development of the left atrium and ventricle and the aortic and mitral valves are usually

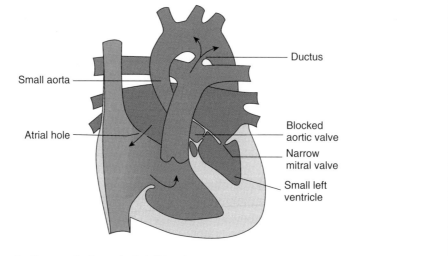

Figure 16.8 Schematic diagram of a hypoplastic left heart.

atretic (Fig. 16.8). The ascending aorta is hypoplastic and blood reaches the systemic circulation retrogradely through the duct. The infant usually develops severe cardiac failure in the first week of life. The pulses are weak and there is often cyanosis with pallor and marked hepatomegaly.

Clinical presentation

Typically this is diagnosed antenatally, after which a specialized neonatal team manages a metabolically stable infant with PGE_1. Alternatively, the infant may present with mild heart failure or a profound circulatory collapse with multiorgan failure and acidosis after the ductus arteriosus closes.

Investigations

Chest radiograph shows a large heart with plethoric lung fields. The ECG, if performed, shows little left ventricular activity and RVH. Echocardiography confirms the diagnosis.

Treatment

Infants with a prenatal diagnosis should be delivered in a cardiac centre. Palliative surgery is offered to establish a viable, haemodynamically stable heart.

This may require a series of operations in the first 2 years of life. In some centres cardiac transplantation is performed following palliative management if the brain and other organs are intact. Before surgical management is considered parents must be fully counselled regarding the mortality risks associated with stage 1 reconstruction (Norwood procedure), followed by two further cardiac operations and very likely a heart transplant and some degree of cognitive impairment.

Coarctation of the aorta

Coarctation of the aorta (CoA) affects 1 in 2500 births. It is an anatomical narrowing of the descending aorta, most commonly at the site of the ductus arteriosus, and is normally associated with bicuspid aortic valve (in 80%) and VSD (in 40%). If outflow obstruction is severe, then cardiac failure occurs in infancy. Blood has to enter the descending aorta retrogradely through the ductus arteriosus, but if the latter closes then the infant rapidly deteriorates, presenting with breathlessness, shock and cardiac failure. The femoral pulses are weak and the BP considerably higher in the arms than in the legs. The right-to-left shunt across the duct means that oxygen saturation measurements are lower in the legs than the right arm (preductal). About half of patients with CoA have a VSD or aortic stenosis, and a murmur is usually audible.

Investigations

Radiographs show a large heart with pulmonary plethora. ECG reveals severe RVH with little evidence of left ventricular activity. Echocardiography can confirm the diagnosis, but excluding CoA is difficult while the PDA is open. MRI is useful in showing the extent of the coarctation, as well as the presence of hypoplasia of the ascending aorta. Balloon angioplasty of the aorta may be remarkably successful.

Treatment

At presentation an infusion of PGE_1 may be life-saving in maintaining ductal flow. Dopamine infusion ($5\,\mu g\,kg^{-1}\,min^{-1}$) will improve compromised renal blood flow. If CoA is suspected antenatally then the child should be delivered in a cardiac centre, where if asymptomatic they may be monitored with serial echocardiography and regular assessment of the femoral pulses as the duct closes.

Aortic stenosis

Aortic stenosis affects 1 in 4500 births, but rarely presents in the neonatal period unless it is very severe, when it is likely to be associated with a hypoplastic left ventricle. The prognosis is poor, although PGE_1 and balloon septostomy or urgent balloon valvotomy may help to stabilize the patient. Critical aortic stenosis has a gradient between the left ventricle and ascending aorta of 60 mmHg or more, and usually there is severe obstruction *in utero* with marked LVH and endocardial fibroelastosis. The presentation is with congestive heart failure and shock due to severe myocardial dysfunction.

Management of congestive heart failure

General management

Supportive treatment consists of oxygen therapy and respiratory support as required, elevation of the head of the cot, correction of metabolic acidosis with sodium bicarbonate and nasogastric tube feeding with high energy milk or supplemented expressed breast milk (EBM).

Blood transfusion

An increase in oxygen to the tissues can best be obtained by ensuring an adequate haemoglobin concentration. The haemoglobin should be maintained at over 12 g/dL in the acute phase. Diuretic cover should be given, if there is already evidence of heart failure.

Diuretics

Furosemide in a dose of 1 mg/kg is the usual diuretic used in acute heart failure. Maintenance diuretic therapy consists of furosemide 2 mg/kg per day and spironolactone 2 mg/kg per day, with electrolyte monitoring. Fluid restriction to 100–120 mL/kg per day will act as an adjunct to other therapies, but calorie intake must be maintained.

Captopril, an ACE inhibitor, can reduce afterload and may be of value in patients who continue to show signs of cardiac failure after maximum diuretic therapy. Captopril causes a fall in BP, which must be carefully monitored.

Dysrhythmias

The newborn infant is subject to disorders of cardiac rate and rhythm, some of which may be detected before birth during antepartum monitoring. Many are transient, especially following birth asphyxia and birth trauma.

The most important dysrhythmias in the newborn are:
- supraventricular tachycardia (SVT)
- congenital atrioventricular block
- ventricular tachycardia and fibrillation.

Supraventricular tachycardia

SVT is the commonest form of tachycardia and is increasingly recognized *in utero* as a result of cardiotocography (CTG) monitoring and real-time ultrasound examinations. Prolonged fetal SVT leads to congestive cardiac failure and hydrops fetalis. If it is considered necessary to treat the fetus medically, the mother may be given an anti-arrhythmic drug such as amiodarone, flecainide or digoxin.

In the newborn SVT may be idiopathic or due to irritation of the sinoatrial node by inadvertent catheterization of the right atrium during central line insertion. Heart failure may develop after a few hours, and treatment includes one of the following:
• Vagal stimulation by application of an ice pack applied to the face.
• Adenosine, by rapid bolus injection via a UVC, is the drug of choice in treating neonatal SVT.
• Synchronized DC cardioversion (0.5 J/kg).

Once sinus rhythm is restored, maintenance treatment may be necessary with flecainide or amiodorone. An interval ECG may demonstrate the Wolff–Parkinson–White syndrome (short P-R interval and a wide QRS complex). All neonates with SVT should be referred to a cardiologist for further investigation.

Congenital heart block

In 50% of cases this is due to a major congenital cardiac anomaly, such as TGA or Ebstein's anomaly. Some cases are associated with maternal systemic lupus erythematosus (see Chapter 4). Heart block is only likely to cause clinical problems in the newborn period if it is complete (third degree) and associated with profound bradycardia (<60 bpm). Treatment is initially with an infusion of isoprenaline to increase the heart rate. A number of cases are transient and recover fully, but in some infants an electronic pacemaker may be necessary.

Ventricular tachycardia and fibrillation

If these occur they must be rapidly recognized and efficiently treated to avoid cerebral ischaemia. The commonest cause of ventricular **tachycardia** is hyperkalaemia (Chapter 18). This occurs spontaneously in some critically ill very low birthweight infants and may develop if the potassium level exceeds 7.5 mmol/L. Treatment of the tachycardia includes
• calcium gluconate (10%) IV under ECG control
• correction of acidosis with sodium bicarbonate infusion

• lidocaine (lignocaine) IV bolus /infusion
• cardioversion (4 J/kg).

Usually calcium gluconate is successful in reverting the ventricular tachycardia to sinus rhythm. The treatment of hyperkalaemia is discussed on p. 234, Chapter 18. Ventricular **fibrillation** should be treated with external cardiac massage and non-synchronized DC cardioversion. The cause (hypothermia, drugs or electrolyte imbalance) must be urgently corrected.

Cardiomyopathy

Dilated cardiomyopathy (heart muscle dysfunction) can arise either secondary to prolonged dysrrythmia (see above) or due to hypoxia (anomalous insertion of the coronary arteries) or as part of a metabolic storage disorder. Infective myocarditis (enterovirus, parvovirus or adenovirus) should also be excluded.

Infants of diabetic mothers may develop severe hypertrophic obstructive cardiomyopathy (HOCM) secondary to high fetal insulin levels. A similar condition develops after prolonged high-dose steroid therapy. Both can cause left ventricular outflow tract obstruction, though this usually resolves over 3–6 months. Autosomal dominant HOCM does not usually present in the neonatal period.

Circulatory maladaptation at birth

The normal changes in the circulation occurring at birth are described in Chapter 1. Interruption of this normal transition in preterm infants commonly leads to persistence of the PDA. In term infants and those with sepsis, maladaptation can result in persistent pulmonary hypertension of the newborn (PPHN).

Persistent pulmonary hypertension of the newborn

Conditions that interfere with normal oxygenation or lung expansion after birth may delay the physiological drop in pulmonary vascular resistance, resulting in PPHN. Failure of the pulmonary vascular resistance to fall, with persistence of the intracardiac shunts, leads to severe hypoxia and cyanosis, which further exacerbates the problem.

The normal tone of pulmonary arterioles is in a fine balance, depending on the opposing influence of vasoconstrictors (e.g. leukotrienes, endothelin-1) and vasodilators (iNO, prostacyclins). It is now recognized that iNO has the major influence on pulmonary vasodilatation after birth. When there is a shunt present (e.g. PDA), pulmonary flow depends on the balance between pulmonary and systemic vascular resistance.

Aetiology

PPHN can have various causes, broadly categorized as primary or secondary: see Table 16.7.

Clinical features

The clinical features depend on the underlying cause, but affected babies usually present shortly after birth with cyanosis and respiratory distress (tachypnoea, grunting and recession). In some cases cyanosis may be delayed by several hours, and may initially be intermittent, with wide fluctuations in PaO_2 from normal to severe hypoxia due to arteriolar lability.

Arterial blood gases show hypoxaemia, acidaemia and variable hypercarbia. These infants resemble those with cyanotic CHD. Untreated, their hypoxaemia may become extreme, despite assisted ventilation with high inspiratory pressures. In the survivors the respiratory distress decreases after some days.

It has been suggested that the conditions listed in Box 16.4 should be satisfied before a diagnosis of PPHN can be made.

Management

Management should be directed towards treating the underlying cause of the PPHN (e.g infection) if this can be identified, as well as strategies aimed to reverse the right-to-left shunting.

General principles

• Correct any hypothermia, hypocalcaemia, hypomagnesaemia or hypoglycaemia.
• Correct metabolic acidosis.

Table 16.7 Aetiology of persistent pulmonary hypertension of the newborn

Aetiology	Examples
Primary (idiopathic)	Primary muscular hypertrophy of pulmonary arterioles. Accounts for 20% Alveolar-capillary dysplasia (V-Q mismatch)
Secondary to lung disease	Diaphragmatic hernia and pulmonary hypoplasia Meconium aspiration syndrome Severe RDS Chronic lung disease (baby develops late onset pulmonary hypertension)
Secondary to infection	Pneumonia Group B streptococcal infection or other systemic perinatal sepsis
Secondary to impaired physiological circulatory transition after birth	Metabolic acidosis secondary to tissue hypoxia (usually following perinatal asphyxia) Hypothermia Metabolic disturbance: hypoglycaemia or hypocalcaemia Polycythaemia with hyperviscocity (PCV >0.65–0.7)
Drug induced	Antenatal or very early postnatal exposure to prostaglandin synthetase inhibitors (e.g. ibuprofen, aspirin)

• Treat polycythaemia (packed cell volume (PCV) >65%) with a partial exchange transfusion.
• Correct systemic hypotension with volume expanders, and inotropes.

Specific management

• Provide sufficient oxygen to maintain PaO_2 at 9–13 kPa (70–100 mmHg). Clinicians frequently target higher PaO_2 levels of >13 kPa (100 mmHg) but there is no evidence for this practice.
• Ventilatory support should be used to treat hypoxia if the PaO_2 is <7 kPa (50 mmHg) in 100%

> ## Box 16.4 Diagnostic criteria for persistent pulmonary hypertension of the newborn
>
> - **Severe hypoxia** (disproportionate to the degree of lung disease):
> PaO_2 <6 kPa (<44 mmHg) in 100% inspired oxygen and appropriate ventilation
>   CXR may show oligaemic lung fields or underlying pathology (e.g. MAS, CDH)
> - **Suprasystemic pulmonary BP:** Can be estimated from ductal flow velocity or tricuspid regurgitation velocity using echocardiography and invasive arterial blood pressure monitoring via UAC
> - **Normal cardiac anatomy:** Cyanotic CHD should be excluded by echocardiography
> - **Evidence of right-to-left shunting:**
>   Bidirectional flow across a PDA or foramen ovale on echocardiography
>   Drop between pre- and postductal oxygen saturation measurements
>
> CDH, congenital diaphragmatic hernia; CXR, chest radiograph; MAS, meconium aspiration syndrome; PDA, patent ductus arteriosus; UAC, umbilical arterial catheter

oxygen. Both respiratory and metabolic alkalosis lower pulmonary vascular resistance in animal models. However, these therapies are controversial in neonates because very low $PaCO_2$ levels are associated with neurodevelopment, sernsorineural hearing loss and volutrauma to lungs. $PaCO_2$ should be kept in the low–normal range and certainly above 4 kPa. Therapeutic metabolic alkalosis is not well studied in neonates. HFOV ventilation (see Chapter 15) is recommended as it can achieve maximal oxygenation with the lowest pulmonary vascular resistance.

- It is vital to ensure an adequate systemic BP. Right-to-left shunting can be reduced by increasing the systemic (left-sided) BP and therefore maintaining a gradient above the pulmonary pressure. Inotrope infusion (dopamine and/or dobutamine) is given to increase the systemic BP by at least 20%, typically to over 50 mmHg in term infants.
- Reduce the pulmonary pressure using pulmonary vasodilators. These are discussed below.
- Extracorporeal membrane oxygenation (ECMO). This therapy is aimed at supporting the cardiorespiratory system until pulmonary hypertension settles. It is therefore only indicated for potentially recoverable conditions. It is not recommended for structural pulmonary hypoplasia but is used in some centres for stabilization of severe pulmonary hypertension associated with diaphragmatic hernia. A randomized study has shown clearly that the outcome in term babies with severe respiratory

failure is twice as good with ECMO than with conventional ventilatory techniques.

> CLINICAL TIP: Boosting the systemic BP with inotropes can be a vital intervention in PPHN, especially if the baby is in a smaller centre that does not have immediate access to nitric oxide. It is as important as pulmonary vasodilatation in reversing right-to-left shunting, but is often overlooked.

Pulmonary vasodilators

The pulmonary artery pressure in PPHN is by definition higher than the systemic pressure, and right-to-left shunting occurs through the ductus arteriosus and/or the foramen ovale for at least part of the cardiac cycle. For therapy to be successful, this shunt must be reduced by selectively reducing the pulmonary vascular resistance while maintaining (or even boosting) systemic vascular resistance.

- **Inhaled nitric oxide (iNO)** is a specific pulmonary vasodilator and has replaced other non-selective agents as the first-line pulmonary vasodilator. iNO is effective in the management of PPHN when given in low concentrations through the ventilator circuit. The therapeutic dose is 5–20 ppm. Careful monitoring is necessary, as methaemoglobinaemia may occur with higher concentrations. Nitric oxide is contraindicated in conditions that rely on right-to-left shunting (e.g. CoA).

• **Other pulmonary vasodilators.** Prostacyclin, tolazaline and magnesium sulphate will all cause pulmonary vasodilatation and are sometimes used in the immediate management of severe PPHN in units that do not have access to iNO. However, due to their intravenous administration their actions are much less specific to the pulmonary circulation and they can cause systemic hypotension which can be counterproductive. Intravenous sildenafil is also being used for severe PPHN, but usually as a follow-on treatment after nitric oxide. Milrinone (a selective phosphodiesterase inhibitor) has been used successfully when PPHN is resistant to nitric oxide.

Up to 70% of major congenital heart lesions are diagnosed antenatally, but the baby with suspected CHD can still present an urgent diagnostic challenge soon after birth. Some regions have embraced screening for duct-dependent CHD by measuring post ductal oxygen saturations in all babies within the first 24 h. Echocardiography conducted by an experienced cardiologist usually provides an accurate diagnosis of neonatal CHD, and increasingly neonatal intensivists are developing basic echocardiography skills to guide their management. If cyanotic CHD is suspected then a PGE$_1$ infusion should be commenced immediately to keep the ductus arteriosus patent and improve pulmonary blood flow. PGE1 infusion may also be life-saving for left heart obstructive lesions by providing systemic blood flow from the right ventricle through the ductus arteriosus. Congestive heart failure needs early recognition, supportive care, diuretic therapy prior to definitive interventional or surgical management. Inhaled nitric oxide is a specific pulmonary vasodilator and has revolutionized the immediate management of PPHN.

SUMMARY

 Now visit **www.essentialneonatalmed.com** to test yourself on this chapter.

CHAPTER 17

Gastrointestinal and abdominal disorders

Key topics

Introduction

Normal structural and functional development of the gastrointestinal tract is essential for life. Malformations can occur anywhere from the mouth to the anus. Many of these can now be identified on antenatal ultrasound and there are some specific abnormalities that only present in the neonatal period. Normal coordination of suck and swallow does not appear until 34 weeks' gestation and as a result feeding difficulties are one of the most common clinical problems encountered in the neonatal nursery. This chapter aims to give a broad overview of the specific conditions that affect the gastrointestinal tract in the neonatal period.

Development of the gastrointestinal tract

The gastrointestinal (GI) tract develops 4 weeks after conception as a tube from mouth to cloaca. The lip is normally fused by 5 weeks and the palate by 8–9 weeks. Part of the foregut differentiates into trachea and oesophagus, and disorders of development at this stage cause oesophageal atresia, usually with tracheo-oesophageal fistula. The lower bowel initially opens into the yolk sac and later forms the vitello-intestinal duct. The midgut forms a loop, which protrudes from the abdominal cavity and then re-enters the abdomen after turning through

270°. Failure of the bowel to re-enter the abdomen causes exomphalos, and failure to twist leads to malrotation. During the sixth week of gestation a septum separates the cloaca into rectum and urogenital sinus. The gut then ruptures through the perineum to form an anus. The liver and pancreas develop from the gut endoderm at the same time as the duodenum is formed. The gut is fully differentiated by 20 weeks.

Functional development

Motility

Bowel motility is present from 16 weeks' gestation but is not fully functional until 36 weeks. The passage of meconium *in utero* is rare before 34 weeks' gestation. Functional intestinal obstruction or paralytic ileus are common findings in premature infants due to this disorganized bowel motility.

Swallowing

The fetus begins to swallow liquor at around 16 weeks' gestation. This is an important factor in the regulation of amniotic fluid volume (see Chapter 1). If the upper gastrointestinal tract is not patent then polyhydramnios will develop. Although the preterm infant can swallow, nutritive suck and swallow does not start to become coordinated until 34 weeks' gestation. Almost all preterm infants will require nasogastric or orogastric tube feeding until their coordinated suck–swallow is established. Gastro-oesophageal reflux is common, especially in the preterm infant, because of low gastrooesophageal sphincter pressures and transient relaxations of the sphincter.

Carbohydrate absorption

Disaccharidase activity in the small bowel is low at term and gradually increases to mature levels by 10 months of age. In the preterm baby maltase is the first disaccharidase to reach reasonable activity, followed by sucrase and then lactase. Lactase deficiency is common before 30 weeks' gestation, with consequent lactose intolerance in these infants.

Fat absorption

Bile salts are essential for fat absorption but are themselves not readily absorbed. Fat malabsorption in the newborn may occur because of reduced bile salts. In infants below 1300 g birthweight, 70–75% of dietary fat is absorbed. Premature infants are better able to absorb polyunsaturated fats (present in excess in human milk) than saturated fats. Some degree of physiological steatorrhoea is therefore normal in preterm infants. Premature infants cope better with the absorption of medium-chain triglyceride fats than long-chain fatty acids.

Secretions

Gastric acid secretion does not occur to any significant degree before 32 weeks' gestation. Pancreatic secretions of lipase are adequate for dietary needs by full term, but trypsin is often deficient, resulting in relative protein malabsorption.

Malformations

Malformations of the gastrointestinal tract can occur anywhere from the mouth to the anus.

Cleft lip and palate

Cleft lip and palate are the most common congenital anomalies of the craniofacial region. Cleft lip or palate may occur in isolation but they are found together in up to 70% of cases. The lip and palate normally fuse by about 6 weeks' gestation. Cleft lip may be unilateral (70% on left side) or bilateral. Clefts in the palate can have one of three forms:

- **Complete**, involving the hard and soft palate, and may involve the alveolar margin. It may be unilateral, bilateral or involve the midline.
- **Submucosal**, a bony defect completely covered by mucosa, and often a bifid uvula.
- **Simple clefts** of the soft palate only.

Cleft lip and palate have been associated with maternal anticonvulsant therapy, and also occur in the fetal alcohol syndrome. Many clefts will be diagnosed on antenatal ultrasound.

CLINICAL TIP: Severe midline facial clefts may be associated with intracranial anomalies, including holoprosencephaly, and are a feature of trisomy 13. In these severe cases, other lesions need to be excluded such as hypoglycaemia, panhypopituitarism and hypothyroidism.

Management

Management is best undertaken by a multidisciplinary team involving plastic surgeons; ear, nose and throat surgeons; orthodontists; speech pathologists; psychologists; audiologists and specialist nurses. If the diagnosis is made antenatally, arrangements should be made to talk to someone from the team before delivery.

The infant often has an unattractive appearance at birth and time must be spent with the parents talking to them about the condition. Photographs of treated cases showing the preoperative and postoperative appearances are particularly helpful in allaying parental anxieties (Fig. 17.1).

Feeding is usually a problem, particularly if there is a cleft palate, because the baby is unable to achieve adequate suction, with resultant regurgitation of milk through the nose. Aspiration of milk can cause recurrent pneumonitis. Feeding can often be successfully facilitated with the help of a speech therapist. A special teat may be required. The careful use of a squeeze bottle aids suction in many infants. In some cases the fitting of an acrylic dental obturator around the edges of the palate is helpful.

Most surgeons prefer to repair the lip in the first 6–12 weeks of life, but very early closure in the first week is recommended by some. Surgical closure of the palate is normally attempted at 9–12 months before speech has developed. Long-term complications of cleft lip and palate are listed in Table 17.1.

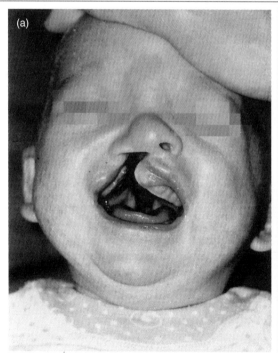
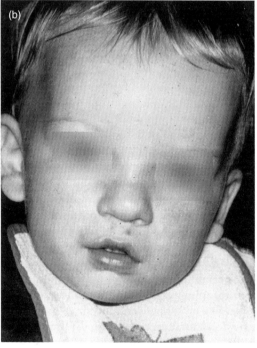

Figure 17.1 Cleft lip. At birth the infant has a right-sided cleft lip (a). The same infant following repair (b).

Table 17.1 Long-term complications of cleft lip and palate	
Speech and language	Problems include nasal escape and articulation. A speech therapist should always be closely involved in the management of these children
Hearing	Eustachian tube function is usually impaired, predisposing the child to middle ear infections. Regular hearing assessment and ENT supervision are essential
Dental	Tooth development is often delayed and there may be malocclusion
Local ulceration	Ulceration may be due to poorly fitting acrylic plates

Reoccurrence risk

It is usually of polygenic inheritance and has a higher frequency in some families. Cleft palate is associated with DiGeorge syndrome which is autosomal dominant with a 50% reoccurrence risk. The risk of recurrence in subsequent pregnancies is about 3–5%. It is more common in the pregnancies of older mothers. Recurrence risk counselling is affected by whether the lesion is unilateral or bilateral, is associated with cleft palate, and if other first-degree relatives are affected. Cleft lip with or without cleft palate is associated with a broader pattern of altered morphogenesis in 35% of cases.

CLINICAL TIP: Pierre Robin sequence is the association of cleft palate (hard or soft) with micrognathia. The small jaw allows the tongue to prolapse backwards, thereby obstructing the airway and leading to cyanotic spells. The infant should be nursed prone to prevent airway obstruction. A nasopharyngeal airway may be required in severe cases.

Intestinal obstruction

The causes of obstruction may be classified depending on the site of blockage (large or small bowel) or whether it is anatomical or functional. Causes of intestinal obstruction are listed in Table 17.2. On occasions it is impossible to be sure of the diagnosis or even the level of obstruction, and laparotomy may be the only way of making a diagnosis in order to treat the condition effectively. Intestinal obstruction occurs in about 1/1000 babies. If the obstruction is in the upper gastrointestinal tract it is often associated with maternal polyhydramnios. If more than 25 mL of fluid is aspirated from the stomach after birth, intestinal obstruction should also be suspected.

CLINICAL TIP: Occasionally, bile-stained amniotic fluid from intrauterine vomiting may be confused with meconium-stained liquor.

Clinical features

The infant with intestinal obstruction may present with some or all of the following features:
- **Bile-stained vomiting.** This is a very important sign that must not be ignored. A history of bile-stained vomiting demands immediate investigation as it suggests obstruction is below the second part of the duodenum. Sporadic bile-stained vomiting suggests partial obstruction caused by malrotation, duplication or annular pancreas.
- **Abdominal distension.** This may not be prominent with a high obstruction.
- **Visible peristalsis.**
- **Delayed passage of meconium.** In cases of low obstruction there may be no passage of meconium at all. With a high obstruction meconium may be passed for a day or two. A changing stool is never seen with congenital bowel obstruction. Anal atresia should be recognized early at routine examination (see below).

Table 17.2 Types of intestinal obstruction in the newborn

Congenital	Acquired	Functional
Intrinsic		
Atresias – oesophageal, duodenal, small bowel, colonic	Necrotizing enterocolitis Intussusception Peritoneal adhesions	Hirschsprung's disease Meconium plug syndrome
Stenoses		
Anorectal malformation		Ileus
Meconium ileus		Peritonitis
Enteric duplications		
Extrinsic		
Volvulus		Intestinal pseudo-obstruction syndrome
Peritoneal bands		
Annular pancreas		
Cysts and tumours		
Incarcerated hernia		

• **Dehydration.** The infant may present with dehydration and collapse as the result of excessive vomiting.

Investigations and management

The following investigations and management options apply in cases of suspected intestinal obstruction.
• Obstetric ultrasound as early as 17–19 weeks might reveal suspicious features such as polyhydramnios, 'double bubble' or echogenic bowel.
• Initial abdominal radiographs should be plain films with infant in the supine and left lateral positions:
    duodenal obstruction shows a 'double bubble'
    distal obstruction shows a series of dilated air- and fluid-filled loops of intestine
    meconium ileus usually has no air/fluid levels but sometimes a 'soap bubbles' appearance.
• Withhold feeds, insert IV and nasogastric replogle (double-lumen) tube.

• Consult paediatric surgeon if obstruction confirmed or suspected.
• If diagnosis is in doubt or meconium ileus suspected, a contrast enema is performed: **microcolon** suggests small bowel atresia or meconium ileus.
• An upper gastrointestinal contrast study is performed if plain film and contrast enema are non-diagnostic.

Malrotation (volvulus neonatorum)

This results from incomplete fixation and rotation of the bowel after it returns to the fetal abdominal cavity from the yolk sac between the eighth and tenth weeks of gestation. The three features of malrotation are:
• the duodenojejunal junction is at or to the right of the vertebral column
• the ileocaecal junction is near the midline and higher than normal
• the bowel is abnormally fixed by avascular (Ladd's) bands, which cross the second part of the duodenum.

These abnormalities cause the small bowel mesentery, in which the superior mesenteric artery lies, to be abnormally mobile and to twist around its axis, leading to a volvulus with rapid impairment of gut blood flow. This may cause intestinal obstruction in one of two ways:

- **strangulation obstruction:** the superior mesenteric artery supplying blood to the bowel is occluded
- **Ladd's bands** obstruct the second part of the duodenum.

Midgut volvulus can occur at any time but 80% of cases occur in the neonatal period or *in utero*.

Diagnosis

This lesion characteristically produces episodic obstruction with abdominal distension, bile-stained vomiting, pallor and a vague abdominal mass in an infant who was previously tolerating feeds well. The baby may rapidly proceed to shock.

Plain radiography of the abdomen in the erect position may show a characteristic double bubble, but gas is seen beyond the duodenum. Contrast studies may show a corkscrew duodenum or an abnormally situated subhepatic position of the caecum. Ultrasound scan may show an abnormal relationship between the superior mesenteric artery and vein strongly suggestive of malrotation.

Treatment

Laparotomy needs to be performed urgently to untwist and relieve the volvulus. It may be difficult to exclude volvulus clinically and, in view of the rapidity with which bowel infarction occurs, an early laparotomy is advisable in suspected cases.

Pyloric stenosis

Vomiting (often projectile) is the predominant symptom in this condition which occurs between birth and 6 months of age. It most commonly presents between weeks 3–5 as vomiting after feeding. The vomitus contains partially digested milk but no bile. Gastric peristalsis may be seen. Preterm infants will often present with pyloric stenosis prior to hospital discharge. The condition is due to hypertrophy of the pylorus. A pyloric mass is sometimes palpable in the right upper quadrant, particularly in cases where diagnosis has been delayed. There is often a family history, and boys are affected four times more often than girls. The cause of the hypertrophy is not known, but may be related to stress in a genetically susceptible infant. Incidence is 1/1000 to 1/3000. The risk for subsequent siblings is about 7%. Diagnosis is made using ultrasound examination and finding the pylorus 3 mm or more in thickness.

Treatment is surgical following adequate restoration of electrolyte and fluid balance and correction of metabolic alkalosis. At surgery the muscle fibres of the hypertrophied pylorus are incised down to the mucosa. This is known as Ramstedt's procedure and is performed via a periumbilical incision or laparoscopically.

Duodenal obstruction

Complete duodenal obstruction presents early with vomiting, which will be bile stained if the obstruction is below the second part of the duodenum. Duodenal obstruction may be due to either intrinsic or extrinsic obstruction (see Table 17.3). Partial duodenal obstruction, such as occurs with malrotation, may be more difficult to diagnose, as vomiting may be intermittent and stools may be normal.

Table 17.3 Causes of duodenal obstruction	
Duodenal atresia	50% are associated with Down's syndrome but other associations include other bowel atresias, and cardiovascular and anorectal malformations
Duodenal stenosis	Septum or membrane
Malrotation	May cause the second part of the duodenum to be obstructed by Ladd's peritoneal bands
Annular pancreas	May cause extrinsic obstruction to the duodenum

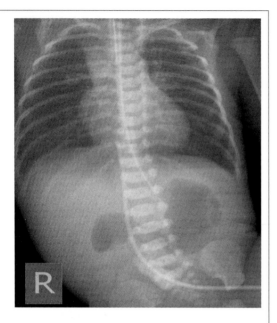

Figure 17.2 Duodenal atresia. Abdominal radiograph showing the 'double bubble' appearance.

Diagnosis

A plain radiograph of the abdomen classically shows a 'double bubble' appearance (Fig. 17.2) in duodenal atresia. If there is no air beyond this double bubble, then the diagnosis of duodenal atresia is certain and no further investigations are required. Small bubbles of air beyond the second part of the duodenum suggest an incomplete bowel obstruction and must be investigated further for malrotation. Duodenal atresia is a common finding in babies with trisomy 21.

Treatment

After resuscitation with fluids and electrolytes, definitive surgical repair is performed. Postoperatively these infants often require prolonged total parenteral nutrition because of poor peristaltic activity across the anastomosis. Often the dilated proximal duodenum is tapered to reduce the duodenal dysmotility. Passage of a transduodeno-duodenostomy feeding tube may facilitate earlier enteral feeding. Presence of duodenal atresia should prompt screening for trisomy 21.

Jejunal and ileal atresia

Half of all intestinal atresias occur in the jejunum or ileum. Rarely they are associated with gastroschisis, intrauterine volvulus or meconium ileus.

The jejunum is the commonest site for intestinal atresia. The atretic segment may be isolated or multiple. The diagnosis is often made on prenatal ultrasound examination. After birth the infant rapidly develops marked abdominal distension, and the radiograph shows loops of dilated bowel with multiple fluid levels. Peritoneal calcification signifies the presence of meconium peritonitis. Treatment is by resection of the atretic segment, but sacrifice of grossly dilated bowel above the stricture may be necessary before primary anastomosis is possible.

Colonic atresia

Less than 10% of bowel atresias occur in the colon; they are probably due to a vascular accident in the mesentery during early pregnancy. The infant usually presents on the second or third day of life presents with vomiting, abdominal distension, abdominal tenderness, and failure to pass meconium. Abdominal radiograph shows dilated bowel with multiple fluid levels. A contrast enema may show a distal microcolon.

Anorectal malformations

An imperforate anus is a perineum without an anal opening. The commonest classification of anorectal malformations is shown in Table 17.4. The arrested development of the anus and rectum may be divided into high lesions (rectal deformities), intermediate and low lesions (anal deformities). The incidence is 1/5000 live births. There is a slight preponderance of cases affecting male infants, in whom there is a higher incidence of the more serious rectal deformities, whereas in females the anal type is more common, with a stenotic ectopic orifice.

Clinical features

This condition should be obvious on examination. Other anomalies, such as genitourinary, vertebral, alimentary tract (especially oesophageal atresia), cardiac and central nervous system, must be care-

Table 17.4 International classification of anorectal malformations

	Female	Male
High (above levator ani)	Anorectal agenesis	Anorectal agenesis
	Rectovaginal fistula	Rectoprostatic fistula
	No fistula	No fistula
	Rectal atresia	Rectal atresia
Intermediate	Rectovaginal fistula	Bulbar fistula
	Rectovestibular fistula	Anal agenesis
	Anal agenesis	
Low (below levator ani)	Anovestibular fistula	Anocutaneous fistula
	Anocutaneous fistula	Anal stenosis persistent cloaca
	Anal stenosis	

Source: Stephens FD, Smith ED. Classification, identification and assessment of surgical treatment of anorectal anomalies. Pediatr Surg Int 1986;1:200–205.

fully excluded. Anorectal anomalies may be one of the features of the VACTERL association.

Defecation and micturition should be observed in these infants. In the female all orifices must be carefully examined and probed for evidence of additional fistulous tracts. Most female infants will decompress their bowel spontaneously via a vaginal fistula. In the majority of males meconium will be seen in the urine owing to a rectovesical or rectourethral fistula.

Investigations

Radiographs of the spine and sacrum will detect any vertebral or sacral anomalies. A cross-table plain film is taken, with the pelvis elevated, after 24 h of age, when adequate gas should have passed to the end of the bowel. A line drawn between the pubic symphysis and the sacrococcygeal junction constitutes the pubococcygeal line. Gas cranial to this line

indicates a high rectal anomaly, whereas gas caudal to this line indicates an anal anomaly.

A renal ultrasound examination will reveal an associated renal anomaly in 25% of cases. A micturating cystourethrogram will demonstrate a rectovesical fistula and vesico-ureteric reflux.

Management and outcome

High lesions will require a colostomy in the neonatal period to decompress the bowel, followed by rectoplasty at 6–12 months of age. High lesions are generally associated with rectal incontinence after treatment. Before closure, a distal colostogram allows for the precise localization of fistula.

The results of surgery in intermediate or low atresia are somewhat better. Generally, about one-third will have normal anal continence, one-third will have acceptable continence with some soiling, and one-third will be totally incontinent. The avoidance of repeated urinary tract infections in males with rectovesical fistula is important. Long-term constipation is a common complication of this disorder.

Hirschsprung's disease (aganglionosis)

This condition results from the absence of ganglion cells in the plexus of Auerbach, which prevents orderly peristaltic activity through the bowel. It is the commonest cause of large bowel obstruction in the newborn and has an incidence of 1/5000. In 20% there are other associated diseases such as Down's syndrome, Waardenburg's syndrome, Smith–Lemli–Opitz syndrome or central hypoventilation syndrome. It is inherited as a polygenic disease with a recurrence risk within families of 12.5%. Hirschsprung's disease may result from mutations in several genes either singly or in combination. These mutations may give dominant, recessive or polygenic patterns of inheritance. There are two distinct types:
- **Short aganglionic segment (85–90%).** This is the most common type, with a male to female ratio of 4:1. It usually affects the rectum and sigmoid colon.
- **Long aganglionic segment (8–10%).** This is rarer and has a 1:1 male to female ratio. This type is more commonly inherited in families.

Only 15% of patients with Hirschsprung's disease present in the newborn period.

Clinical features

The most common presentation in the newborn period is with acute obstruction. The infant vomits and has a distended abdomen, with failure to pass meconium. Rectal examination may reveal an explosive gush of meconium, to be followed by progressive constipation and further signs of obstruction. In older infants chronic constipation may develop with 'spurious diarrhoea', which is not seen in the neonate. It may be difficult to distinguish Hirschsprung's disease from cystic fibrosis and meconium plug syndrome.

Investigations

A plain radiograph of the abdomen may show dilated bowel loops and fluid levels, and lateral radiography of the pelvis may show the air-filled cone. Contrast studies may show the dilated normal bowel above a tapering transitional zone with distal microcolon. The definitive diagnosis is made by biopsy. This may be either a suction biopsy of the rectal mucosa and submucosa (less invasive), or a formal full-thickness strip biopsy of the bowel under a general anaesthetic. Histology reveals the absence of ganglia in the nerve plexus. Some centres use cholinesterase staining techniques to confirm the histological findings.

Management

Definitive management is surgical repair, but there are three alternatives for initial treatment: rectal irrigation, colostomy or primary repair.

Irrespective of whether repair is done using one or two operations, the classic operation is the 'pull through', consisting of excision of the aganglionic segment and pulling the normally innervated bowel down to the anus.

Meconium plug syndrome

This may occur with intrauterine growth restriction, Hirschsprung's disease, meconium ileus, or as an isolated condition. The infant fails to open his/her bowels in the first 24 h and may develop clinical and radiological signs of obstruction. A white plug of meconium is passed spontaneously or following rectal examination or contrast enema, and the signs of obstruction settle down. These infants require careful follow-up in order to detect those with Hirschsprung's disease or cystic fibrosis.

Meconium ileus

Meconium ileus is a form of intestinal obstruction caused by failure to pass meconium in the first few days of life. About 10–15% of infants with cystic fibrosis present with meconium ileus owing to pancreatic insufficiency with inspissated meconium, and 90% of infants with meconium ileus have cystic fibrosis. In about half, meconium ileus is complicated by ischaemia, volvulus, stenosis and malrotation, or meconium peritonitis with intraperitoneal calcification and pseudocyst formation, secondary to intrauterine perforation.

Diagnosis

A plain film of the abdomen shows multiple fluid levels and typically a foamy pattern of air bubbles trapped around inspissated meconium. A Gastrografin enema shows a microcolon. All children with meconium ileus should have investigations for cystic fibrosis. Diagnosis of cystic fibrosis may be made by the identification of two gene mutations. Over 1000 genes have been identified, but most tests will only search for 10–20 of the commonest mutations. If none or only one mutation is identified using genetic probes, sweat testing at 1–3 months of age is essential to exclude cystic fibrosis.

CLINICAL TIP: A raised immunoreactive trypsin (IRT) on a heel-prick blood specimen is a sensitive method for diagnosing cystic fibrosis and is used in the neonatal screening test. After operation for meconium ileus the IRT level may rapidly fall despite the child having cystic fibrosis. Even if the IRT is low, all infants with meconium ileus need to be investigated for cystic fibrosis.

Treatment

The decision as to whether the bowel obstruction is to be managed medically or surgically will be made by the surgeon. Management with Gastrografin enemas under fluoroscopic control may be initially diagnostic and subsequently therapeutic by softening the meconium so that it can be passed normally. Surgical decompression is often necessary in complicated cases, and is done in conjunction with Gastrografin washouts of the bowel. The baby with cystic fibrosis will also require lifelong treatment with appropriate antibiotics, chest physiotherapy, salt replacement, pancreatic extracts and fat-soluble vitamins. Genetic counselling is essential for this autosomal recessive condition.

Abdominal wall defects

Exomphalos (omphalocoele) and gastroschisis are both eviscerations of gastrointestinal contents: an exomphalos emerges through the umbilicus, whereas gastroschisis is through a right paramedian abdominal cleft.

Omphalocoele or exomphalos

The terms omphalocoele and exomphalos are used interchangeably. Omphalocoele occurs in 1/4000 live births. The exact cause is unknown however it results from a failure of the bowel to re-enter the abdomen before 12 weeks' gestation. The extra-abdominal bowel is covered by peritoneum and the umbilical cord is at the apex of the omphalocoele. Giant omphalocoeles may rupture before delivery, giving the appearance of no peritoneal covering. It is associated with other anomalies in 60–80% of cases, particularly when the defect is small. These include congenital heart disease, Beckwith–Wiedemann syndrome (exomphalos, large tongue and hypoglycaemia) or chromosomal disorders (e.g. trisomy 13, trisomy 18).

The diagnosis is often made on antenatal ultrasound examination after 14 weeks' gestation and elevated maternal serum alpha-fetoprotein. Fetal chromosome analysis is recommended, together with careful surveillance for other congenital malformations. On occasion, the peritoneal sac rup-

tures *in utero* and exposes bowel loops to amniotic fluid, with resultant matting of bowel loops.

Management

At birth, sac and contents should be kept warm and moist by use of plastic wrap. A nasogastric tube is inserted, the stomach is decompressed and IV fluids commenced. Operative repair is recommended within 2–4 h after birth.

Small lesions, with abdominal defects of less than 5 cm, can generally be treated surgically with primary closure. Larger defects may not be amenable to primary closure and the eviscerated bowel is protected by a Teflon silo, which is progressively reduced in size to allow reduction of the hernia. A vacuum device to facilitate the reduction of bowel contents and wound healing can also be used in some cases.

> **CLINICAL TIP:** If the intra-abdominal compartment is too small to accommodate the bowel and a primary closure has been attempted, possible complications include respiratory distress, hypotension, bowel ischaemia, and renal failure.

Gastroschisis

Gastroschisis is the herniation of abdominal contents through an abdominal wall defect, usually to the right of the umbilical cord. In contrast to exomphalos, gastroschisis has no peritoneal covering and the bowel is loose within the amniotic cavity. Consequently, it becomes scarred and bound with adhesions, with resultant stenosis, strictures, atresias and poor intestinal motility. There is often intrauterine growth failure, possibly associated with a short bowel syndrome, failure to thrive and steatorrhoea.

The incidence of gastroschisis is increasing worldwide and is currently 1/3800 births in Australia. It is usually associated with young mothers of low gravidity. Unlike exomphalos, it is rarely associated with other congenital malformations. There is no satisfactory embryological explanation for gastroschisis, but a vascular lesion related to intrauterine interruption of the omphalomesenteric artery seems most plausible.

Management

At birth the bowel must be handled very carefully to avoid further trauma. The baby can either be placed in a sterile plastic bag (up to the armpits) or the bowel can be covered in plastic wrap. This helps to both avoid hypothermia and prevent excessive fluid loss. Primary repair is possible if the defect is small, but repair becomes more difficult when there is massive evisceration. A silo may be necessary before the abdomen can be fully closed. For selected cases, reduction of the gastroschisis can be successfully undertaken in the neonatal intensive care unit shortly after birth, without general anaesthesia, by a paediatric surgeon. Following abdominal repair severe respiratory embarrassment may occur as the result of diaphragmatic splinting secondary to raised intra-abdominal pressure. Prolonged mechanical ventilation is often required postoperatively. Unlike in exomphalos, the bowel tends to show prolonged dysfunction in the absence of any anatomical abnormality. This may require long-term parenteral nutrition.

Congenital ascites

Congenital ascites (see Fig. 17.3) often presents as part of generalized oedema such as occurs in hydrops fetalis. Occasionally it is isolated and can occur where there is an obstruction to lymph flow from the gut or abnormal development of the lymphatic system from the gut (lymphangectasia and lymphatic hyperplasia).

Necrotizing enterocolitis

Necrotizing enterocolitis (NEC) is the most important acquired bowel abnormality occurring in the newborn period. The aetiology is poorly understood but is probably due to a combination of factors including mucosal injury, enteral feeding, associated inflammatory response and invasion of bowel organisms. It most commonly affects the terminal ileum or sigmoid colon.

The overall incidence of NEC varies between 0.2 and 3/1000 births. The incidence increases as

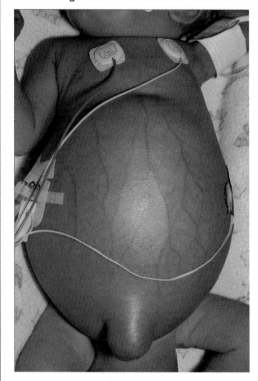

Severe congenital ascites with umbilical hernia

Figure 17.3 Congenital ascites.

birthweight decreases with approximately 5% of very low birthweight infants developing NEC. The overall mortality is 10–30%, higher in infants of less than 28 weeks' gestation, and surgery is required in 25–50% of survivors.

In full-term infants, causes of gut ischaemia such as congenital heart disease, perinatal asphyxia, Hirschsprung's disease or an endocrine disorder, must be sought as the possible cause of NEC.

The radiographic appearance of intramural gas (pneumatosis intestinalis) is generally considered confirmatory evidence of the disease. A definitive diagnosis can only be made at autopsy or on pathological examination of surgical specimens.

Pathogenesis

Loss of integrity of the gut mucosa is an important factor in the development of NEC. This may be due to the immaturity of the mucosal defences, invasion of pathogenic organisms or ischaemia of the mucosa (see Box 17.1). Supporting the possible contribution of ischaemia in the pathogenesis is the finding that NEC is twice as common in infants with a patent ductus arteriosus (PDA) compared to controls. Enteral feeding seems to be an important initiating factor as NEC is very rare in infants who have not been fed. NEC is more common in formula-fed babies. Although the leucocytes and

immunoglobulins in breast milk are thought to protect an infant from this disease, NEC does occasionally occur in exclusively breastfed infants. NEC occurs less commonly in institutions with established feeding protocols for at-risk babies. Although infection is probably not the direct cause, some enteric organisms predispose to the development of this condition. Many organisms have been implicated, including coliforms, staphylococci, clostridia and rotavirus. A schema to illustrate this process is shown in Fig. 17.4.

Box 17.1 Predisposing factors for NEC

Mucosal injury

- Immaturity of the mucosal defences
  Increasing immaturity with increasing prematurity
- Abnormal blood flow to the gut mucosa, as occurs in:
  Asphyxia
  Patent ductus arteriosus
  Polycythaemia
  IUGR with abnormal Doppler studies (absent or retrograde diastolic flow)
  Exchange transfusion
  Umbilical venous and arterial catheter use
  Cyanotic heart disease
  A complication of Hirschsprung's disease due to local mucosal ischaemia

Enteral feeds

- The risk of NEC may be due to the effect of milk on bacterial proliferation, or the volume of feed
- NEC is also more common where hyperosmolar feeds and formula feeds rather than breast milk are used

Infection

- May be the initiating factor for mucosal injury or may be secondary to decreased mucosal defences
- There is invasion of gas-producing bacteria, which causes pneumatosis coli

Source: Weaver LT. Digestive system development and failure. *Semin Neonatol* 1997;**2**:221–230.

Clinical features

The early signs of NEC are often non-specific, with lethargy, apnoea, bile-stained aspirates and failure to maintain body temperature. These features are common in preterm infants, but the early cessation of feeding under these circumstances may prevent

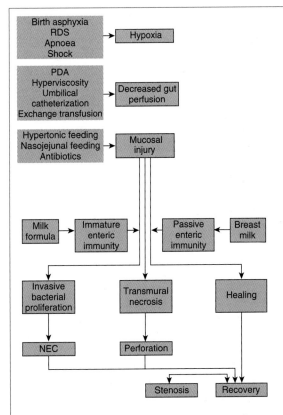

Figure 17.4 Schema for the development of NEC.

the progression to full-blown NEC. The signs may progress to include abdominal distension, blood and mucus in the stool, and circulatory collapse. Apnoea, bradycardia, shock, poor urine output and metabolic acidosis are commonly seen in severe cases. The severity of NEC is staged using Bell's criteria (Table 17.5).

CLINICAL TIP: The classic clinical triad for the presentation of NEC is abdominal distension, bloody mucous stools and bile-stained aspirates.

Investigations

The main avenues of investigation in cases of NEC are:
• **Abdominal radiographs (erect and cross-table).** Initially, there may be signs of an ileus with distension of bowel loops or fluid levels. Late signs include ascites, intramural gas (pneumatosis intestinalis), portal vein gas, and pneumoperitoneum (see Fig. 17.5).

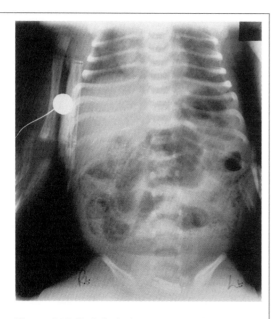

Figure 17.5 Radiological appearance of NEC. The image shows extensive intramural gas in the bowel and dilated loops of small bowel.

• **Ultrasound examination.** Increasingly being used in the diagnosis of NEC. The finding of intramural or intrahepatic gas is diagnostic.
• **Full blood count.** This shows a neutropenia or neutrophilia, a shift to the left of the leucocytes, toxic granulations in the neutrophils and thrombocytopenia.
• **C-reactive protein (CRP).** Will often be greatly elevated in cases of NEC and can be used to monitor resolution of the inflammatory process.
• **Coagulation studies.** Disseminated intravascular coagulation (DIC) is a common finding in severe cases of NEC.
• **Microbiological investigation.** Blood and occasionally faeces should be cultured. Many organisms have been associated with NEC, including Gram-negative bacteria, Gram-positive bacteria, fungi and viruses.

Prevention

Various strategies have been suggested to reduce or eliminate the risk of NEC. These are listed in Table 17.6. The most useful of these appear to be antenatal steroids, probiotics and breast milk. Probiotics are dietary supplements that contain potentially beneficial bacteria or yeast. They can be added to the enteral feeds of preterm infants. Compelling evidence exists that probiotics significantly reduce the incidence of NEC and the risk of dying. Controversy remains over the choice of probiotic and to which patient groups they should be given. Proposed mechanisms of action include direct competition with pathogenic bacteria, protection of the intestinal mucosa and enhanced host immune responses. The use of breast milk compared with formula feeds decreases the risk of NEC; this is one of the reasons why some people advocate the use of donor breast milk if maternal milk is not available in preterm infants. Small volumes of breast milk and breast milk mixed with formula also appear to lower the risk.

Treatment

At the first sign of gastrointestinal intolerance feeds are stopped in order to rest the bowel. Cultures should be collected and broad-spectrum antibiotics

Table 17.5 Modified Bell's staging criteria for necrotizing enterocolitis

Stage	Systemic signs	Intestinal signs	Radiological signs	Treatment
I: Suspected				
A	Temperature instability, apnoea bradycardia	Elevated pregavage residuals, mild abdominal distention, occult blood in stool	Normal or mild ileus	NPO, antibiotics × 3 days
B	Same as for IA	Same as for IA, plus gross blood in stool	Same as for IA	Same as for IA
II: Definite				
A: Mildly ill	Same as for IA	Same as I, plus absent bowel sounds, abdominal tenderness	Ileus, intestinal pneumatosis	NPO, antibiotics × 7–10 days
B: Moderately ill	Same as for I, plus mild metabolic acidosis, mild thrombocytopenia	Same as I, plus absent bowel sounds, abdominal tenderness, abdominal cellulites, right lower quadrant mass	Same as for IIA, plus portal vein gas, with or without ascites	NPO, antibiotics × 14 days
III: Advanced				
A: Severely ill, bowel intact	Same as for IIB, plus hypotension, bradycardia, respiratory acidosis, metabolic acidosis, DIC, neutropenia	Same as for I and II, plus signs of generalized peritonitis, marked tenderness, and distension of abdomen	Same as for IIB, plus definite ascites	NPO, antibiotics × 14 days, fluid resuscitation, inotropic support, ventilator therapy, paracentesis
B: Severely ill, bowel perforated	Same as for IIIA	Same as for IIIA	Same as for IIB, plus pneumoperitoneum	Same as for IIA, plus surgery

DIC, disseminated intravascular coagulation; NPO, nil per os (nil by mouth).

Table 17.6 Strategies used in the prevention of necrotizing enterocolitis	
Antenatal steroids	These have shown a dramatic effect in reducing the risk of NEC. This is most likely to be related to the reduced risk of RDS and the lower likelihood of gut ischaemia secondary to this
Probiotics	Probiotics have been shown to significantly decrease the incidence of NEC in preterm infants as well as significantly decrease all-cause mortality. It is unknown as to what dose and duration is most effective. It is unknown if the same benefits apply to ELBW infants
Prebiotics	Prebiotics are substances that stimulate the growth of non-pathogenic bacteria. Their role in the prevention of NEC is yet to be determined
Delay milk feeding in babies at high-risk of NEC (e.g. IUGR with abnormal Doppler flow)	There is no evidence to suggest delaying feeds decreases the incidence of NEC. There is a decreased risk of NEC in nurseries that have standardized feeding regimes
Breast milk	Breast milk decreases the risk of NEC compared with formula feeds. Small volumes of breast milk and breast milk mixed with formula also appear to lower the risk
Human milk fortifier	Milk fortifiers which are added to increase the caloric and nutritional content of breast milk may slightly increase the risk of NEC but are generally recommended in preterm infants to improve weight gain and growth
Oral antibiotic therapy	This has been shown to reduce the risk of NEC in a number of small studies. However, the Cochrane Review suggested that this is not recommended at present because of the risk of antibiotic resistance
Oral immunoglobulin (IgA and IgG)	These have been suggested to decrease the risk of NEC. The Cochrane Review did not support this finding and they are not recommended

ELBW, extremely low birthweight; IUGR, intrauterine growth retardation; NEC, necrotizing enterocolitis; RDS, respiratory distress syndrome.

commenced (gentamicin, ampicillin and metronidazole), or third-generation cephalosporins for 7–10 days. Total parenteral nutrition (TPN) is started and fluid, electrolyte and acid–base disorders must be corrected. Sometimes aggressive fluid resuscitation is required to manage the septic shock. Transfusions with fresh whole blood and correction of coagulopathy may be necessary.

Infants with proven NEC are best managed conservatively. The indications for surgical intervention include:

- pneumoperitoneum – free air in the peritoneum, indicating bowel perforation
- clinical deterioration during conservative management – this should be carefully assessed with a view to surgical intervention
- failure to improve on medical management.

Surgical intervention includes peritoneal drainage or formal laparotomy. The former may be done under general anaesthetic or in the newborn unit with a cannula under local anaesthesia. Laparotomy is best done in a specialist neonatal surgical centre. Fashioning an ileostomy in a healthy bowel with peritoneal drainage is usually the best form of treatment, and necrotic bowel is often not resected as a primary procedure. A second laparotomy may be

Table 17.7 Complications of necrotizing enterocolitis

Acute	Death
	Septicaemia
	Gangrenous bowel
	Bowel perforation
	DIC
	Acute renal failure
	Hypotension
	Lactose intolerance and malabsorption in the recovery period
Chronic	Death
	Bowel obstruction secondary to stricture formation
	Intrahepatic cholestasis secondary to inflammation and parenteral nutrition
	Short bowel syndrome

DIC, disseminated intravascular coagulation.

necessary when the baby has recovered from the acute NEC.

Complications

Acute and long-term complications of NEC are listed in Table 17.7; 50% of survivors will develop some form of long-term complications. Short bowel syndrome is one of the major complications and is discussed further below. Lactose intolerance caused by damage to the brush border of the mucosa, arises in 5–10% of infants after NEC. Semi-elemental formulas are recommended when the gut is rechallenged after recovery from extensive disease. Stricture formation occurs in approximately 15% of infants following NEC; the descending colon is the most commonly affected site. NEC reoccurs in up to 10% of babies; in these cases Hirschsprung's disease must be considered as an aetiological factor.

Short bowel syndrome

If there is insufficient bowel length to allow the adequate absorption of nutrients for normal growth then the baby is referred to having short bowel syndrome. Causes include significant intestinal atresia, gut ischaemia, and extensive NEC. These babies will be dependent on long-term parenteral nutrition to allow adequate growth or in some centres, small bowel transplantation may be successful in selected cases. Long-term parenteral nutrition carries significant risks including septicaemia and liver failure. Generally, if the small bowel is less than 40 cm in length in a term infant and there is no ileocaecal valve, short bowel syndrome will develop. In cases where there is an intact ileocaecal valve, as little as 25 cm of small bowel in a term infant may be sufficient to eventually establish successful enteral feeding.

Rectal bleeding

Blood and mucus in the stool is a common finding in the neonatal period, but the sight of blood on the nappy of a newborn infant is alarming for a mother. It is important to distinguish whether the blood is fresh or altered, confined to the outside of the stool or mixed throughout. Other symptoms, such as constipation, abdominal distension or pain, may assist with the diagnosis. The causes of rectal bleeding are listed in Box 17.2.

Investigations

The clinical history and examination will elucidate the cause in most cases. Most infants with blood and mucus in their stool will settle spontaneously without any obvious cause being found on investigation.

The following investigations may be useful:
• Apt's test will distinguish fetal from maternal blood.
• Plain radiographs of the abdomen may confirm NEC.
• Upper GI contrast study may be required to exclude malrotation.
• Faecal cultures and examination of the stool for human rotavirus or other infectious agents will confirm the clinical diagnosis of gastroenteritis.
• The ectopic gastric mucosa in a bleeding Meckel's diverticulum or bowel duplication may be demonstrated with a technetium radioisotope scan.
• The bleeding and prolonged prothrombin time in an infant with haemorrhagic disease of the newborn are corrected by a dose of vitamin K intramuscularly.

Box 17.2 Causes of blood in the stools in neonates

- Swallowed maternal blood
- Rectal or anal fissure (secondary to constipation or trauma)
- NEC
- Benign haemorrhagic colitis. This is one of the commonest causes of blood in the stool. It is usually associated with mucus and occurs most commonly in formula-fed infants. It may be due to cows' milk protein intolerance and recurs when cows' milk protein is reintroduced in the feeds
- Malrotation
- Intussusception
- Meckel's diverticulum and bowel duplication with ectopic gastric mucosa
- Gastroenteritis: human rotavirus, shigella, salmonella, enteropathogenic *Escherichia coli*
- Rectal polyp
- Haemorrhagic disease of the newborn (Vitamin K deficient bleeding)

SUMMARY

Normal structural and functional development of the gastrointestinal tract is essential for life. Many of the malformations that affect the gastrointestinal tract are identified on antenatal ultrasound. Appropriate paediatric surgical management in the newborn period will allow most babies to have an excellent long-term outcome. Preterm infants are unable to coordinate their suck and swallow until 34 weeks' gestation and as a result all will require intragastric feeding. NEC is in an infrequent but significant problem that causes significant morbidity.

Now visit **www.essentialneonatalmed.com** to test yourself on this chapter.

CHAPTER 18
Renal disorders

Key topics

Introduction

Many renal disorders are now diagnosed on routine antenatal ultrasound. Some of these conditions are fatal, others require active management and some will need conservative observation only. This chapter discusses the basic physiology of the kidney, its role in amniotic fluid, presentation and investigation of renal disease, and specific conditions which may affect the renal tract.

Role of amniotic fluid

Amniotic fluid volume is regulated from a number of fetal pathways including urine production, lung fluid secretion and fetal swallowing. The fetal kidney is the major contributor to the volume of amniotic fluid. Ultimately all amniotic fluid is derived via the placenta. Some of the roles of amniotic fluid are described in Box 18.1.

Essential Neonatal Medicine, Fifth Edition. Sunil Sinha, Lawrence Miall, Luke Jardine.
© 2012 John Wiley & Sons, Ltd. Published 2012 by John Wiley & Sons, Ltd.

Box 18.1 Roles of amniotic fluid

Amniotic fluid has a number of important roles, including:

- Providing space for fetal growth and movement
- Cushioning the umbilical cord against compression
- Protecting the fetus against trauma
- Providing protection against infection
- Maintenance of fetal temperature
- Providing nutrients, hormones and growth factors
- Development of respiratory, gastrointestinal and musculoskeletal systems

---

CLINICAL TIP: Decreased amniotic fluid volume (e.g. oligohydramnios or anhydramnios) can lead to lung hypoplasia. Severity depends on the cause, duration and timing of onset and degree of volume loss. Infants with hypoplastic lungs will present with respiratory distress at birth.

Renal physiology

The first permanent nephrons appear at around 8 weeks' gestation and nephrogenesis is complete by 36 weeks' gestation. The increase in renal mass thereafter is predominantly tubular growth. The human has approximately 1 million nephrons. Urine production commences shortly after the first nephrons develop; however, the fetus does not depend on the kidney to excrete waste products as the placenta performs this function. Renal function in the newborn depends on both gestational and postnatal age. Renal function rapidly matures within the first week after birth.

The newborn baby is largely water. The total body water (TBW) is 75% of body weight at term. The TBW is 80–90% in preterm infants of 26–30 weeks' gestation.

The size of the extracellular fluid compartment (ECF) decreases steadily throughout life from approximately 65% of body weight at 26 weeks to approximately 40% at term and 20% by 10 years of age. Adaptation to the *ex utero* environment requires rapid loss of excess fluid. The net water and sodium balance is negative in the first few days of

life and this is the most important reason for babies losing weight in the first week of life. Normal weight loss can be up to 10% in term babies, and 15% in preterm infants.

CLINICAL TIP: Excess fluid administration to preterm infants is associated with increased morbidity from PDA, NEC, and chronic lung disease.

Glomerular filtration rate

The newborn infant has a very low glomerular filtration rate (GFR) being approximately 20% of adult values. Preterm infants have lower GFR than term infants. After 34 weeks' gestation, and in response to birth, there is a marked increase in GFR. Although maturation of GFR is most rapid in the first month of life, it continues into the second year. The measurement of serum creatinine is the most convenient index of GFR in infants. Creatinine measured in the first 24 h after birth is not clinically useful as it is more likely to reflect maternal renal function. Plasma urea is also unreliable in neonates as it increases with catabolism even in the presence of normal renal function. The normal limits of creatinine for preterm infants for preterm infants in the first 4 days of life are shown in Table 18.1.

Tubular function

The concentrating ability of the developing kidney increases throughout gestation and improves rapidly

Table 18.1 Upper limit for normal serum creatinine levels (µmol/L) in neonates

Gestational age (weeks)	Age of infant (days)			
	1	2	3	4
23–26	145	200	200	185
27–28	150	175	150	110
30–32	105	145	80	70
33–35	95	95	70	50

These numbers represent approximately the 95th centile of normality for gestational age (Miall 1999).

after birth. This is due partly to elongation of the collecting tubes and partly to a hormonal effect (see below).

Tubular function can most easily be assessed by measuring the fractional excretion of sodium (FES); in the newborn this should be less than 2.5%.

Sodium conservation

The fetus has a very poor ability to conserve (reabsorb) sodium. In adults 80–90% of filtered sodium is reabsorbed in the proximal convoluted tubule. Sodium potassium adenosine triphosphatase (Na^+,K^+-ATPase) creates the electrical chemical gradient for transport. Sodium that enters the distal convoluted tube and collecting ducts is reabsorbed under the influence of aldosterone. Premature babies have decreased Na^+,K^+-ATPase in the proximal tubule and therefore higher sodium loads are delivered to the distal tubules. They also have limited aldosterone responsiveness at the distal tubule (and therefore less sodium absorption). Maturation of the system appears to be increased by the stress of delivery. Birth causes an increase in the Na^+,K^+-ATPase, upregulation of transporter proteins and increasing responsiveness of the distal tubule to aldosterone.

CLINICAL TIP: Antenatal steroids increases the abundance of Na^+,K^+-ATPase mRNA in both kidneys and lungs and therefore enhance maturation of renal tubular transport.

Hormonal function

The kidney is influenced by a number of hormones.

Antidiuretic hormone

Antidiuretic hormone (ADH) increases water reabsorption from the collecting ducts. It is present from early in fetal life but the fetal kidney is relatively insensitive to it. After birth the collecting ducts become more sensitive. ADH is active in very premature infants, and even the most immature infant is capable of concentrating the urine to a remarkable extent within days of birth.

Renin–aldosterone

Renin levels are higher in newborn infants than in adults and increase in response to sodium loss. However, the adrenal does not respond with high aldosterone levels and consequently sodium retention is poor, but matures in response to birth.

Normal urine output

Due to the reduced renal concentrating ability the maximum flow rate is 300 mL/kg per day and the minimum is 25 mL/kg per day. Over 90% of normal infants pass urine in the first 24 h of life, and 98% have voided by 48 h from birth. On day 1 of life, the urine output is approximately 0.5 mL/kg per hour, thereafter it is 2–3 mL/kg per hour. Neonates often do not completely empty their bladder on voiding.

CLINICAL TIP: Care needs to be taken when interpreting potassium values in neonates as:

- Haemolysis can falsely elevate (especially if collected via heel prick)
- Tissue serum (particularly in oedematous patients) can also falsely elevate
- Delay in processing can elevate.

If the baby has a normal urine output, high potassium levels are unlikely to cause clinical concern.

Investigation of renal disease

Ultrasound

This is the mainstay of investigating the structure of the renal tract both before and after birth (Fig. 18.1). Renal Doppler can be used to assess blood flow in and out of the kidney.

MAG 3 renogram

A MAG 3 (mercaptoacetyltriglycine) renogram is a kinetic scan that involves intravenous injection of a radioactive tracer, which is taken up by the kidney thereby enabling excretion curves to be plotted and obstruction to be visualized. Delay in excretion of isotopes from the kidney is suggestive of obstructive uropathy such as pelvi-ureteric junction (PUJ) obstruction. It is also possible to estimate differential kidney function using this scan prior to the excretion phase.

DMSA scan

A dimercaptosuccinic acid (DMSA) radionuclide scan is a static scan that delineates renal scarring or dysplasia and allows better estimation of differential renal function. It may show false-positive results if done during or soon after an episode of acute urinary tract infection.

Micturating cystourethrogram

The micturating cystourethrogram (MCUG) is the investigation of choice for vesicoureteric reflux. It involves urethral catheterization with the injection of radio-opaque dye into the bladder and observation of whether the dye refluxes into the ureters on micturition. It is an invasive procedure and prophylactic antibiotics are often recommended before and after the procedure.

Presentation of renal disease

Most significant structural renal anomalies are detected antenatally as the result of routine fetal anomaly scanning. Some diagnoses are so severe (e.g. renal agenesis) that termination of pregnancy or palliative care may be offered to the parents. In other cases the neonatal team will be notified before delivery of a baby with a renal anomaly and a variety of investigations will be required after birth. Genitourinary disease in the newborn may present in a number of different ways. These are discussed separately.

Potter's syndrome

Potter's syndrome refers to the association of dysmorphic clinical features and bilateral renal agenesis. The incidence of this condition is 1/4000 births,

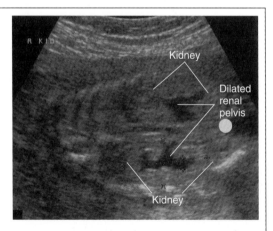

Figure 18.1 Longitudinal ultrasound view of fetal abdomen showing bilateral renal pelvocalyceal dilatation. Courtesy of Dr R Cincotta.

with a male predominance. Failure of renal development is associated with oligohydramnios and abnormal lung development. These infants usually have severe lung hypoplasia, are severely asphyxiated at birth and, although often resuscitated, die within several hours owing to their lung hypoplasia. The oligohydramnios also gives rise to characteristic facial features, including a beaked nose, low-set abnormal ears, prominent epicanthic folds and up-sloping palpebral fissures. The syndrome is usually considered to be sporadic, but may be polygenic with a recurrent risk of unilateral or bilateral renal agenesis of approximately 1%.

Facial features identical to those seen in Potter's syndrome are seen in other causes of oligohydramnios due to urinary outflow obstruction, sometimes referred to as pseudo-Potter's syndrome. In these cases large kidneys are usually palpable.

Renal pelvis dilatation

The most common abnormal feature detected by prenatal scanning is renal pelvis dilatation and is found in approximately 1% of antenatal scans. The majority will be transient or physiological however pathological causes include PUJ obstruction and vesico-ureteric reflux (VUR) and these are discussed below. The size of the pelvic dilatation and whether or not it is unilateral or bilateral, determines the pathway for investigation (see Fig. 18.2).

Obstructive uropathy

Causes of urinary obstruction are listed in Box 18.2. The diagnosis of uropathy is often suspected antenatally as described above. Infants may present with an abdominal mass (bladder and/or kidney) or

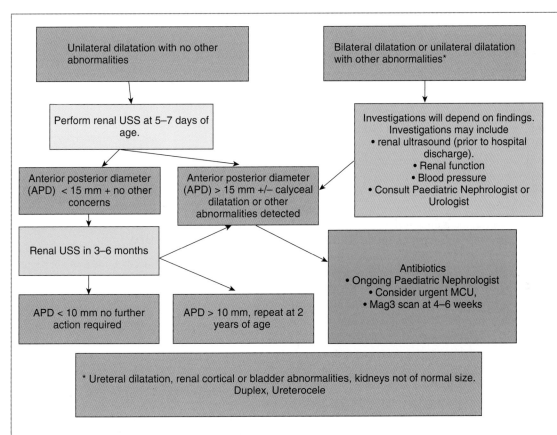

Figure 18.2 Management of renal pelvis dilatation.

Box 18.2 Causes of obstructive uropathy in the newborn

- PUJ obstruction
- Posterior urethral valves
- Urethral meatal stenosis in males
- Neurogenic bladder
- Ureterocoele
- Prune-belly syndrome

dribbling urine. If obstruction has been severe, the infant may be born with the facial appearances of Potter's syndrome and lung hypoplasia. **Prune-belly syndrome** is another clinical presentation of obstructive uropathy and is an absence of the musculature of the anterior abdominal wall. It is probably due to degeneration of the abdominal musculature as a result of a distended bladder. The penis should be examined carefully for a normal meatus. The spine should be inspected for meningomyelocoele.

Pelvi-ureteric junction obstruction

This is the most common form of obstructive uropathy and occurs equally in both males and females. PUJ obstruction is usually unilateral, but in 25% of cases is bilateral. It is most often diagnosed on antenatal ultrasound but if not detected may present clinically as a unilateral mass in the loin. PUJ obstruction may be found with other abnormalities such as horseshoe kidney or CHARGE syndrome. Most cases will resolve spontaneously, and conservative management is all that is warranted. Indications for surgery may include poor renal function, deteriorating renal function, and increasing hydronephrosis. There is no clear evidence that prophylactic antibiotics improve outcome but recommendations will vary between centres.

Posterior urethral valves

In this condition mucosal folds arise within the lumen of the male urethra producing a valve-like obstruction. Obstruction to urinary flow causes dilatation and hypertrophy of the urethra, bladder, ureter and kidneys. Diagnosis is most often made on antenatal ultrasound. Cases that are not diagnosed antenatally may present clinically with urine dribbling from the penis and a hard muscular bladder felt suprapubically. Severe cases may present with olighydramnios and pulmonary hypoplasia at birth. Renal dysplasia is often associated with posterior urethral valves and 20% of patients will eventually progress to end-stage renal failure. Ultrasound will confirm the presence of a hypertrophied bladder and establish the degree of upper tract involvement. MCUG is required to confirm the diagnosis and identify any vesicoureteric reflux.

If the lesion is mild, surgical ablation of the valves through a cystoscope is all that is necessary. In more severe cases a vesicostomy will be required. Antenatal diagnosis and the insertion of a vesico-amniotic catheter into the fetal bladder are indicated in highly selected cases of severe obstruction.

Ureterocoele

This is a ballooning of the distal terminal ureter into the bladder, which obstructs the drainage of the kidney on that side. They are more common in females and in white babies. A duplex collecting system is frequently associated. The ureterocoele tends to occur on the ureter that drains the upper pole of the kidney. Diagnosis is generally made by antenatal ultrasound. MCUG is required to identify vesicoureteric reflux. The ureterocoele should be excised and the ureter reimplanted to avoid urinary reflux.

Acute renal failure

Acute renal failure may occur as the result of numerous disease processes, many of which are detected on antenatal ultrasound; these can be divided into prerenal, renal and postrenal causes (Table 18.2). Prerenal failure is the commonest variety and usually occurs with severe respiratory disease or as a postoperative complication.

Clinical features

The clinical features of acute renal failure are listed in Box 18.3. Severe complications of acute renal failure are listed in Box 18.4.

Table 18.2 Causes of renal failure in the neonate

Prerenal	Renal	Postrenal
Dehydration	Cystic disease	Obstructive uropathy (see Box 18.2)
Hypotension due to:	Acute tubular necrosis	
Haemorrhage	Cortical necrosis	
Infection	Disseminated intravascular coagulation	
Cardiac dysrhythmia	Infection (pyelonephritis)	
Asphyxia	Haemolysis	
Hypothermia	Venous thrombosis Congenital nephrotic syndrome Drugs (aminoglycosides)	

Box 18.3 Clinical signs and symptoms of acute renal failure in the newborn

- Oliguria (urine output <1.0 mL/kg per hour)
- Oedema
- Rising serum creatinine and blood urea
- Metabolic acidosis (decreased pH, decreased bicarbonate)
- Increased potassium
- Increased phosphate
- Decreased sodium,
- Decreased calcium
- Decreased magnesium
- Cardiac dysrhythmias may develop as a result of hyperkalaemia

Box 18.4 Complications of acute renal failure

- Hyperkalaemia (>7.5 mmol/L). Insulin and dextrose may be necessary to drive potassium into the cells. A single dose of IV salbutamol can also briefly reduce serum potassium
- Severe metabolic acidosis (pH < 7.20)
- Fluid overload with severe oedema and congestive cardiac failure
- Hypertension, usually due to fluid overload
- Severe uraemia with central nervous system (CNS) depression

Under these circumstances peritoneal dialysis may be indicated.

Oliguria may be difficult to detect early in the infant's life as the passage of urine may have occurred unnoticed or may not have been recorded. Abdominal ultrasound may also be useful in showing whether there is urine in the bladder. If oliguria is suspected, insertion of a urinary catheter will allow accurate determination of urine output.

In oliguric infants there may be difficulty in distinguishing prerenal from renal failure; FES Na may be used in such cases. In prerenal failure the urine is concentrated and the serum and urinary creatinine measurements are high. If doubt still exists, a fluid bolus with a dose of furosemide should resolve the issue. The obstructive uropathy causes of acute renal failure must be excluded in postrenal failure (see Box 18.2).

Pathological examination of the kidneys of infants dying with acute renal failure shows acute tubular necrosis, acute cortical necrosis or bilateral renal vein thrombosis. With renal vein thrombosis, loin masses are generally palpable and the baby has haematuria.

Management

In established renal failure the underlying cause should be treated wherever possible. Consultation with a paediatric nephrologist is often helpful. The measures listed below are usually sufficient to maintain homeostasis until renal function recovers.

Fluid restriction

Water intake should be restricted so that only sensible (e.g. urine output) and insensible losses (e.g. respiration and perspiration) are replaced. These losses are calculated separately. Insensible loss depends on the infant's birthweight and gestational age. Insensible losses fall quickly in the first few days of life as the stratum corneum layer in the skin matures. Daily weighing is an accurate way of assessing fluid balance.

Protein and potassium restriction

Potassium should not be given unless the infant is hypokalaemic. To avoid endogenous protein breakdown and fluid overload, a high-carbohydrate infusion (e.g. 15–20% dextrose) should be given. The volume depends on the infant's output (see above).

Correction of electrolyte imbalance

Hyponatraemia is usually due not to sodium depletion but rather to fluid overload. Water should be restricted until this is corrected.

Metabolic acidosis

Sodium bicarbonate is carefully administered if the pH falls below 7.25. Care is necessary to avoid hypernatraemia.

Urinary tract infection

The incidence of symptomatic urinary tract infection in the neonatal period is 1%. The symptoms of urinary tract infection in the newborn are generally non-specific, with jaundice, vomiting, failure to thrive, temperature instability, lethargy and poor feeding. Specific symptoms of dysuria, frequency and abdominal discomfort are rarely seen. Urinary

---

Box 18.5 Interpretations of neonatal urine results

Microurine

- A white cell count of more than 30,000/mL suggests infection and a count of less than 10,000/mL is probably normal
- NB: Some normal newborn infants have up to 30,000 white cells/mL, even on a bladder tap aspirate of urine
- White cell counts in urine specimens from collecting bags are high and should be interpreted carefully, and only in conjunction with colony counts

Culture

- A pure growth of more than 100,000 organisms/mL indicates a significant infection
- Less than 10,000/mL or mixed organisms suggests contamination
- Counts between 10,000 and 100,000/mL indicate that the urine sample should be repeated
- Any growth of organisms obtained on bladder tap is significant
- The presence of budding hyphae in the urine strongly suggests systemic fungal infection (see Chapter 10)

---

tract infections in the newborn are more common in the male and may be blood borne, ascending or secondary to an abnormality of the urinary tract. In the neonatal period pyelonephritis is usually due to blood-borne infection. Investigations include an adequate urine specimen sent for microscopy and culture. Interpretation of urinalysis is provided in Box 18.5.

CLINICAL TIP: A 'clean voided' bag sample of urine is used only as a screen and is never the basis for a definitive diagnosis. If the bag sample suggests a urinary tract infection or if the baby is sick and in need of urgent treatment, either a 'clean catch', suprapubic aspiration or a urinary catheter sample will be necessary.

Treatment

Antibiotics that are excreted in the urine should be started immediately in an infant for whom there is a strong clinical suspicion of urinary tract infection. This is particularly important in pyelonephritis. In the presence of severe or suspected infection, therapy is usually commenced with an intravenous aminoglycoside (e.g. gentamicin) and ampicillin. Once cultures and sensitivities are known, any inappropriate antibiotic may be stopped. Co-trimoxazole (Septrin) may be used after the first week of life. Other suitable antibiotics include cefalexin (cephalexin), ceftriaxone or cefotaxime (cephotaxime). Treatment is continued for 10 days, when repeat urine microscopy and culture are performed.

Ultrasound examination together with a micturating cystourethrogram (MCU) are indicated in all neonates with proven urinary tract infection. Other investigations include MAG 3 (see p. 230) and a DMSA scan, which allows estimation of differential renal function and delineates renal scarring or dysplasia. Severe reflux may be associated with renal scarring even in the absence of infection. Specimens of urine should be regularly checked during the first year of life to ensure that reinfection does not occur.

Renal masses

Normal kidneys, especially the right, may be just palpable in the newborn infant. If a renal mass is easily felt, the kidney is probably pathologically enlarged. Differentiation of the mass can be achieved using ultrasound. The causes of a renal mass are listed in Box 18.6.

Box 18.6 Causes of a renal mass in the newborn period

- Hydronephrosis (bilateral)
- PUJ obstruction (unilateral)
- Cystic disease of the kidneys
- Renal vein thrombosis
- Wilms' tumour (nephroblastoma)
- Adrenal haemorrhage

Box 18.7 Renal cystic disease affecting neonates

- Cystic dysplastic (multicystic) kidneys
- Autosomal dominant polycystic kidney disease (ADPKD)
- Autosomal recessive polycystic kidney disease (ARPKD)
- Cysts secondary to obstructive uropathy (see Table 18.2)
- Simple renal cysts

Cystic disease of the kidneys

There is a great variety of cystic conditions of the kidney in the newborn. Congenital renal cystic diseases are a genetically and clinically diverse group of disorders with the common pathological finding of diffuse bilateral cystic structures without dysplasia. Many hereditary malformation syndromes are associated with renal cysts. Renal cystic diseases affecting the neonate are listed in Box 18.7.

Autosomal dominant polycystic kidney disease

Autosomal dominant polycystic kidney disease (ADPKD) is the commonest inherited renal disease, with an incidence of 1/200–1/1000. It was originally known as 'adult-onset PKD' because of the usual clinical presentation in the third to fifth decades, although the disease can manifest itself *in utero* or at any time thereafter. It may be diagnosed on perinatal ultrasound with the finding of enlarged or cystic kidneys. Clinically the disease can present along a spectrum, from the severe neonatal form with renal failure and Potter's syndrome, to the asymptomatic unilateral renal cyst found on renal ultrasound.

Autosomal recessive polycystic kidney disease

Originally known as 'infantile PKD' because of its more common perinatal presentation, autosomal recessive polycystic kidney disease (ARPKD) can present at any time from *in utero* to adulthood. It is due to mutations in the *PKHD1* gene which encodes a protein called fibrocystin. It is often diagnosed on antenatal ultrasound with the finding of enlarged kidneys and increased echogenicity. The cysts are very small (<3 mm) and are due to dilatation of the renal collecting ducts. There will always be some degree of biliary dysgenesis with periportal fibrosis. ARPKD is associated with oligohydramnios and often severe pulmonary hypoplasia. End-stage renal failure is common in early childhood.

Familial juvenile hyperuricaemic nephropathy

This is a spectrum of diseases all involving a mutation in the uromodulin gene. Conditions have been used to describe this mutation include medullary cystic kidney disease type 2 (MCKD2), glomerular cystic kidney disease (GCKD) and uromodulin-associated kidney disease. Uromodulin is a protein produced in the thick ascending limb of the loop of Henle. Abnormalities lead to accumulation of the protein and eventual cell death. They are inherited in an autosomal dominant pattern. Although most patients will not present until adulthood with hyperuricaemia and end-stage renal disease, it may present in the newborn with palpable enlarged kidneys.

Cystic dysplastic (multicystic) kidneys

This is a sporadic condition producing a non-functioning kidney and is usually unilateral as bilateral cases are fatal. It tends to occur on the left side and is more common in males. Most cases are identified on antenatal ultrasound. The kidney shows multiple small and large cysts, there may be no normal renal tissue identifiable. There is little or no renal function on the affected side. Hypertension and possible malignancy in the dysplastic kidney are long-term complications. Renal ultrasound is often performed after birth to confirm the diagnosis and ensure the other kidney is normal. Conservative management is all that is required in most cases however occasionally surgical excision is indicated.

Isolated renal cysts

These are a common incidental finding. Patients with isolated cysts will have normal renal function and no renal dysplasia. Long-term follow-up for simple cysts is not required.

Haematuria

In the first few days of life the presence of red cells in the urine is not uncommon, but after this haematuria is an important finding and must be further investigated. Box 18.8 lists causes of haematuria. Investigations include urinalysis, clotting studies, creatinine and ultrasound examination. Treatment depends on the underlying cause.

> CLINICAL TIP: Haematuria must be differentiated from the presence of urates in the urine, a benign condition that produces pink staining of the nappy/diaper.

Congenital abnormalities

Hypospadias

In this condition the urethral meatus opens on to the undersurface of the glans penis, the penile shaft or the perineum. It is one of the most common abnormalities of male infants, with an incidence of 1/350 male births. Frequently there is a dorsal hood

---

Box 18.8 Neonatal renal disorders associated with haematuria

- Acute tubular necrosis
- Infection
- Renal vein thrombosis
- Bleeding disorders
- Cystic renal disease
- Obstructive uropathy
- Tumours

to the penis and a ventral curvature of the glans (**chordee**). It may be classified as glandular, penoglandular, penile, penoscrotal or perineal, depending on the site of the urethral opening. Chromosome studies are indicated with undescended testes and severe penoscrotal or perineal lesions. Mild types are repaired in a one-stage procedure in the first 6 months, but severe types require several staged operations. The infant must not be circumcised, otherwise definitive surgical treatment will be made more difficult. **Epispadias** refers to the urethra opening on the dorsal surface of the penis and has a worse prognosis.

Ectopia vesicae (bladder exstrophy)

This is a complex disorder of the abdominal wall, bladder and pelvis. The mucosa of the bladder herniates through a deficient lower abdominal wall. There is a deficient pelvic floor and wide separation of the pubic symphysis. It is more common in male than in female infants. In the male there is total epispadias, undescended testes and a deficient penis. In the female the two halves of the clitoris are separate and the vagina is duplicated.

The surgical management of this complex disorder is extremely difficult and continues over many years. Urinary continence is rarely achieved.

SUMMARY

Adequate renal function is essential for the development and survival of the neonate. Many renal disorders are diagnosed on routine antenatal ultrasound. Renal disorders have a wide variety of clinical presentations ranging from non-survivable pulmonary hypoplasia at birth to being asymptomatic. Appropriate investigation and follow-up is required for many of these disorders with the ultimate aim being to preserve normal renal function.

 Now visit **www.essentialneonatalmed.com** to test yourself on this chapter.

CHAPTER 19
Jaundice

Key topics

Introduction

Jaundice is a yellow discolouration of the skin, sclera and mucous membranes due to the deposition of bilirubin. Neonatal jaundice is the most common problem encountered in the newborn. About 50% of all full-term infants and 85% of preterm infants are visibly jaundiced within the first week of life. In most infants the jaundice is physiological as there is no underlying disease. Physiological jaundice results from increased bilirubin production (due to increased haemoglobin levels at birth and a shortened red cell lifespan), and decreased bilirubin excretion (due to low concentrations of the hepatocyte binding protein, low activity of glucuronosyl transferase, and increased enterohepatic circulation). Unconjugated bilirubin, which is elevated in the most common forms of neonatal jaundice, can pass through the blood–brain barrier and is neurotoxic. High levels in the brain can cause acute or chronic encephalopathy if not treated appropriately. Conjugated hyperbilirubinaemia is much less common than unconjugated jaundice in the newborn, but has a much more serious prognosis.

Physiology of bilirubin metabolism

Fetal

In the uterus, the fetal liver is relatively inactive. The placenta and maternal liver metabolize the bilirubin from worn-out red blood cells. The fetus is capable of conjugating bilirubin in small amounts and when haemolysis occurs *in utero* (as in severe rhesus isoimmunization), bilirubin conjugation increases and high levels may be measured in the umbilical cord blood.

Essential Neonatal Medicine, Fifth Edition. Sunil Sinha, Lawrence Miall, Luke Jardine.
© 2012 John Wiley & Sons, Ltd. Published 2012 by John Wiley & Sons, Ltd.

Newborn

The metabolism of bilirubin in the newborn is summarized in Fig. 19.1. Each of the steps in the metabolism of bile will be discussed in turn.

Bilirubin production

Most of the daily bilirubin production comes from ageing red blood cells. The red cells are destroyed in the reticuloendothelial (RE) system and the haem is converted to unconjugated bilirubin. One gram of haemoglobin will produce 600 μmol (35 mg) of unconjugated bilirubin. Haemolysis may be increased by maternal drugs such as salicylates, sulphonamides, phenacetin and nitrofurantoin. Twenty-five per cent of the daily production of bilirubin comes from sources other than the red cells, such as haem protein and free (tissue) haem.

Transport and liver uptake

Most of the unconjugated bilirubin in the blood is bound to serum albumin and is transported to the liver as a bound complex. This binding is extremely important and may be altered by many factors. Factors that decrease albumin binding ability include low serum albumin, asphyxia, acidosis, infection, prematurity and hypoglycaemia. In addition, there are many competitors for bilirubin binding sites, and these include

- non-esterified (free) fatty acids produced by starvation, cold stress or intravenous fat emulsion
- drugs (sulphonamides, cephalosporins, sodium benzoate (present in diazepam), frusemide and thiazide diuretics).

When bilirubin is bound to albumin it is probably non-toxic, but free unbound unconjugated bilirubin is fat soluble and can be transported across the blood–brain barrier and be deposited in certain neurons causing damage. Hepatocytes lining the liver sinusoids are able to extract unconjugated bilirubin from the blood and this is then accepted in the liver cell by the Y and Z proteins (ligandins).

Conjugation and excretion

The unconjugated bilirubin is conjugated in the liver and the reaction involves the conversion of insoluble unconjugated bilirubin to direct-reacting bilirubin (water soluble). Each molecule of bilirubin is conjugated with two molecules of glucuronic acid in a reaction catalysed by the enzyme glucuronyl transferase. The conjugated bilirubin is excreted into the bile, and subsequently into the duodenum. In the older child the bilirubin is reduced to stercobilinogen by bacteria in the small bowel, but in the newborn with a relatively sterile bowel and poor peristalsis much of the conjugated bilirubin may be hydrolysed by glucuronidase back to unconjugated bilirubin. This is then absorbed in the bowel, re-entering the circulation for further liver metabolism, a process called enterohepatic circulation.

This may be important in pathological situations, and reinforcement of the enterohepatic circulation will increase unconjugated bilirubin levels in prematurity, small bowel obstruction, functional bowel obstruction and pyloric stenosis.

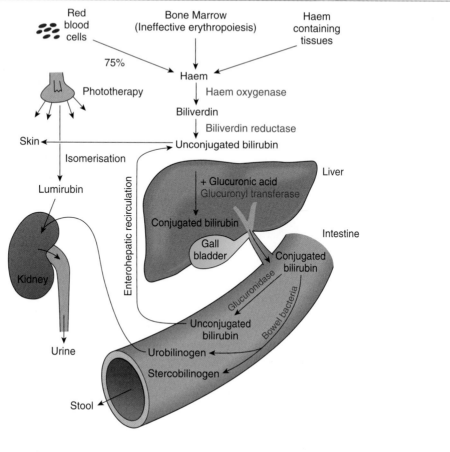

Figure 19.1 Summary of neonatal bilirubin metabolism.

Clinical assessment of the jaundiced infant

Jaundice can be detected clinically once the serum bilirubin result (SBR) is above 90 μmol/L. As jaundice is common it is essential to have a clinical method for determining its severity. Proper lighting (ideally daylight) is important for detecting subtle levels of jaundice.

An older method of assessing the degree of jaundice is the use of Kramer's rule (Kramer 1969). This technique depends on the blanching of the infant's skin with the examiner's finger at standard zones (1–5) and observing the colour in the blanched area.

CLINICAL TIP: Caution must be taken when applying Kramer's rule (particularly in non-white babies) as high bilirubin levels may be found even with jaundice in zone 1.

A non-invasive method of assessment is the use of transcutaneous bilirubinometry (TcB). It can provide a useful screening test in babies 35 weeks or more and more than 24 h of age. If the TcB suggests a high bilirubin a SBR should be collected. TcB has good correlation with total serum bilirubin, but may have limitations in specific situations.

CLINICAL TIP: Bilirubin in the urine (tested by a 'stick' test) indicates that a component of the serum bilirubin is conjugated. Pale stools might suggest that the normal passage of bile from the liver into the duodenum is blocked. These are important clinical signs suggestive of obstructive jaundice. Stool charts are available for parents to describe the stool colour against.

Management

The first investigation in any jaundiced newborn is to take a careful history. Important considerations in history taking are listed in Box 19.1. The next step is to perform a complete physical examination. Clinical findings that may help to delineate the cause are listed in Box 19.2.

Box 19.1 Required history when assessing for causes of neonatal jaundice

- Events in pregnancy, e.g. suspected infection, maternal diseases (e.g. thyroid disorders, diabetes), maternal drugs
- Maternal blood group, and presence of antibodies
- Family history, e.g. ethnic origin, previous jaundiced infant requiring treatment, red cell morphological disorders (spherocytosis, elliptocytosis, stomatocytosis, pynknocytosis), red cell enzyme disorders (thalassaemia, G6PD, pyruvate kinase), thyroid disorders, galactosaemia, cystic fibrosis
- Birth history, e.g. traumatic delivery, condition at birth
- Gestational age and birthweight of the infant
- Current postnatal age of the infant and when baby first became clinically jaundiced
- Current clinical condition of the infant (feeding, stooling, urine output)
- Has the baby received any treatment since birth, e.g. phototherapy, medications, etc.?

Box 19.2 Clinical findings that may help to determine the cause and severity of neonatal jaundice

- Extravascular blood, e.g. extensive bruising, purpura, petechiae
- Plethora or pallor
- Hepatosplenomegaly
- Evidence of intrauterine infection, e.g. small for gestational age, cataracts, microcephaly
- Evidence of infection, e.g. umbilicus, skin, urine
- Neurological signs: hypertonia, opisthotonus, fits, abnormal eye movements, abnormal cry
- Abdominal distension: associated with bowel obstruction, bowel stasis or hypothyroidism

In assessing the significance of jaundice in a newborn infant the following guidelines may be useful. Investigations should be carried out under the following circumstances:
- Any infant who is visibly jaundiced in the first 24 h of life.
- Any jaundiced infant whose mother has rhesus antibodies.
- A preterm infant whose estimated serum bilirubin is greater than 150 μmol/L.
- A term infant whose estimated serum bilirubin exceeds 200 μmol/L.
- Any infant who has the clinical signs of obstructive jaundice (dark urine, pale stools).
- Prolonged hyperbilirubinaemia beyond 1 week in term infants and beyond 2 weeks in preterm infants.

First line tests should include:
- unconjugated bilirubin
- direct antibody test
- blood group
- full blood count (FBC) and red cell morphology

Directed tests may include:
- infection screen (e.g. TORCH, septicaemia)
- glucose-6-phosphate dehydrogenase assay
- thyroid function
- conjugated bilirubin
- liver USS
- erythrocyte galactose uridyl transferase activity if considering galactosemia.

Once this basic information has been collected the possible aetiology, and therefore the investigations that should be collected, will often be obvious. Table 19.1 lists the common causes of jaundice and the timing of their presentation.

Repeated total serum bilirubin estimations should be performed in infants with a rapid and early rise of (unconjugated) bilirubin so that treatment for hyperbilirubinaemia can be instituted. Bilirubin in the urine indicates that the conjugated fraction of bilirubin should be estimated in the laboratory and causes of conjugated hyperbilirubinaemia considered.

Unconjugated hyperbilirubinaemia

Causes

The causes (and timing of onset) of unconjugated hyperbilirubinaemia are shown in Table 19.1. In any baby presenting with jaundice in the first 24 h of life it is important to exclude a haemolytic cause for the unconjugated hyperbilirubinaemia. The most common causes are 'physiological jaundice' and 'jaundice of prematurity' and these usually present between day 2 and day 5. Breastfeeding infants are more likely to develop jaundice secondary to a lower caloric intake and increased enterohepatic circulation of bilirubin. The causes of prolonged (lasting >10 days) or late-onset unconjugated hyperbilirubinaemia are shown in Box 19.3.

Table 19.1 Possible causes of jaundice presenting at different times in the neonatal period

Day	Unconjugated jaundice	Conjugated jaundice
1	Haemolytic disease assumed until proven otherwise	Neonatal hepatitis Rubella CMV Syphilis
2–5	Haemolysis Physiological Jaundice of prematurity Sepsis Extravascular blood Polycythaemia Glucose-6-phosphate dehydrogenase deficiency Spherocytosis	As above
5–10	Sepsis Breast milk jaundice Galactosaemia Hypothyroidism Drugs	As above
10+	Sepsis Urinary tract infection	Biliary atresia Neonatal hepatitis Choledochal cyst Pyloric stenosis

CLINICAL TIP: Jaundice presenting in the first 24 h of life may be secondary to haemolysis. The important causes are rhesus isoimmunization and ABO incompatibility. These conditions can lead to rapid rises in the bilirubin level and often need early and aggressive treatment to prevent complications.

Box 19.3 Causes of prolonged unconjugated hyperbilirubinaemia

- Rhesus and ABO incompatibility
- Hereditary spherocytosis
- Glucose-6-phosphate dehydrogenase deficiency
- Septicaemia and TORCH infection
- Extravasated blood and excessive bruising
- Twin-to-twin transfusion
- Prematurity
- Dehydration
- Hypothyroidism
- Breast milk jaundice
- Delayed passage of meconium

Physiological jaundice

Physiological jaundice is a term used by clinicians to describe jaundice for which no underlying cause is identified and is therefore a diagnosis of exclusion. The major cause is increased bilirubin production (due to increased haemoglobin levels at birth and a shortened red cell lifespan). Decreased bilirubin excretion (due to low concentrations of the hepatocyte binding protein, low activity of glucuronosyl transferase, and increased enterohepatic circulation) also contributes to the development of physiological jaundice.

Infection

Bacterial infections, particularly septicaemia and urinary tract infections, may cause unconjugated hyperbilirubinaemia. Occasionally severe bacterial infection may cause hepatocellular damage with a conjugated form of jaundice. TORCH infections may cause either type of hyperbilirubinaemia, but the conjugated form is most frequently seen.

Breastfeeding and jaundice

Breastfeeding-associated jaundice is the term used to refer to the increased bilirubin levels seen during the first week of life in almost two-thirds of infants who are breastfed. It is probably due to calorie and fluid deprivation in the first few days of life and delayed passage of stools, as it can be reduced by an increased frequency of breastfeeding during the first few days of life.

Breast milk jaundice is prolonged jaundice that extends until the first 3 months of life. Characteristically it is a form of non-haemolytic, unconjugated hyperbilirubinaemia and should be diagnosed primarily by exclusion of other aetiologies in a thriving infant and by its time course. The enzyme β-glucuronidase has been shown to be elevated in some women's breast milk. Excess of this enzyme causes increased enteric absorption of bilirubin, thus increasing the hepatic bilirubin load. In this respect, breast milk jaundice can be thought of as an extension of physiological jaundice, and the greater the consumption of this enzyme in milk, the higher is the concentration of neonatal serum bilirubin. Breast milk jaundice does not require any treatment and is not an indication to abandon breastfeeding, but babies with high bilirubin levels should be kept under review.

Delayed passage of meconium

This increases the risk of jaundice due to increased enterohepatic absorption of bilirubin.

Gilbert's syndrome

This is a common cause of unconjugated hyperbilirubinaemia in young adults, but rarely causes problems in the neonatal period. It is due to a single gene mutation affecting a hepatic bilirubin enzyme uridine diphosphate glucuronyltransferase (UDPGT), and in the newborn is associated with mild unconjugated hyperbilirubinaemia (<85 μmol/L). The prognosis is excellent.

Crigler–Najjar syndrome

This group of conditions has been shown to be due to multiple gene defects and causes very severe hyperbilirubinaemia potentially leading to kernicterus. There is little effective treatment other than prolonged phototherapy. Liver transplantation has been successful in some severe cases; in milder cases phenobarbitone may lower the serum bilirubin.

Investigations

The initial investigations for jaundice were discussed above. The aim is to identify the infant at risk of acute bilirubin encephalopathy and thereby prevent it occurring by commencing appropriate treatment. Prolonged unconjugated hyperbilirubinaemia requires additional investigation when present for more than 10 days in a term infant, and for more than 14 days in a premature one. Box 19.4 lists the investigations for prolonged unconjugated hyperbilirubinaemia.

Management

Prevention

Early feeding reduces the incidence of jaundice by preventing dehydration and the elevation of free

Box 19.4 Investigations in an infant with prolonged unconjugated hyperbilirubinaemia

- Indirect- and direct-acting bilirubin
- Haemoglobin
- Blood film for red cell morphology
- Maternal and infant blood group
- Direct antibody test
- Maternal antibodies
- Infection screen
- Urine-reducing substances
- Erythrocyte galactose uridyl transferase activity if galactosaemia a possibility
- Glucose-6-phosphate dehydrogenase assay
- Serum thyroxine and thyroid-stimulating hormone

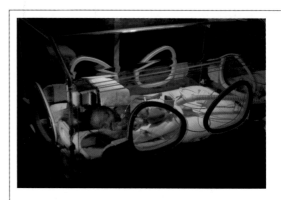

Figure 19.2 Phototherapy for hyperbilirubinaemia.

fatty acids. The maintenance of an adequate fluid intake is an essential part of the care of a jaundiced baby. In addition, feeding will overcome bowel stasis and minimize the effects of the enterohepatic bilirubin circulation. Breastfeeding-associated jaundice is minimized by frequent, early breastfeeding in the first 3 days of life.

Phototherapy

Phototherapy causes isomerization in the skin of the bilirubin molecule to lumirubin which is water soluble and can be excreted in the urine (Fig. 19.2). The conversion process is rapid, but the excretion of the molecule out of the skin is slow. Phototherapy is the standard of treatment and has resulted in a decline in the number of exchange transfusions being performed.

CLINICAL TIP: Do not use sunlight as phototherapy for hyperbilirubinaemia. Even relatively short durations of exposure to sunlight can cause burning and increases the long-term risk of developing skin cancer.

Phototherapy can be delivered from either overhead or underneath the baby (or both). A number of different types of phototherapy devices have been studied including conventional incandescent, quartz halogen, fluorescent, light-emitting diode (LED). Devices essentially differ in their colour spectrum, energy output and total dose of light delivered. Given equivalent light sources, other factors that might influence the effectiveness of phototherapy include the number of lights, the distance from the light source to the infant, the time spent in phototherapy and the surface area of skin exposed. LED phototherapy may have an advantage in reducing dehydration.

Various thresholds for commencing phototherapy and for monitoring at risk infants have been developed by different organizations, commonly used charts are found in the NICE neonatal jaundice guideline (see Fig. 19.3) and the American Academy of Pediatrics guideline (see Further Reading). A general approach to the management of a jaundiced infant is provided in Fig. 19.4.

Once therapy has been commenced serum bilirubin estimates will be necessary to assess the severity of jaundice because the skin colour becomes unreliable. In cases of severe jaundice, the SBR will need to be repeated 4–6h after initiating

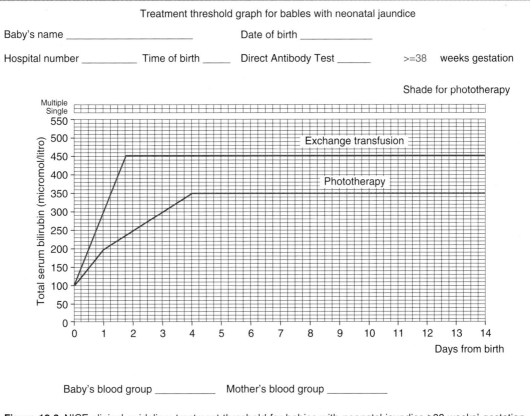

Figure 19.3 NICE clinical guideline: treatment threshold for babies with neonatal jaundice ≥38 weeks' gestation.

phototherapy and then every 6–12 h once it is stable or falling.

Phototherapy can be stopped once the SBR has fallen below the phototherapy threshold (the NICE guideline recommends at least 50 μmol/L below).

A rebound SBR should be collected (12–24 h) after stopping phototherapy. Babies do not necessarily have to remain in hospital for this to be done.

Some complications of phototherapy are listed in Box 19.5.

General care of the baby during phototherapy includes eye protection, monitoring the baby's temperature and fluid balance, and supporting the parents by educating them and encouraging them to interact with their baby.

Early discharge and home management of jaundice

The introduction of early discharge programmes for healthy term infants has resulted in the need for jaundice to be treated at home. The resurgence of kernicterus is probably also related to the combination of early discharge and breastfeeding. This may result in dehydration if the baby feeds poorly and there is a lack of recognition of severe hyperbilirubinaemia. The NICE and AAP (see Fig. 19.5) guidelines can be used to estimate the risk of an infant developing jaundice that may require treatment. Predicting which infants might require treatment using direct and indirect techniques of measuring serum bilirubin at age 24 h has been suggested, but more research is required to identify sensitive

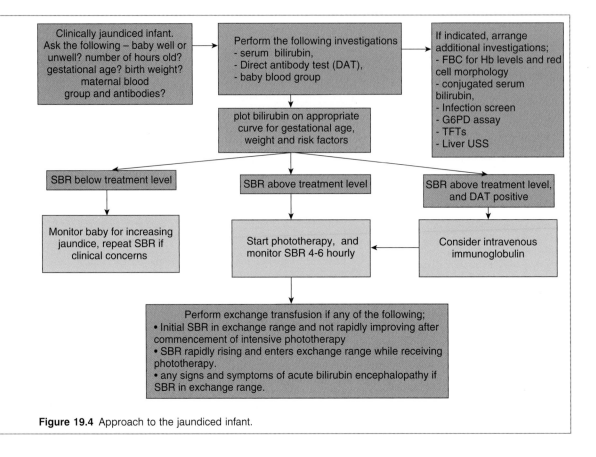

Figure 19.4 Approach to the jaundiced infant.

Box 19.5 Some complications of phototherapy

- **Temperature instability**
- **Dehydration**: regular assessment of the baby's fluid balance (monitor weight and urine output) and early management may be required
- **Diarrhoea**: phototherapy decreases bowel transit time and induces lactose intolerance; both are important causes of diarrhoea and consequent fluid loss
- **Retinal damage**: the eyes are thought to be vulnerable to phototherapy but this has never been proved. It is, however, a wise precaution to protect the infant's eyes from the light by a suitable eye shield

methods. Home treatment has been facilitated by the introduction since 1990 of the BiliBlanket (MedNow Inc., Eagle, Idaho, USA) using a fibreoptic phototherapy system. The infant is placed on a mat containing fibreoptic strands which flood the body with therapeutic light while the infant is normally clothed.

Exchange transfusion

Although there are no randomized controlled trials on exchange transfusion versus no treatment, it is generally accepted that exchange transfusion is beneficial in the treatment of severe hyperbilirubinaemia. The exchange transfusion allows
- removal of unconjugated bilirubin
- removal of the antibody causing haemolysis (if present)

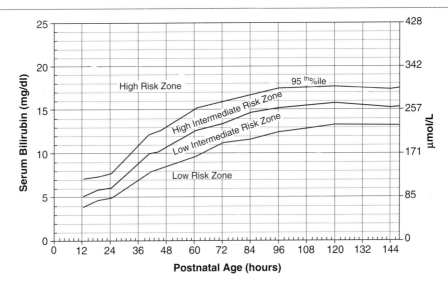

Figure 19.5 Algorithm for the management of jaundice in the newborn nursery. Reproduced with permission from *Pediatrics* 2004;**114**:297–316, copyright © 2004 by the AAP.

- replacement of sensitized red cells with cells that cannot be haemolysed as easily
- restoration of blood volume and correction of anaemia
- provision of free albumin for bilirubin binding.

Exchange transfusions may be required in conjunction with phototherapy for infants with severe jaundice, especially when due to rhesus iso-immunization. The indications for exchange transfusion depend on the infant's gestational age, postnatal age and state of health. Metabolic compromise with acidosis predisposes to brain damage due to bilirubin toxicity. The level at which bilirubin damages the brain is not known, and the indications for exchange transfusion are therefore arbitrary. Different charts are used in different centres to guide treatment. The NICE neonatal jaundice guideline provide recommendations as to the bilirubin level at which exchange transfusion should be performed for infants of different gestations. The AAP guideline also has similar recommendations.

The technique of exchange transfusion is described in Chapter 29. Complications associated with exchange transfusions are listed in Box 19.6.

Box 19.6 Complications associated with exchange transfusions

- Death (reported mortality rates between 5 and 10%)
- Electrolyte disturbance (hypocalcaemia, hyperkalaemia)
- Blood glucose disturbance – initially hyperglycaemia followed by rebound hypoglycaemia, especially in rhesus immunization
- Infection – viral (CMV, hepatitis B, HIV) or bacterial (*Staphylococcus aureus* and streptococcus) due to contaminated blood
- Embolism of either air or thrombosed blood
- Necrotizing enterocolitis (NEC)
- Fluid overload or rarely hypovolaemia
- Acidosis, hypoxia, bradycardia, cardiac arrest
- Benign intrahepatic cholestasis in severely growth-restricted infants
- Haemorrhage

Adjunct therapy

Immunoglobulin

Intravenous immunoglobulin (IVIG) given to infants at high risk of severe hyperbilirubinaemia secondary to rheusus isoimmunization is effective in reducing the need for exchange transfusion and the total number of exchange transfusions required. There is no evidence to suggest that it prevents mortality or neurodevelopmental sequelae. IVIG appears to be safe and well tolerated, but supplies are limited. Rare complications of IVIG administration include haemolysis, renal failure and sepsis. More research is required into the long-term effects, which patients are most likely to benefit, dosing and timing of administration.

A number of additional treatment methods for hyperbilirubinaemia have been described (see Box 19.7). There is insufficient evidence to justify their use.

Bilirubin encephalopathy and kernicterus

Unconjugated bilirubin can penetrate the blood–brain barrier in newborn babies. Unconjugated bilirubin is potentially neurotoxic and can cause both short-term and long-term problems. On postmortem specimens, bilirubin is seen as yellow staining in the basal ganglia, hippocampus and subthalamic nuclei and this is referred to as kernicterus.

Acute bilirubin encephalopathy is a spectrum of features due to the acute toxic effects of bilirubin on the brain. It consists of lethargy, irritability, high-pitched cry, abnormal muscle tone (initially hypotonia followed by hypertonia), opisthotonus, fever, apnoea and seizures. This is followed by death in 50% of the affected infants.

Kernicterus refers to the yellow staining of the brain, but historically the term has also been used to describe the chronic form of bilirubin encephalopathy. Chronic bilirubin encephalopathy includes the following signs and symptoms; choreoathetoid cerebral palsy, high-frequency deafness, intellectual impairment, and paralysis of upward gaze (Parinaud's sign). Preterm infants may manifest more subtle bilirubin brain damage consisting of mild disorders of both motor function and cognitive function (minimal cerebral dysfunction) without demonstrating any of the acute clinical features of bilirubin encephalopathy. High-tone frequency hearing loss is the commonest feature of the bilirubin encephalopathy syndrome and is most commonly seen in premature infants.

The levels at which unconjugated bilirubin causes brain damage are not known, and it is probably only free (non-protein-bound) bilirubin that is dangerous, although bound bilirubin has been reported to cross a leaky blood–brain barrier. Acidosis, asphyxia, prematurity and drugs that compete for bilirubin binding sites predispose infants to kernicterus, possibly by opening the blood–brain barrier to bilirubin molecules, and the indication for exchange transfusion is at a lower level of unconjugated bilirubin in these babies. Unfortunately, by the time that symptoms of bilirubin encephalopathy appear, brain damage has probably already started.

Box 19.7 Previous treatments for hyperbilirubinaemia now NOT recommended

- Agar
- Albumin
- Barbiturates
- Charcoal
- Cholestyramine
- Clofibrate
- D-Penicillamine
- Glycerin
- Manna
- Metalloporphyrins (Including tin mesoporphyrin)
- Riboflavin
- Traditional Chinese medicine
- Acupuncture
- Homeopathy

Conjugated hyperbilirubinaemia

Conjugated hyperbilirubinaemia is much less common than unconjugated jaundice in the newborn, but has a much more serious prognosis. Conjugated forms of neonatal jaundice are due to intra- or extrahepatic obstruction (also called cholestasis). It usually presents in the second week of life or later and is associated with greenish skin discoloration, dark bile-stained urine and pale acholuric stools. Hepatosplenomegaly is commonly present and the infant often fails to thrive. Occasionally, conjugated hyperbilirubinaemia is present at birth as a result of TORCH infections or rhesus isoimmunization. The timing of presentation of causes of conjugated hyperbilirubinaemia are shown in Table 19.1 above.

Causes

The causes of conjugated hyperbilirubinaemia are listed in Table 19.2. Biliary atresia and neonatal hepatitis account for 80% of the cases of conjugated hyperbilirubinaemia in term infants whereas cholestasis secondary to prolonged parenteral nutrition administration is the most common cause in preterm infants.

Investigations

The diagnostic dilemma is to distinguish biliary atresia from neonatal hepatitis. Box 19.8 lists the investigations that are of value in distinguishing these conditions. Liver biopsy, radionuclide scanning and further management should be carried out in a specialist children's liver centre.

Biliary atresia

At birth these infants have absent or atretic bile ductules involving the main bile ducts or the main branches of the bile ducts. The deeper in the liver substance that the ducts are abnormal, the more severe is the condition. The commonest variety is extrahepatic biliary atresia. The pathogenesis is unknown. In up to 30% of cases, biliary atresia may be associated with other malformations including renal anomalies, heart malformations, asplenia, polysplenia, malrotation and situs inversus. The onset of jaundice may be delayed by up to 4 weeks

Table 19.2 More common causes of conjugated hyperbilirubinaemia	
Bile duct abnormalities	Biliary atresia Inspissated bile Choledochal cyst
Idiopathic	
Infection	Systemic (e.g. septicaemia) Hepatic TORCH Hepatitis B HIV
Metabolic	Alpha-1-antitrypsin deficiency Galactosaemia Cystic fibrosis Fructosaemia Tyrosinaemia Alagille's syndrome Dubin–Johnson rotor syndrome
Endocrine	Hypothyroidism Hypopituitarism
Toxic	Parenteral nutrition

Adapted from McKiernan PJ. Neonatal cholestasis. *Semin Neonatol* 2002;**7**:153–165.

Box 19.8 Investigations to detect the cause of neonatal conjugated hyperbilirubinaemia

- Liver enzymes
- Alkaline phosphatase
- Serial bilirubin levels
- Alpha-Fetoprotein
- Alpha-1-antitrypsin screen and phenotype
- ^{123}I Rose Bengal excretion test
- Abdominal ultrasound
- Sweat test
- TORCH serology
- Amino acid screen
- Percutaneous liver biopsy
- Radionuclide (HIDA) scan (injection of radioactive hydroxyiminodiacetic acid which is taken up in the liver and excreted in the biliary system)

Box 19.9 Main causes of neonatal hepatitis

- **Infection**: most commonly due to TORCH infections contracted in the first trimester, but other viruses may also produce hepatitis. If a mother is positive for hepatitis B, the infant should be protected from infection by immunization (see Chapter 10)
- **Metabolic causes**: fructosaemia and tyrosinaemia may cause severe neonatal hepatitis. Galactosaemia more commonly presents with unconjugated hyperbilirubinaemia, but affected infants later develop cholestasis
- **Alpha-1-antitrypsin deficiency**: this is an autosomal recessive condition and causes a relatively common form of conjugated hyperbilirubinaemia. Only infants who are homozygous for the PiZZ type are at risk of neonatal hepatitis. There is no specific treatment, and up to 50% of affected children improve and may recover fully. Death due to liver failure occurs in the other half, and liver transplantation may be life-saving in this group
- **Severe intrauterine growth restriction.** This results in a benign intrahepatic cholestasis
- **Long-term TPN use** (e.g. gastroschisis, short gut syndrome)
- **Chronic hypoxic–ischaemic damage to liver** (i.e. recovery from multiorgan failure but liver failure persists)

from birth. It is a surgically operable condition, but because progressive obliteration of the bile ducts occurs rapidly with advancing age, early diagnosis is essential for successful treatment. If surgery is attempted before 60 days of age, there is an 80% chance of achieving biliary drainage by the portoenterostomy operation, known as the Kasai procedure. Serum bilirubin falls rapidly after successful surgery, but many children develop ascending cholangitis, which is the most serious postoperative complication. Approximately two-thirds of survivors will require liver transplantation by 10 years of age.

Neonatal hepatitis

This is a non-specific condition with a variety of causes, which are discussed below; the prognosis depends on the underlying cause. In general, approximately one-third of cases deteriorate and develop hepatic cirrhosis, one-third have evidence of chronic liver disease and one-third recover fully. The prognosis for idiopathic neonatal hepatitis is good and more than 90% resolve by 1 year of age.

The main causes of neonatal hepatitis are listed in Box 19.9.

Inspissated bile syndrome

High and prolonged levels of unconjugated bilirubin may cause a condition in which the bilirubin produces cholestasis with progressive conjugated hyperbilirubinaemia. Ultrasound scanning may show sludge in the gallbladder. It is usually a self-limiting condition but ursodeoxycholic acid (UDCA) may be an effective therapeutic option.

Dubin–Johnson syndrome

This is a rare and benign condition in which the neonate may develop low-grade conjugated and unconjugated hyperbilirubinaemia.

Jaundice is the most common clinical condition presenting in the newborn period. In most infants the jaundice is physiological as there is no underlying disease. Jaundice presenting in the first 24h may be due to haemolysis and always requires investigation. Physiological jaundice, which commonly presents between day 2 and day 5 of life, is a diagnosis of exclusion. Unconjugated bilirubin is neurotoxic in high levels and can cause acute or chronic encephalopathy if not treated appropriately. Conjugated hyperbilirubinaemia is much less common than unconjugated jaundice in the newborn, but has a much more serious prognosis.

SUMMARY

 Now visit **www.essentialneonatalmed.com** to test yourself on this chapter.

CHAPTER 20

Haematological disorders

Key points

Introduction

Haematological disorders in the fetus and newborn infant arise from the conditions which primarily affect blood constituents such as red blood cells (RBCs), haemoglobin and platelets. Some of the conditions are inherited and amenable to prenatal diagnosis or screening at birth. Symptoms in affected infants may start either *in utero* or after birth. Diagnosis of some of the haematological conditions may be complex, requiring interpretation by a paediatric haematologist. Treatment includes prevention and specific therapies. It should be borne in mind that the normal haematological indices in newborns are different from those in older children and vary according to postnatal age.

Placental transfusion

The blood volume and red cell mass at birth and in the neonatal period depend on the volume of the placental transfusion and subsequent readjustments of blood volume.

This occurs within 3 min of delivery and can contribute up to 25% of the total neonatal blood volume. This amount will be increased in the following situations:
- elevated maternal blood pressure
- use of oxytocic drugs

Essential Neonatal Medicine, Fifth Edition. Sunil Sinha, Lawrence Miall, Luke Jardine.
© 2012 John Wiley & Sons, Ltd. Published 2012 by John Wiley & Sons, Ltd.

- late clamping or milking of the cord
- infant held in a low, dependent position at birth.

On the other hand, the amount will be reduced by early cord clamping, or holding the infant above the level of the attached placenta.

The average blood volume of a newborn infant is 85–90 mL/kg, but ranges from 75 to 100 mL/kg. The practice of delay in clamping the umbilical cord or milking the cord from the placenta to the baby may have both advantages and disadvantages. Although this can result in improved blood volume and reduced iron deficiency in childhood, there may be associated disadvantages too as inadvertently high red cell mass can result in symptomatic pulmonary plethora and hyperbilirubinaemia. This subject of 'early' versus 'late' (i.e. physiological) clamping of umbilical cord is still a matter of debate. The UK Resuscitation Council recommends delaying cord clamping for 1 min in uncompromised babies.

Anaemia

Anaemia is usually defined by a haemoglobin (or haematocrit) level and classed as mild if the haemoglobin level (Hb) is 10–12, moderate if it is between 8–10 and severe if it is less than 8 g/dL. The causes of neonatal anaemia are shown in Box 20.1 and broadly fall under the following headings:

- physiological
- haemorrhage
- haemolysis
- hypoplasia or aplasia (diminished production).

Box 20.1 Causes of neonatal anaemia

- Physiological anaemia
- Anaemia of prematurity
- Haemorrhage
    - Antepartum haemorrhage
    - Fetomaternal transfusion
    - Twin-to-twin transfusion
    - Neonatal internal haemorrhage
- Haemolysis (see Box 20.2)
- Aplasia: Blackfan–Diamond syndrome

Physiological anaemia

The full-term infant is born with a haemoglobin concentration in the range 15–23.5 g/dL, whereas in the premature infant the haemoglobin level is slightly lower. Initially there is a slight increase due to haemoconcentration, but then haemoglobin gradually drops and remains low for most of the first year of life (Fig. 20.1). This is known as physiological anaemia.

Anaemia of prematurity

In the preterm infant physiological anaemia occurs earlier, is more severe and prolonged than in the term infant, and is termed anaemia of prematurity. It is caused by a number of factors.

Lack of erythropoietin
At birth the infant moves from a relatively hypoxic fetal state to become relatively hyperoxic. This suppresses erythropoietin secretion for the first 7–8 weeks of life. In addition the bone marrow is probably more resistant to the stimulatory effect of erythropoietin. When this ends, reticulocytes start appearing in the peripheral blood film.

Repeated blood sampling
The preterm infant is often subjected to daily repeated blood sampling for laboratory investigation. This is the commonest cause of anaemia in babies admitted to neonatal units.

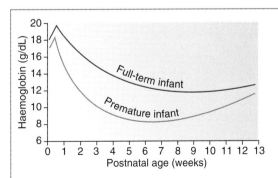

Figure 20.1 Physiological anaemia. The two graphs show the normal fall in haemoglobin with postnatal age in mature and premature infants.

Relative haemodilution

There is an increase in plasma volume over the first months of life and, together with poor red cell production, the haemoglobin falls. This is referred to as 'early anaemia'.

Iron deficiency

The full-term infant is born with sufficient iron stores for the first 4 months of life, but in preterm infants these stores are low and exhausted more quickly because of the infant's rapid growth rate. An infant of 1.5 kg at birth has half the iron stores of a 3.0 kg neonate. Iron deficiency mostly causes the 'late anaemia' that accounts for low haemoglobin levels after 4 months of age, characterized by hypochromic red cells seen on a blood film.

Haemolysis

Haemolysis may occur in preterm infants as a result of vitamin E deficiency. Administration of vitamin E may reduce the extent of late anaemia of prematurity but is not used in practice.

Treatment

A daily dose of elemental iron is associated with a good response in most cases, but routine iron supplementation from an early age to 'prevent' anaemia is controversial and not practised universally.

Transfusion (10–20 mL/kg) may be necessary in premature infants if the haemoglobin falls below 7–8 g/dL and the infant is symptomatic. Symptoms include breathlessness with feeds, tachycardia, apnoea and bradycardia or failure to gain weight. However, blood transfusion can also suppress erythropoietin activity, and hence if the infant shows a reticulocyte count of more than 5%, transfusion should be delayed if possible, depending on the infant's condition. Premature infants receiving intensive care do end up receiving repeated blood transfusions. In such situations, exposure to multiple blood donors can be avoided by using the same batch blood from a single donor and stored in mini packs. Donor blood should be screened for blood-borne viruses, particularly cytomegalovirus (CMV).

The following formula may be used to calculate the volume of blood to be transfused for an anaemic infant (Hct is the haematocrit):

$$\text{Donor blood required (mL)} = \frac{(\text{desired Hct} - \text{actual Hct}) \times \text{body weight (Kg)} \times 90}{\text{donor Hct}}$$

The administration of subcutaneous recombinant human erythropoietin to preterm infants has been shown to stimulate red blood cell production, thereby avoiding the need for frequent blood transfusions. But this treatment has not been shown to be cost-effective and is not widely used.

Haemorrhage

Causes are listed in Box 20.2 and investigations in Box 20.3.

Treatment

Acute blood loss, if significant, is more likely to present with signs of hypovolaemia and shock as the initial manifestation such as changes in blood pressure, heart rate, tissue perfusion and urine output. In acute haemorrhage, the haemoglobin may be normal in the beginning as enough time has not passed for haemodilution to occur.

Severe haemorrhage may present as a neonatal emergency and require immediate transfusion with blood or blood substitute (such as crystalloid or 4.5% albumin) to prevent irreversible shock. In an

---

Box 20.2 Causes of haemorrhage

- Haemorrhage before and during delivery from:
  Placental – placenta praevia, placental abruption, incision into the placenta during caesarean section
  Fetal–fetomaternal or twin-to-twin transfusion
  Cord – rupture or torn vessels on insertion into the placenta
- Neonatal haemorrhage:
  - Trauma – bleeding may occur into skull, brain, lung, peritoneum or bowel
  - Haemorrhagic disease of the newborn

Box 20.3 Investigations to determine cause of haemorrhage

These will depend on the likely diagnosis, but include:

- Haemoglobin and haematocrit
- Kleihauer's test (to assess the presence of fetal cells in maternal blood, indicating fetomaternal transfusion)
- Coagulation studies (indicated if a bleeding diathesis is suspected)
- Investigations to determine site of bleeding (e.g. ultrasound of head or abdomen)

Box 20.4 Causes of immune and non-immune neonatal haemolysis

Immune haemolysis (positive Coombs' test)

- Rhesus incompatibility
- ABO incompatibility
- Minor blood group incompatibility (e.g. Kell, Duffy, Kidd)
- Maternal autoimmune diseases (e.g. SLE)

Non-immune haemolysis (negative Coombs' test)

- Congenital infection
- Disseminated intravascular coagulation (DIC)
- G6PD deficiency
- Pyruvate kinase deficiency
- Hereditary spherocytosis (HS)
- α-Thalassaemia
- Infantile pyknocytosis
- Vitamin E deficiency

emergency, unmatched group O rhesus-negative blood may be used, but formal cross-matching should be done whenever possible. Remember babies rarely die of anaemia; hypovolaemia is much more damaging.

Haemolysis

The causes of neonatal haemolysis are shown in Box 20.4. Haemolysis is usually associated with unconjugated hyperbilirubinaemia and reticulocytosis. Causes of haemolytic anaemia can be broadly divided into two groups; immune and non-immune.

Rhesus haemolytic disease

This occurs because the mother's immune system has been sensitized by rhesus-positive cells from her fetus. Sensitization may be due to
- fetomaternal transfusion (during previous delivery or from miscarriage)
- rhesus-incompatible transfusions.

The rhesus factor is complex, comprising CDE/cde antigens. The commonest antigen is D, and this accounts for 95% of cases. Approximately 83% of the population are D positive, that is, rhesus positive (Rh +ve). If sensitization occurs, maternal immunoglobulin G (IgG) crosses the placenta to cause haemolysis of 'foreign' fetal erythrocytes. IgG remains present in the neonatal circulation for up

to 3 months and neonatal haemolysis may continue to occur for some weeks after birth.

Prevention

Rh IgG prophylaxis (anti-D gammaglobulin) is indicated in the management of all non-immunized pregnant women who are Rh negative. Current recommendations include the routine administration of IgG at 28 weeks' gestation to all pregnant women who are RhD negative, and within 72 h of delivery to all rhesus-negative women who give birth to rhesus-positive infants. If antibodies are already present anti-D is not required. The standard dose of 300 μg is sufficient for protection for up to 30 mL of fetal blood. This provides satisfactory prophylaxis for 99% of all term deliveries.

Anti-D gammaglobulin should also be given to at-risk rhesus-negative women after every sensitizing event, such as miscarriage, termination of pregnancy or amniocentesis.

Anti-D gammaglobulin is ineffective against non-D rhesus antigen (usually C, E). If a large transfusion of fetal blood occurs, the standard dose of 300 μg/kg may be insufficient. In women at high risk, a Kleihauer–Berke smear test can be performed to quantitate for the fetal blood present. For every 30 mL of fetal blood detected, an additional 300 μg of IgG can be administered.

Management during pregnancy

This includes routine testing for antibodies, monitoring of antibodies, assessment of bilirubin in amniotic fluid, monitoring of fetal well-being and monitoring for signs of fetal complications.

- **Routine testing.** Rhesus-negative women should be screened for rhesus antibodies at their first antenatal visit, and at subsequent visits according to local guidelines. If antibodies are detected at any of these times, more frequent testing will be necessary.
- **Antibodies present.** If antibodies are present, then depending on the level and/or whether the titre is rising, an amniocentesis should be performed. Amniocentesis is commonly done at 30–32 weeks but may be performed earlier, depending on the level of antibodies, and particularly on the history of previous pregnancies. A Kleihauer test is done before and after amniocentesis. The timing of delivery will depend on the antibody levels, amniocentesis result and previous history of affected infants.
- **Assessment of bilirubin in liquor.** Fetal rhesus disease is now a relatively rare condition, and affected pregnancies should be managed in recognized regional centres experienced in treating these women and their babies.
- **Assessment of fetal well-being.** High-resolution ultrasound is an essential adjunct to the assessment of isoimmunized pregnancies. It allows early detection of hydrops, assessment of fetal behaviour (biophysical profile, which provides important evidence of fetal well-being), and interventions such as fetal blood samplings and transfusion. Ultrasound is used to assess the amniotic fluid index, hepatomegaly, subcutaneous oedema, ascites and increases in middle cerebral artery blood flow velocity.

Management of the rhesus-immunized infant

The baby should be assessed for maturity, pallor, jaundice, hepatosplenomegaly, oedema, ascites, ecchymoses, heart failure and respiratory distress. The placenta is examined for the presence of oedema, weighed and sent to the pathology department for confirmation of the diagnosis.

- **Investigations at birth.** Cord blood is taken for grouping, direct Coombs' test, haemoglobin and platelet count and total bilirubin estimation. The Coombs' test is always positive in rhesus incompatibility, unless an intrauterine transfusion with rhesus-negative blood has recently been performed. The more positive the Coombs' test, the more severely affected the infant is likely to be.
- **Indications for exchange transfusion** are listed in Box 20.5.

Interval exchange transfusion is done to prevent the serum unconjugated bilirubin reaching a potentially dangerous level (e.g. 450 in >38 weeks and 350 at 35 weeks). This is usually carried out as an adjunct to phototherapy, and guideline graphs are useful (see Chapter 19).

Exchange transfusion is performed with warmed (37 °C) **whole** blood less than 5 days old. The infant is given a double-volume exchange (180 mL/kg). The blood should be rhesus negative and ABO compatible with the mother's blood. The method for exchange transfusion is described in Chapter 29.

Complications of rhesus incompatibility are detailed in Box 20.6.

Box 20.5 Indications for exchange transfusion

Principal indications for immediate exchange transfusion

- Cord haemoglobin <8 g/dL* (recent *in utero* transfusion may lead to falsely reassuring Hb)
- Hydrops fetalis.

Indications for early exchange transfusion

- Cord bilirubin >85 μmol/L (5 mg/100 mL)
- Cord haemoglobin 8–12 g/dL
- Rapidly rising serum bilirubin that crosses the level for exchange transfusion on the charts (see Chapter 19)
- A very strongly positive Coombs' test

Box 20.6 Complications of rhesus incompatibility

The complications include:

- Kernicterus and bilirubin encephalopathy (see Chapter 19)
- Hyaline membrane disease
- Beta-cell hyperplasia of the pancreas, resulting in hypoglycaemia
- Hypoalbuminaemia and lung oedema
- Thrombocytopenia and DIC
- Complications of exchange transfusion (see Chapter 19)
- Anaemia. This results from ongoing haemolysis and require monitoring by checking haemoglobin levels and reticulocyte counts. Treatment includes folic acid administration and 'top-up' transfusions. Iron therapy is not necessary unless the infant is born prematurely

ABO incompatibility

Haemolytic disease caused by ABO incompatibility is now the commonest cause of isoimmune haemolytic anaemia, but is generally less severe than that caused by rhesus incompatibility.

The naturally occurring anti-A or anti-B antibody is of the IgM type, which does not cross the placenta. Approximately 10% of women carry 'immune' anti-A or anti-B antibodies of the IgG class. It is in the pregnancies of these women that ABO incompatibility occurs, as the IgG crosses the placenta to haemolyse fetal red cells. Women with blood group O are most likely to have anti-A and anti-B IgG agglutinins, and it is this maternal blood group that accounts for the vast majority of ABO incompatibility. This may occur in the first pregnancy, and subsequent pregnancies may be relatively unaffected.

ABO incompatibility generally occurs with the blood group combinations listed in Table 20.1.

Clinical features

The usual presentation is with jaundice on the first day or two of life. Kernicterus is an unusual complication, and hydrops fetalis has only occasionally

Table 20.1 Blood group combinations causing ABO incompatibility

Mother	Infant	Frequency
O	A or B	Common
A	B or AB	Rare
B	A or AB	Rare

been reported. Unlike rhesus disease, late anaemia is seldom a problem but folic acid is recommended because of ongoing haemolysis.

Investigations

ABO incompatibility is usually suspected in the presence of maternal blood group O and when the infant is either blood group A or, less commonly, group B.

- The direct Coombs' test on the infant's blood is usually negative or only weakly positive, but the indirect Coombs' test may be positive.
- A blood smear from the infant may show features of haemolysis, often with microspherocytes. Spherocytes are rarely seen in rhesus disease.
- If the mother's serum causes haemolysis of adult A or B cells, this strongly suggests that she carries α or β haemolysins. Maternal blood should be examined for haemolysins.
- Immune anti-A or anti-B may be eluted from fetal RBCs or cord blood.

Treatment

This is as for rhesus haemolytic disease, but intrauterine fetal transfusion is much less likely to be required.

Minor blood group incompatibilities

Rarely blood group incompatibilities are caused by Duffy, Kell, Kidd and C and E antibodies. They usually present with mild jaundice, but hydrops fetalis has been reported.

Glucose-6-phosphate dehydrogenase deficiency

This disease is inherited in an X-linked recessive manner and is due to a deficiency of the enzyme glucose-6-phosphate dehydrogenase(G6PD) within the RBCs, thereby rendering the cells more susceptible to haemolysis. More than 100 million people throughout the world, mainly Chinese, southern Mediterranean, black American or black African, have this abnormality. It usually occurs in males, although the heterozygote female may manifest mild features of the disease. There are many variants of this condition, some requiring an oxidizing agent to trigger haemolysis and others that cause haemolysis spontaneously. Some infants with the enzyme deficiency develop jaundice in the newborn period without exposure to oxidant drugs, but in other variants of the condition oxidant drugs are required to trigger haemolysis. In later years otherwise healthy children may become acutely ill with anaemia when exposed to drugs.

Box 20.7 lists drugs that commonly cause haemolysis in susceptible neonates. Some drugs excreted in breast milk are liable to haemolyse red cells in G6PD-deficient infants, including nitrofurantoin, sulfonamides and sulfasalazine. In addition, respiratory viruses, viral hepatitis and fava beans cause haemolysis in susceptible infants. Routine administration of vitamin K to G6PD-deficient infants is safe.

Clinical features

Haemolysis may occur spontaneously or after exposure to infection or drugs. Jaundice and pallor may be the only clinical signs. It may be severe and require exchange transfusion. Hepatosplenomegaly is uncommon.

Investigations

Anaemia with spherocytosis, reticulocytes and crenated red cells is seen. Heinz bodies are another feature of the haemolytic anaemia. A screening test for G6PD deficiency is available and is reliable in infants of Chinese and Mediterranean extraction. In black infants, once haemolysis has occurred, a population of young red cells may remain with normal enzyme activity, and this makes the screening test unreliable. Black infants and those positive on the screening test should have the enzyme level directly assayed.

Treatment

Infants born into families known to have G6PD deficiency should not be exposed to agents likely to cause haemolysis. Spontaneous haemolysis may occur, and the treatment is as for any cause of unconjugated hyperbilirubinaemia. Anaemia may require transfusion.

Pyruvate kinase deficiency

This is an autosomal recessive condition affecting glucose metabolism within the red cell membrane. Spontaneous haemolysis occurs in the neonatal period with anaemia and jaundice. Splenomegaly is always present. Diagnosis is made by enzyme assay.

Hereditary spherocytosis

Hereditary spherocytosis (HS) is an autosomal dominant condition that may cause neonatal haemolysis. The blood film shows spherocytes with little splenomegaly initially. ABO incompatibility may present in a similar way, and a family history of HS is an important diagnostic point. The spherocytes show an increased osmotic fragility, although this may not be apparent in the first few months of life. Severe haemolysis with very high levels of hyperbilirubinaemia may occur suddenly.

Thalassaemia

Classic β-thalassaemia major does not affect neonates because most of the haemoglobin is in the

---

Box 20.7 Drugs that may cause haemolysis in infants with G6PD deficiency

- Antimalarials (primaquine, quinine)
- Nitrofurantoin
- Sulfonamides
- Phenacetin
- Aspirin (acetylsalicylic acid)
- Nalidixic acid
- Methylene blue
- Naphthalene
- Vitamin K (large doses)
- Chloramphenicol

fetal (HbF) form. α-Thalassaemia is a rare and severe condition that causes hydrops and severe anaemia.

Infantile pyknocytosis

This is a rare cause of neonatal haemolysis and is diagnosed by finding large numbers of small distorted 'pyknocytes' in the peripheral blood film. The greater the numbers of pyknocytes, the greater the tendency to haemolysis. This condition may be due to vitamin E deficiency and is self-limiting.

Hydrops fetalis

This term is used to describe an infant who shows severe and generalized oedema and fluid in at least two visceral cavities (pleural effusions, ascites, pericardial effusions) irrespective of the cause.

Causes

There are many causes of hydrops fetalis which can be broadly categorized as immune and non-immune (Table 20.2).

Investigations

Investigations are done to determine the cause of the hydrops fetalis and include:
- Coombs' test and full blood count
- Haemoglobin electrophoresis
- Maternal Kleihauer test
- TORCH/syphilis/parvovirus serology
- Placental examination
- Chest radiograph
- Detailed ultrasound examination of chest and abdomen
- Echocardiography
- Total serum proteins and serum albumin
- Chromosomal analysis
- Dysmorphology evaluation
- Autopsy.

Treatment

This may include paracentesis of the abdomen and chest, transfusion, intubation and positive-pressure ventilation, plus diuretic and intravenous albumin therapy. Despite intensive treatment, prognosis for non-immune hydrops remains poor, particularly if there are structural defects or its cause is not known, compared with cases caused by isoimmunization.

Table 20.2 Causes of hydrops fetalis	
Immune	**Non-immune**
Severe haemolytic disease of the newborn (rhesus, ABO, minor blood groups).	**Severe chronic anaemia *in utero*:** fetomaternal haemorrhage, homozygous α-thalassaemia, chronic fetomaternal transfusion, twin-to-twin transfusion
	Cardiac failure: severe congenital heart disease, large atrioventricular malformation (haemangioma), fetal supraventricular tachycardia
	Hypoproteinaemia: renal disease congenital nephrosis, renal vein thrombosis, congenital hepatitis
	Intrauterine infections: syphilis, toxoplasmosis, CMV, parvovirus B19[a]
	Congenital malformations: cystic adenomatoid malformation of the lung, obstructive uropathy, pulmonary lymphangiectasia
	Genetic abnormality: trisomy 21, 18 and 13; Turner's syndrome (45XO); triploidy; Noonan's syndrome
	Idiopathic[b]

[a] This usually causes hydrops secondary to severe anaemia.
[b] This may account for up to 50% of cases where no obvious cause is found after extensive investigations.

Aplasia

Impaired RBC production is an unusual cause of anaemia in the newborn. The most common cause is the Diamond–Blackfan syndrome, also known as congenital hypoplastic anaemia.

Polycythaemia

Polycythaemia in the newborn is common and is defined as a venous haematocrit of 65% or more (approximating to a haemoglobin of 22 g/dL), during the first week of life. Polycythaemia does not mean the blood is hyperviscous. Blood viscosity depends largely on packed cell volume (haematocrit), but the deformability of RBCs and the plasma viscosity may also be significant factors. The relationship between viscosity and haematocrit is linear below a haematocrit of 60–65%, but increases exponentially above this level. Viscosity is much greater in small vessels than in large ones.

Polycythaemia should only be diagnosed on a free-flowing venous specimen and not from a heel-prick sample.

The causes of polycythaemia are listed in Box 20.8.

Clinical features

The infant looks plethoric, and polycythaemia may cause problems in a number of organ systems owing

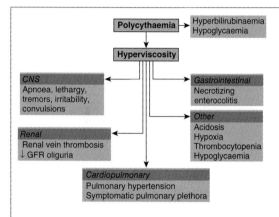

Figure 20.2 The interrelationship between polycythaemia and hyperviscosity and their contribution towards clinical signs. CNS, central nervous system; GFR, glomerular filtration rate.

to diminished blood flow through small vessels. The clinical signs associated with polycythaemia/hyperviscosity are illustrated in Fig. 20.2.

Management

Infants at risk of polycythaemia should have a haematocrit measured on free-flowing venous blood. Babies with a haematocrit greater than 75% even if asymptomatic should have a dilutional exchange transfusion. When symptoms are present, dilutional exchange should be considered even at a lower haematocrit level (>65%).

A dilutional exchange (which should not be confused with exchange transfusion as in rhesus disease) is performed with plasma and is aimed at reducing the haematocrit (Hct) to about 50% by the following formula:

$$\text{Volume (mL) to be exchanged} = \frac{(\text{actual Hct} - \text{desired Hct}) \times \text{body weight (Kg)} \times 90}{\text{actual Hct}}$$

where 90 refers to the blood volume (in mL) per kg.

Box 20.8 Causes of neonatal polycythaemia

- Chronic intrauterine hypoxia:
  SGA infants
  Postmaturity
- Excessive transfusion of blood
  Placental transfusion due to delayed clamping
  Twin-to-twin transfusion
  Maternofetal transfusion
- Infants of diabetic mothers
- Down's syndrome
- Neonatal thyrotoxicosis
- Congenital adrenal hyperplasia
- Beckwith–Wiedemann syndrome

Bleeding and coagulation disorders

These may be due to thrombocytopenia, clotting factor deficiency, abnormal capillaries or a combination of these. Coagulation is a complicated process and is relatively less efficient in the newborn (particularly premature infants) than in older children.

When the vascular endothelium is damaged specific factors are released that cause platelet aggregation, upon which thrombus is deposited. This induces fibrin formation, which further induces platelets to be deposited, leading to the creation of a platelet–fibrin syncytium that prevents further bleeding. Thrombin is formed from prothrombin by the action of factor X. Factor X may be activated by either the intrinsic or the extrinsic pathway to precipitate a cascade of clotting factors, culminating in the production of fibrin. Plasminogens act to remove fibrin (fibrinolysis), and in the healthy state this system is balanced with the clotting mechanism by a series of inhibitors.

Clinical features

Bleeding may be overt, from venepuncture sites or the umbilical stump. Bruising (ecchymoses), purpura or petechial haemorrhages may be present at birth or develop in the neonatal period.

A careful maternal history should be taken, including a family history of bleeding, drugs (warfarin, aspirin), idiopathic thrombocytopenic purpura (ITP) and recent viral illness

Neonatal examination includes:
• site of bleeding: examination will determine the origin of bleeding, such as the gastrointestinal tract, umbilicus or circumcision
• presence of purpura suggesting thrombocytopenia
• hepatosplenomegaly suggesting possible: infection (TORCH, bacterial)
• presence of other congenital anomaly, e.g. giant haemangioma, thrombocytopenia with absent radii (TAR) syndrome.

Investigations

Platelet count

A platelet count less than $100 \times 10^9/\text{mm}^3$ is usually classified as thrombocytopenia. A useful guide to severity is

• 50–100,000: mild thrombocytopenia (bleeding with surgery)
• 25–50,000: moderate thrombocytopenia (bleeding with minor trauma)
• <25,000: severe thrombocytopenia (spontaneous bleeding is likely).

Infants with long-standing thrombocytopenia may have no spontaneous bruising even with platelet concentrations as low as $10,000/\text{mm}^3$.

Coagulation profile

• **Bleeding time.** This measures the time to stop bleeding after a standard small wound, as from an Autolet device. The upper limit of normal for this test in the neonate is 3.5 min. Prolonged bleeding time is seen in thrombocytopenia, von Willebrand's disease and disseminated intravascular coagulation (DIC).
• **Prothrombin time (PT).** This assesses the extrinsic clotting pathway (factors II, V, VII and X). It is not markedly affected by heparin.
• **Partial thromboplastin time (APTT).** This assesses the intrinsic clotting pathway (most factors except VII and XII) but is prolonged by heparin contamination. It is the most sensitive test for coagulation disturbances.
• **Thrombin clotting time.** This assesses fibrinogen activity and requires calcium for activation.
• **Fibrin degradation products (FDPs).** Fibrin is deposited during coagulation and is simultaneously degraded by plasminogens to FDPs. The presence of increased levels of FDPs or elevated D-dimer indicates that fibrinolysis is occurring, usually following thrombosis or as part of DIC.
• **Clotting factor analysis.** Specific factors can be assayed individually, but interpretation may be difficult because of uncertainty as to the normal range in very immature infants.

The normal ranges for some of these tests are shown in Table 20.3.

Thrombocytopenia

Petechiae and ecchymoses, which may be present at birth or appear after birth, are the characteristic lesions produced by platelet deficiencies. Whereas bleeding may occur from any site, intracranial

Table 20.3 Normal results for some of the more commonly used tests of coagulation

Test	Preterm (30–36 weeks)	Term
PT (s) (I, II, V, VII, X)	13–23	13–17
Thrombotest (TT;%) (II, VII, IX, X)	15–50	15–60
APTT (s) (I, II, V, VII, IX, X, XI, XII)	35–100	35–70
Thrombin time (s)	12–24	12–18
Reptilase time (s)	18–30	18–24
Fibrinogen concentration (g/L)	1.2–3.8	1.5–3.5

Box 20.9 Causes of neonatal thrombocytopenia

- Infection:
    Any bacterial infection
    TORCH infections
- Isoimmune
- Maternal disease:
    Severe toxaemia of pregnancy
    Idiopathic thrombocytopenic purpura (ITP)
    Systemic lupus erythematosus
    Drug induced (hydralazine, thiazides)
- Neonatal drug exposure:
    Thiazide diuretics
    Quinine
    Sulphonamides
- DIC
- Thrombocytopenia with absent radii (TAR syndrome)
- Giant haemangioma (Kasabach–Merritt syndrome)
- Fanconi's anaemia
- Leukaemia
- Pancytopenias

haemorrhage is the most devastating complication. Box 20.9 lists the causes of neonatal thrombocytopenia.

Alloimmune thrombocytopenia

This is analogous to rhesus isoimmunization but is a much rarer condition. A transfusion of fetal A1 antigen-positive platelets into the maternal circulation may produce maternal IgG antibodies if the mother is platelet A1 antigen negative. The mother has normal numbers of platelets. Thrombocytopenia in the neonate may be severe, but is usually transient. The disease presents with intracranial haemorrhage (often fatal) in 20%. *In utero* treatment consists of fetal platelet transfusion and regular gammaglobulin therapy. Neonatal treatment is valuable, using platelet transfusions, gammaglobulin and steroids.

Maternal idiopathic thrombocytopenia

Transplacental maternal antibodies cause thrombocytopenia in the neonate and the mother will usually have thrombocytopenia. The lower the concentration of maternal platelets, the more severely affected the infant may be. Prenatal administration of corticosteroids or high-dose intravenous IgG (IVIG) has been advocated to reduce the incidence and severity of neonatal thrombocytopenia, but the response to these treatments is uncertain and unpredictable. The use of IVIG in the thrombocytopenic neonate may cause the platelet count to increase rapidly.

It has been suggested that delivery by caesarean section should be undertaken in severely thrombocytopenic fetuses to avoid trauma, but recent evidence suggests that intracerebral bleeds may occur before the onset of labour.

Prednisolone may be given to the severely affected neonate, but the condition is transient, lasting at most 12 weeks. Treatment of severe thrombocytopenia includes platelet transfusion (10 mL/kg). Serious neonatal haemorrhage does not occur if the platelet count is above 50,000/mm^3.

Haemorrhagic disease of the newborn

Classic haemorrhagic disease of the newborn is caused by a deficiency of the vitamin K-dependent clotting factors. Its incidence has reduced considerably since routine supplementation with vitamin K (IM or by mouth) at birth became mandatory. Vitamin K is produced by the bacterial flora of the gastrointestinal tract, but as the newborn infant has a sterile bowel at birth there is little production from this source in the first weeks of life.

Clinical features

Spontaneous bleeding can occur from any site but is usually gastrointestinal (producing haematemesis or melaena), umbilical or associated with circumcision. It occurs late in the first week of life, especially in the breastfed infant owing to the low vitamin K levels in human milk, and nowadays almost only occurs if vitamin K prophylaxis has been missed or declined.

Gastrointestinal bleeding in the infant must be differentiated from swallowed maternal blood from antepartum haemorrhage, episiotomy or cracked nipples.

The Apt test, which depends on the resistance of haemoglobin F (fetal red cells) to denaturation by sodium hydroxide, will distinguish the infant's blood (predominantly fetal) from maternal blood (adult blood). Most centres will now perform Hb electrophoresis to identify if it is predominantly fetal or adult haemoglobin to identify the source of bleeding.

Investigations

The diagnosis is confirmed by a prolonged PT but a normal APTT.

Treatment

Vitamin K (IM or IV) is given after blood has been obtained for investigations. Whole-blood transfusion (30 mL/kg) will be indicated for hypovolaemic shock.

Vitamin K prophylaxis

Routine administration of intramuscular vitamin K to all newborn babies will prevent bleeding from vitamin K deficiency. However, concerns about the safety of intramuscular vitamin K, in particular the

risk of cancer, were raised in the early 1990s and although there are few data to support this, a small risk of leukaemia cannot be excluded. In order to avoid the potential risk of IM injection a number of countries have recommended oral administration of vitamin K in all healthy full-term infants.

Konakion MM paediatric drops are licensed in the UK for use in healthy neonates of 36 weeks' gestation and older. The recommended dosage regimen is a dose orally shortly after birth, a further dose at 4–7 days and, if the baby is exclusively breastfed, a third dose should be given at 1 month of age. Failure to give a complete dosage regimen appears to be the reason for the re-emergence of serious late-onset vitamin K deficiency haemorrhage. In rare situations where haemorrhagic tendency still persists after administration of vitamin K, one should exclude the possibility of *cystic fibrosis and α_1-antitrypsin deficiency.*

Disseminated intravascular coagulation

DIC is an acquired coagulation disorder characterized by the intravascular consumption of platelets and clotting factors II, V, VIII and fibrinogen. Widespread intravascular coagulation results from the deposition of thrombi in small vessels and the consumption of clotting factors, with consequent haemorrhage. DIC is recognized as a complication of an increasing variety of neonatal conditions (see Box 20.10).

Box 20.10 Neonatal conditions of which DIC is a complication

- Septicaemia
- Severe shock
- Severe perinatal asphyxia
- Hyaline membrane disease in very low birthweight (VLBW) infants
- Severe rhesus disease
- TORCH infections
- Hypothermia
- Maternal DIC with a transplacental effect; this occurs secondary to antepartum haemorrhage, a dead twin fetus or amniotic fluid embolism

Investigations

- Blood film showing haemolysis with fragmented and distorted red cells
- Thrombocytopenia
- Prolonged PT, PTT and thrombin time
- Low fibrinogen
- Increased FDPs.

Not all these features are necessary to make the diagnosis, but the presence of three or more makes DIC very likely.

Treatment

This is a complex disorder and haematological consultation will often be necessary. Treatment consists of:
- Treating the underlying disease process.
- Treatment of the haematological abnormality, including exchange transfusion with fresh whole blood and/or replacement of clotting factors with fresh frozen plasma, platelet concentrates and cryoprecipitate. Heparinization is unlikely to be of any benefit.

Inherited disorders of coagulation

These include haemophilia, Christmas disease and von Willebrand's disease. Coagulation factors are not transferred from the maternal circulation to the fetus. Severe forms of haemophilia A (factor VIII deficiency) and Christmas disease (factor IX deficiency) account for the majority of haemorrhagic problems of the newborn caused by congenital coagulation abnormalities. Bleeding in these X-linked recessive diseases occurs when male infants are subjected to surgical procedures such as circumcision, or from either birth trauma or routine sampling of capillary blood. The diagnosis is confirmed by a prolonged APTT, normal PT and decreased factor VIII assay. Factor XI deficiency (haemophilia C) is inherited as an autosomal recessive disease and is not usually diagnosed in the neonatal period. Excessive bleeding typically occurs in the post-traumatic or postoperative settings such as after circumcision. Factor XI deficiency has been described as a common finding in Noonan's syndrome.

von Willebrand's disease does not usually present in the neonatal period. However, because von Willebrand factor (vWF) serves as a carrier for factor VIII, those who are symptomatic in early infancy often have signs and symptoms associated with low factor VIII. Laboratory testing requires determination of vWF antigen and vWF activity and a platelet function test in addition to ascertaining factor VIII activity.

Management

A specific diagnosis may be difficult to make at birth because in the healthy infant many of the clotting factor assays are low. Expert advice should be sought. Treatment is only required if there is active bleeding or the baby is extremely preterm and at risk of intraventricular haemorrhage (IVH), otherwise anti-factor VIII antibodies (inhibitors) may develop.

Congenital deficiency of anticoagulant proteins (hypercoagulable states)

The anticoagulant proteins, protein C, protein S, antithrombin III and heparin cofactor II, are all inherited in an autosomal dominant manner. Homozygous protein C or protein S deficiency causes serious thrombotic events in the postnatal period. The parents, who are usually asymptomatic, are heterozygous for deficiency of the suspected protein. Factor V Leiden, a mutation in coagulation factor V that renders it resistant to cleavage by activated protein C, is now the most common abnormality found in patients with excessive venous thrombosis such as in cases of neonatal stroke or peripheral ischaemia. Such patients may require anticoagulation such as with low molecular weight heparin especially if they develop life/limb-threatening thrombosis.

SUMMARY

The common haematological disorders affecting newborn infants include:

- Anaemia resulting from lack of RBCs and haemoglobin due to diminished production (viz. iron deficiency anaemia) or excessive destruction (haemolytic anaemias). Excessive blood loss either *in utero* (such as feto-maternal or twin-to-twin transfusion) and at birth through accidental bleeding from umbilical cord or trauma to the organs such as liver or skull, is another important cause for anaemia in newborn infant and should be suspected even though it is not externally obvious.
- Haemoglobinopathies resulting from a molecular abnormality of haemoglobulin structure result in conditions such as thalassemias and sickle cell anaemia.
- Genetic disorders of RBC membrane (such as congenital spherocytosis) or RBC metabolism (G6PD deficiency) make the red cells fragile and cause haemolytic episodes.
- Disorders of platelets or coagulation factors (coagulopathies) resulting in abnormal haemostasis are common and can be either primary defect or secondary to other conditions (consumption coagulopathy) such as in DIC. On the other hand, congenital deficiency of certain anticoagulant factors (such as protein-C or S) may make the blood hypercoagulable which predisposes to thrombosis and blockage of important blood vessels such as in kidneys or brain (neonatal stroke).
- Newborn babies are deficient in vitamin K which is an essential part of coagulation process. Vitamin K deficiency can lead to lethal haemorrhage and hence it is now a global policy to supplement all babies, particularly those fed on breast milk with vitamin K; the regime may however differ from one unit to another.

 Now visit **www.essentialneonatalmed.com** to test yourself on this chapter.

CHAPTER 21
Endocrine and metabolic disorders

Key topics

Introduction

Some endocrine and metabolic disorders present acutely in the newborn period and can be life-threatening. They must be included in the differential diagnosis of any serious or unexplained illness. Prompt diagnosis and treatment is life-saving. In other cases, clinical presentation may not be so acute but if undiagnosed and left untreated, can cause serious problems such as growth failure, developmental delay and poor cognitive (intellectual) development. Neonatal screening for conditions which can have serious consequences, and for which treatment is available, is undertaken in most developed countries. Investigation and treatment of endocrine and metabolic diseases can be complex and requires specialist input. Some are readily and successfully treated whilst for others, specific treatment is not available. Babies with endocrine and metabolic problems require long-term treatment and follow-up by a specialist team.

Essential Neonatal Medicine, Fifth Edition. Sunil Sinha, Lawrence Miall, Luke Jardine.
© 2012 John Wiley & Sons, Ltd. Published 2012 by John Wiley & Sons, Ltd.

Glucose homeostasis and its abnormalities

The fetus has a continuous supply of glucose from the mother via the placenta, and consequently fetal blood glucose levels are the same as the mother's. At birth the newborn's blood glucose rapidly falls to approximately 75% of the maternal blood glucose level and the infant has to switch rapidly to endogenous gluconeogenesis until feeding is established.

Glucose and oxygen are the main metabolic substrates of the mature brain, but in the neonate the brain can use alternative metabolic fuels such as lactate and ketones. Birth at full term is characterized by a vigorous ketogenic response, but this is impaired in preterm infants and infants who experi-ence intrauterine growth restriction (IUGR). This is why the brain can function normally, or near normally, despite very low levels of blood glucose. Profound neurological compromise and irreversible damage occur if the brain is deprived of glucose and alternative metabolic substrates.

Glucose metabolism

Figure 21.1 summarizes the main metabolic pathways involved in gluconeogenesis.
• **Glycogen production and glycogenolysis.** These occur largely in the liver and muscles, but only if liver glycogen is available for rapid breakdown to glucose.

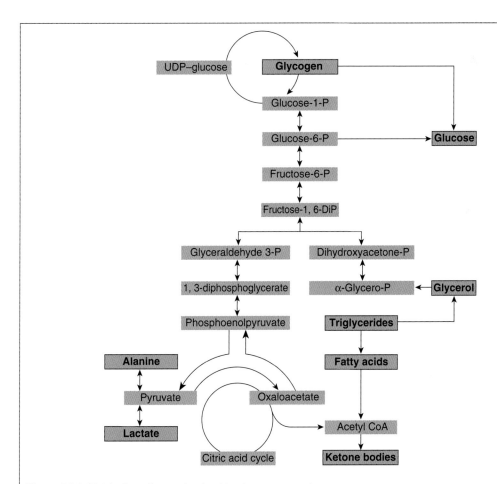

Figure 21.1 Metabolic pathways involved in gluconeogenesis.

• **Gluconeogenesis.** The most important sub-strates are amino acids (particularly alanine), lactate, pyruvate and glycerol. The points at which these are metabolized are shown in Fig. 21.1.

• **Lipolysis.** Glycerol is metabolized from adipose tissue and can be directly utilized in gluconeogenesis metabolism. Other products of lipolysis (fatty acids and triglycerides) are metabolized to ketone bodies, which may be used directly in energy production, particularly by the brain. Ketone body production is stimulated by infant feeding, particularly by breast milk.

These mechanisms are under the control of the endocrine system and are affected by insulin, glucagon, cortisol and growth hormone. Therefore, so that neonates can regulate blood sugar within the physiological range, they must be endowed with adequate liver glycogen, lipid stores and effective metabolic pathways including glycogenolysis and gluconeogenesis, as well as overall endocrine control. Hypoglycaemia will rapidly develop if any of these processes are disturbed.

Measurement of blood glucose

It is essential to measure blood glucose rapidly and accurately in high-risk infants, and a variety of techniques have been developed to give cotside values. Glucose concentrations in plasma or serum are 10–15% higher than in whole blood, and many bedside techniques rely on whole-blood methods, whereas the laboratory techniques are more likely to measure serum glucose levels.

CLINICAL TIP: In the neonatal unit strip reagents are most widely used, but these are generally unreliable particularly in the presence of low blood glucose, which is the range of most importance in the newborn. More recently, portable biosensing devices for measuring glucose at or near the cotside have been introduced which appear to be more reliable. Nonetheless, low levels of blood sugar recorded in the nursery should always be confirmed by sending a specimen to the laboratory for blood glucose analysis.

Hypoglycaemia

The definition of hypoglycaemia has been gradually refined over the last 30 years and higher values for blood sugar are now accepted as normal than was the case in the past. Hypoglycaemia is defined as a blood sugar concentration falling below a predetermined reference value, but this is not usually helpful in a clinical setting. A more important question is what the lowest acceptable level is in an individual baby before physiological compromise occurs. As discussed above, neonatal cerebral function may continue normally despite very low levels of blood sugar because an alternative energy substrate is available.

Attempts have been made to define the level of blood sugar at which cerebral dysfunction occurs and then to set 'normoglycaemia' levels above this. This is based on observational studies in which premature infants (birthweight <1850 g) with blood sugar levels less than 2.6 mmol/L were found to be at increased risk of lower neurodevelopmental scores, particularly when blood sugar values were below this figure on repeated occasions. It has also been shown that a deterioration in neurological function (measured by evoked potentials) occurred with a blood sugar level below 2.6 mmol/L. On the basis of these studies we can define the lower limit of 'normoglycaemia' as 2.6 mmol/L although levels below this do not necessarily mean that damage will occur; however, we recommend maintaining the blood sugar of preterm infants and term infants who are at risk of hypoglycaemia (see below) above 2.5 mmol/L.

Who should be monitored for hypoglycaemia?

The majority of babies who are prone to hypoglycaemia can be predicted on the basis of easily identifiable risk factors (Box 21.1). Careful monitoring of these babies' blood sugar will alert the clinician to the onset of hypoglycaemia and enable management aimed to prevent symptomatic hypoglycaemia.

In babies at risk of hypoglycaemia an early and frequent feeding regimen should be instituted with regular blood sugar monitoring for the first 24 h. 'At-risk' infants should be fed within 2 h of birth.

Box 21.1 At-risk infants for hypoglycaemia

- Infants of diabetic mothers
- Growth-restricted infants
- Premature infants
- Birth asphyxia
- On rewarming after hypothermia
- Infection
- Polycythaemia
- Beckwith–Wiedemann syndrome

Box 21.2 Major and minor symptoms of hypoglycaemia

- **Major.** Apnoea, convulsions and coma. Rarely, prolonged hypoglycaemia may cause congestive heart failure or persistent pulmonary hypertension
- **Minor.** Jitteriness, irritability, tremors, apathy, cyanotic spells and temperature instability

It is not possible to confidently diagnose neonatal hypoglycaemia clinically as the symptoms are non-specific and similar to those of infection.

CLINICAL TIP: Hypoglycaemia may remain entirely without clinical signs or symptoms, and this is referred to as **asymptomatic** hypoglycaemia. It is unusual for a newborn with hypoglycaemia to have a classic autonomic nervous system response, with sweating, pallor and tachycardia, as occurs in adults. A low blood sugar detected by a stick test should be checked by a laboratory blood assay for glucose.

starting immediately before the second feed. More frequent measurements are required in the presence of actual hypoglycaemia. When blood sugar levels are satisfactory, the frequency of heel-prick estimations is reduced before ceasing.

Symptoms of hypoglycaemia

The symptoms of hypoglycaemia in the newborn can be divided into major and minor (see Box 21.2).

Breast feeding is recommended with a frequent administration of expressed breast milk. Formula and IV dextrose may be needed if early breast milk is insufficient. A suitable regimen would be full-strength formula given 2 hourly, although if the mother is adamant that she wants to feed breast milk only an intravenous 10% glucose infusion can be used. Small for gestational age (SGA) infants often tolerate up to 100 mL/kg on day 1 of life. If asymptomatic hypoglycaemia fails to be corrected by early, frequent feeds, an infusion with 10% dextrose will be necessary.

Blood sugar estimates should be made immediately before the feed, as this is the time when the blood sugar is likely to be at its lowest point. In view of the unreliability of reagent strip tests, it may be preferable to undertake more accurate measurement of blood sugar less frequently: one regimen recommends once or twice daily laboratory measurements

Causes of hypoglycaemia

These can be considered under five major headings, which are summarized in Table 21.1.

Management

The major emphasis should be to prevent hypoglycaemia developing, and this is done by recognizing babies who are at higher risk of this condition and giving early and appropriate feeding (see above).

In babies with persistently low glucose level despite feeding, an IV infusion of 10% dextrose at a rate of 80–100 mL/kg per 24 h should be started. If the blood glucose estimate is still less than 2.6 mmol/L (40 mg/100 mL), the dextrose concentration may need to be increased to 15% dextrose. Up to 12.5% dextrose may be infused via a peripheral IV line. If higher concentrations are required, a central IV line will be necessary. Where possible oral feeding should be continued.

Table 21.1 Causes of neonatal hypoglycaemia

Decreased substrate availability	SGA infants (see Chapter 12) Premature infants Multiple birth, especially if growth retarded
Increased glucose utilization	Hyperinsulinaemia Infant of a diabetic mother Rhesus isoimmunization Nesidioblastosis (hypertrophy of pancreas) Islet cell tumour Beckwith–Wiedemann syndrome Polycythaemia
Inability to utilize glucose	Glycogen storage disease Galactosaemia Fructose intolerance Inborn errors of metabolism
Iatrogenic	Inappropriate infusion of glucose
Miscellaneous	Birth asphyxia Endocrine deficiencies (e.g. Congenital Adrenal Hyperplasia) Hypopituitarism

Resistant (or persistent) hypoglycaemia

Rarely, the above regimen fails to control hypoglycaemia and hyperinsulinaemia should be suspected. Under these circumstances other forms of treatment are necessary to control the hypoglycaemia including:

- hydrocortisone
- glucagon
- diazoxide
- somatostatin analogue SMS-201-995 (useful in the short-term management of neonatal hyperinsulinism)

- laparotomy and subtotal pancreatectomy when an insulinoma is strongly suspected.

Investigations

Hypoglycaemia in most infants resolves spontaneously within a few days, but it is sometimes more severe or fails to resolve rapidly. Hyperinsulinaemia is suspected clinically when a baby with severe non-ketotic hypoglycaemia requires a glucose infusion rate exceeding 10 mg/kg per minute to maintain normoglycaemia. These babies have a very brisk response to glucagon injections, with the blood glucose increasing to >1.7 mmol/L above baseline. The definitive diagnosis of hyperinsulinism is made by measurement of serum insulin (>10 mU/mL) during an episode of hypoglycaemia (<2.2 mmol/L). The plasma should be separated and frozen immediately after taking the sample if reliable results are to be obtained. A screen for inborn errors of metabolism may be necessary in some cases. A detailed ultrasound of abdomen and exploratory laparotomy may be necessary in infants suspected of having islet cell tumours. Inborn errors of metabolism or endocrine problems such as hypopituitarism may rarely cause hypoglycaemia, and if these are considered to be a possible cause, appropriate investigations should be undertaken to diagnose or exclude these conditions.

Prognosis

Severe symptomatic hypoglycaemia carries a very poor prognosis. Approximately half of these babies will die and half of the survivors will have severe neurodevelopmental abnormalities, including cognitive delay, convulsions, generalized hypertonia and microcephaly. The prevention of symptomatic hypoglycaemia is one of the most important factors in preventing brain damage in the whole of neonatal medicine.

It is widely believed that infants with asymptomatic hypoglycaemia are not at risk of adverse neurodevelopmental outcome. However, some studies do suggest that neural dysfunction can occur with blood sugar levels below 2.6 mmol/L, even though the baby may not show clinical symptoms. This argument is unresolved.

Specific causes of hypoglycaemia

Infants of diabetic mothers

Maternal diabetes is classified as follows:
- pregestational
- type 1: the basic cause is beta-cell destruction
- type 2: this is due to insulin resistance with an insulin secretory defect
- gestational diabetes.

    Infants of diabetic mothers (IDMs) have unique problems and require specialized neonatal care. The prognosis for the diabetic pregnancy depends on the severity of the diabetes and the quality of diabetic control during pregnancy.

    The two main factors determining whether maternal diabetes will have an effect on the fetus and baby are the vascular complications that the diabetes causes in the mother, and the blood glucose control during pregnancy.
- **Vascular disease.** Mothers with vascular complications as a result of diabetes are much more likely to develop hypertension in pregnancy, which may affect fetal growth and well-being.
- **Glucose control.** The outcome of pregnancy in diabetic women also depends on glucose control both before conception and during gestation. Diabetic women should have their diabetes very care-fully managed before conception, and combined care through pregnancy by a physician and obstetrician is essential. The blood sugar should be maintained below 8 mmol/L with soluble insulin if necessary, and hypoglycaemia avoided. On this regimen the complications for the fetus are reduced and may be avoided completely. A variety of congenital malformations are particularly common in women with diabetes, and the risk appears to depend on the mother's prepregnancy blood sugar levels.

Clinical features of infants of diabetic mothers

Complications to the fetus are likely to occur in diabetic women in whom glucose control has been less than adequate. The frequencies of complications in IDM and in gestational diabetic mothers are given in Table 21.2. Complications include:
- **Congenital malformations.** The most frequent congenital abnormalities in IDM are:
  - congenital heart disease, especially ventricular septal defect, transposition of the great vessels, coarctation of the aorta
  - renal vein thrombosis
  - sacral and coccygeal agenesis (caudal regression syndrome)

Table 21.2 Frequency of complications (percentages) in infants of diabetic mothers and infants of gestational diabetic mothers. Complications are related to the quality of glucose control in pregnancy

Complications	IDM (%)	IGDM (%)
Uneventful course	50	80
RDS	30	10
Hypoglycaemia (asymptomatic and symptomatic)	60	16
Symptomatic hypoglycaemia	20	10
Hypocalcaemia	25	15
Polycythaemia	40	30
Hyperbilirubinaemia	50	25
Congestive heart failure	10	Unknown
Congenital abnormalities	10	3

IDM, infants of diabetic mothers; IGDM, infants of gestational diabetic mothers; RDS, respiratory distress syndrome.

○ left microcolon

○ hypertrophic cardiomyopathy – this mainly affects the intraventricular septum and may cause ventricular outflow obstruction; it is a transient condition that resolves in the first few months of life; inotropic drugs such as digoxin should be avoided.

• **Stillbirth.** There is an increased risk of intrauterine fetal death during pregnancy.

• Infants born to mothers with diabetic vascular disease are more likely to be **SGA**.

• **Macrosomia.** Insulin is a major trophic hormone influencing fetal growth, and hyperinsulinaemic fetuses become macrosomic. These infants are plethoric, obese and 'Cushingoid' in appearance, and have an enlarged heart, liver and spleen (Fig. 21.2).

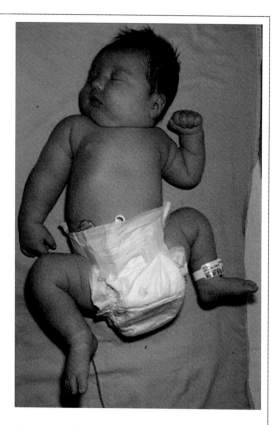

Figure 21.2 Characteristic appearance of the macrosomic infant of a poorly controlled diabetic mother. Note right sided brachial plexus injury.

They have excessive fat stores and inhibition of lipolysis and β-oxidation resulting from hyperinsulinaemia. The large size predisposes to birth-related problems, including:

birth trauma from cephalopelvic disproportion, difficult instrumental delivery and shoulder dystocia; injuries include intracranial haemorrhage, fractured bones and nerve palsies

birth asphyxia, which may occur in a poorly controlled diabetic pregnancy and may be related to cephalopelvic disproportion.

• **Neonatal hypoglycaemia.** Chronically elevated maternal glucose levels cause hyperplasia of the islet beta cells in the fetal pancreas with fetal hyperinsulinism. Once the baby is born the high circulating insulin causes neonatal hypoglycaemia lasting for several days. There are three common patterns:

• transient hypoglycaemia, which lasts 1–4 h, followed by a spontaneous rise in the blood sugar

• prolonged initial hypoglycaemia lasting 24–48 h

• rarely there may be a mild initial hypoglycaemia, followed in 12–24 h by more severe hypoglycaemia, which may be symptomatic.

• Insulin has an **antagonistic effect on surfactant development** and hyperinsulinaemic babies are at much greater risk of developing respiratory distress due to surfactant deficiency, retained lung fluid or polycythaemia, even at full term.

Management

Careful control of diabetes during pregnancy decreases many of the complications. Management of the pregnancy involves obsessional diabetic control, planned delivery in a suitably equipped hospital, examination for congenital abnormalities and screening for anticipated complications, especially hypoglycaemia.

Prognosis for infants of diabetic mothers

This depends on the quality of glucose control in pregnancy. Published studies give perinatal mortality rates of about 30/1000 for diabetic pregnancies, but this has improved considerably with counselling during the periconception period and better antenatal surveillance of diabetic mothers.

Congenital hyperinsulinism

This is due to a group of disorders in the regulatory function of pancreatic beta cells resulting in unregulated secretion of insulin and severe neonatal hypoglycaemia. Specific gene defects have been identified as the cause in 50% of cases. The term nesidioblastosis was previously used to describe congenital hyperinsulinism, but the histological features of it are seen in the normal pancreas and the term is no longer used. Congenital hyperinsulinism should be considered in infants who require glucose infusion exceeding 15 mg/kg/min to prevent hypoglycaemia and confirmed by showing high levels of insulin during hypoglycaemia. Few ketone bodies are produced during the hypoglycaemic episodes.

Severe resultant hypoglycaemia can be temporarily reversed by glucagon and/or octreotide, an analogue of somatostatin. The main drug used in the long-term management of this condition is diazoxide. Those who fail to respond to medical therapy will require surgery. Occasionally the hyperinsulism is due to a localized insulinoma, and full excision of this is curative. More commonly the pancreas is diffusely abnormal, requiring near-total pancreatectomy with removal of up to 95% of the pancreas.

Beckwith–Wiedemann syndrome

This refers to the association of macroglossia, umbilical hernia (or exomphalos) and macrosomia. The infants almost invariably show a crease or fissure in their earlobes. There is often hyperinsulinaemia due to beta-cell hyperplasia. Hypoglycaemia occurs in the neonatal period in about a third of cases. Later malignant disease occurs in about 6% of cases.

Iatrogenic hypoglycaemia

This occurs most commonly in infants at risk of hypoglycaemia in whom low blood sugar is detected and aggressive treatment started. Treatment with rapid intravenous injection of concentrated (25% or 50%) dextrose will cause a rapid increase in blood glucose, and in the presence of hyperinsulinism there may be a rebound hypoglycaemia. When the blood glucose is next measured, hypoglycaemia

is found as a result of this rebound effect, and another rapid infusion of concentrated dextrose is given with similar effect.

Rapid or concentrated injections of dextrose are rarely necessary and should be avoided if possible. When absolutely necessary, they should be followed by a continuous infusion to avoid rebound hypoglycaemia. Effort should be made to maintain normoglycaemia with enteral feeds.

When insulin is used to treat hyperglycaemia or hyperkalaemia, hypoglycaemia may be induced. Regular blood glucose measurements must be performed on all infants receiving insulin.

Hyperglycaemia

Hyperglycaemia is usually defined as a blood sugar concentration greater than 9 mmol/L, at which level glycosuria may occur. Hyperglycaemia frequently occurs in the preterm infant who is receiving 10% dextrose intravenously, or in any infant receiving parenteral nutrition.

Usually hyperglycaemia responds to a reduction in the glucose concentration or the infusion rate. Hyperglycaemia must be considered to be a sign of septicaemia. A full infection screen should always be performed on neonates with high glucose levels or glycosuria. Glycosuria induces an osmotic diuresis and may cause electrolyte imbalance. Very severe hyperglycaemia (>40 mmol/L) is rarely seen, but an increasing number of case reports have shown this to be due to inadvertent infusion of large volumes of dextrose solution or incorrectly made up parenteral feed regimens. If a baby has a blood sugar level above 20 mmol/L then all the baby's infusions should immediately be changed to 5% glucose solution and all the solution formulations and pumps that were used on discovery of the hyperglycaemia should be checked.

Rarely insulin is required to treat hyperglycaemia. Soluble insulin should be given intravenously and repeated as necessary to keep the blood sugar below 9 mmol/L.

Transient neonatal diabetes mellitus

This is very rare and occurs in severely growth-retarded infants. Non-ketotic hyperglycaemia develops as a result of inadequate insulin production by the pancreatic beta cells. Treatment is by correction of electrolyte disturbances and the administration of insulin intravenously. Later, oral hypoglycaemic agents such as sulfonylurea can be substituted for insulin until normal pancreatic function develops.

Disorders of calcium, phosphate and magnesium metabolism

The metabolism of these three electrolytes is interrelated and not completely understood.

- **Calcium.** Half the total serum calcium is in ionized form and half is protein bound. Ionized calcium is the most physiologically active. Fetal calcium levels are higher than maternal levels but drop rapidly, reaching a low point 18–24 h after birth, largely as a result of calcitonin. This fall in serum calcium stimulates parathormone (PTH), with resultant bone reabsorption and an increase in serum calcium to approximately adult levels.
- **Phosphate.** Most inorganic phosphate is in ionic form (PO_4^{3-}) or complexed as either HPO_4^{2-} or $H_2PO_4^-$ ions.
- **Magnesium.** Half the total body magnesium is in bone and most of the rest is intracellular. Neonatal levels are higher than maternal levels. Low levels of magnesium inhibit parathyroid hormone secretion, and hypomagnesaemia is commonly found together with hypocalcaemia.
- **Parathormone (PTH).** This is secreted from the parathyroids in response to low ionized calcium levels. PTH increases serum calcium and lowers serum phosphate levels by the following actions:
    increasing the reabsorption of calcium and phosphate from bone
    increasing tubular reabsorption of calcium and reduces the reabsorption of phosphate
    stimulating the production of renal 1,25-dihydroxyvitamin D.
- **Vitamin D.** This compound requires skin, liver and renal metabolism. Oral cholecalciferol is converted in the liver to 25-hydroxyvitamin D and then further metabolized in the kidney to 1,25-dihydroxyvitamin D. 1,25-Dihydroxyvitamin D increases the intestinal absorption of calcium and phosphate. Low maternal vitamin D levels cause the fetus to be born with relatively low levels.
- **Calcitonin.** This hormone is produced in the thyroid and is secreted in response to a high ionized calcium level. Calcitonin reduces serum calcium and phosphate levels.

Hypocalcaemia

Hypocalcaemia is usually defined as a serum calcium concentration less than 1.8 mmol/L (7.5 mg/dL). It is the ionized fraction that determines whether symptoms occur, but few laboratories routinely measure ionized calcium. Some neonatal intensive care units (NICUs) have blood gas analysers that measure ionized calcium along with other electrolytes. Furthermore, acidosis causes more calcium to be ionized and alkalosis decreases ionized calcium. For these reasons, infants may exhibit few or no symptoms of hypocalcaemia despite low serum calcium levels, provided ionized calcium is normal. This is particularly common in hypoproteinaemic states.

Hypocalcaemia may present early or late.

Early hypocalcaemia

This occurs within the first 72 h of life, although the reasons for this are not fully understood. It is most liable to occur in the following cases:
- prematurity
- associated with respiratory distress syndrome (RDS)
- birth asphyxia
- IDM
- neonatal sepsis.

    Persistent hypocalcaemia is due to hypoparathyroidism. This is a rare condition and may be inherited in either an X-linked or an autosomal recessive manner. It also occurs in the DiGeorge syndrome. Hypocalcaemia is associated with hyperphosphataemia and requires lifelong vitamin D treatment.

Late hypocalcaemia

This is often referred to as neonatal 'tetany' and occurs after the first week of life, but is now rarely seen with adapted infant milk formulas.

Rarely, late hypocalcaemia is due to maternal hyperparathyroidism. Maternal hypercalcaemia causes fetal hypercalcaemia with suppression of the fetal parathyroid. This predisposes the infant to hypocalcaemia in the second or third week of life. It is a transient condition.

Iatrogenic hypocalcaemia

This may occur following exchange transfusion with citrated blood or as a result of inadequate vitamin D supplementation.

Clinical features

Low ionized calcium levels produce neuromuscular irritability. Tremors, tetany, jitteriness and convulsions may occur. Seizures may be identical to those due to hypoglycaemia or other cerebral causes. Occasionally, bradycardia and apnoea may be due to hypocalcaemia.

Diagnosis

Serum calcium and magnesium levels should be measured in 'at-risk' or symptomatic infants. An electrocardiogram (ECG) will show a prolonged Q-T interval (this needs to be corrected for heart rate).

Management

• **Asymptomatic hypocalcaemia**. The low serum calcium should be corrected with oral calcium gluconate supplements or, if there is an intravenous line *in situ*, by IV calcium gluconate.
• **Abnormal movements or apnoea** due to hypocalcaemia should be corrected by a slow infusion of 10% calcium gluconate over 20 min, with ECG monitoring.

Severe and resistant hypocalcaemia, as occurs in congenital hypoparathyroidism, may require vitamin D supplementation in the form of 1-α-vitamin D.

Some cases of hypocalcaemia will not respond to calcium gluconate infusion and require magnesium sulphate (see below).

Prognosis

Most children with neonatal hypocalcaemia recover completely with no adverse neurodevelopmental sequelae (compare hypoglycaemia). Severe enamel dysplasia is seen in the primary dentition of some infants with tetany due to hypocalcaemia.

Metabolic bone disease (rickets or osteopenia of prematurity)

This condition, also referred to as osteopenia of prematurity, was formerly known as rickets of prematurity. Rickets implies a deficiency or abnormality of vitamin D metabolism, which is now known not to be an important factor in metabolic bone disease, hence 'rickets' is a term that is no longer appropriate. It is now a very rare condition as a result of more appropriate feeding regimens in very low birthweight infants. Copper and zinc deficiency causes a condition indistinguishable from the osteopenia due to phosphate deficiency.

The diagnosis is made on radiography of a long bone (Fig. 21.3). The main feature of this condition is bone undermineralization (osteopenia). Skeletal deformities involving the rib cage or alteration in head shape may occur and, in its most severe form, fractures and frank rickets may be present, but these latter abnormalities are now uncommonly seen radiographically. The most sensitive biochemical abnormality is raised alkaline phosphatase (ALP) – usually more than three times the upper normal range – and repeated ALP testing is used to monitor the progress of this disease.

The key to this condition is its prevention. Metabolic bone disease can be avoided by appropriate dietary intake of phosphate. All enterally fed preterm infants should receive 2 mmol/kg per day of phosphate. A baby on full milk feeds of an adapted low-birthweight formula will receive this intake. Premature babies exclusively fed with breast milk will become phosphate deficient and, in these, supplementation with phosphorus is necessary. This is most easily done with a powdered breast milk fortifier. Additional phosphate supplementation is recommended for the first 6 months of life if the baby remains on breast milk alone. Babies on total parenteral nutrition also need phosphate supplementation.

The treatment of established metabolic bone disease is to increase phosphate intake so that serum phosphate levels are normal and phosphorus is

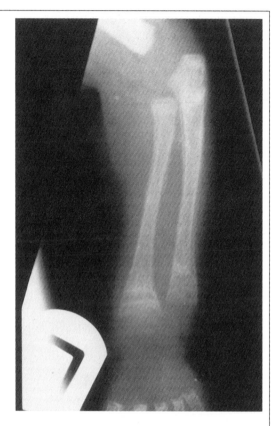

Figure 21.3 Radiograph of an infant's forearm and wrist showing the metaphyseal flaring of neonatal rickets.

excreted in the urine. In some cases additional calcium will also be required. There is no need to give more than 1000 IU/day of vitamin D (cholecalciferol) unless there is evidence of liver disease.

Hypercalcaemia

Hypercalcaemia is defined as a serum calcium concentration greater than 2.75 mmol/L (11 mg/dL). This is often iatrogenic due to the excessive use of calcium gluconate in intravenous fluid therapy. Other rare causes include renal failure, inappropriate antidiuretic hormone secretion, hyperparathyroidism, vitamin D intoxication and Williams' syndrome (idiopathic hypercalcaemia with elfin facies and often supravalvar aortic stenosis or peripheral pulmonary stenosis).

Disorders of magnesium metabolism

Hypomagnesaemia

Hypomagnesaemia is defined as a serum magnesium concentration less than 0.6 mmol/L (1.5 mg/dL). It is always associated with hypocalcaemia. Sometimes hypocalcaemia will not respond to calcium gluconate infusion, but serum calcium levels rapidly increases following magnesium sulphate injections.

Hypermagnesaemia

Hypermagnesaemia is defined as a serum magnesium level greater than 1.5 mmol/L, and it may be associated with hypotonia, bradycardia and apnoea. It may occur as the result of magnesium sulphate administration to the mother for severe maternal pre-eclampsia or to the baby for pulmonary hypertension.

Disorders of sodium and potassium metabolism

Sodium metabolism

The full-term newborn infant requires 2–3 mmol/kg of sodium per day. Preterm infants have greater requirements because of the immaturity of renal tubular reabsorption. Requirements in these infants are in the order of 5–6 mmol/kg per day in the first week of life.

Hyponatraemia

The lower limit of normal for serum sodium is 133 mmol/L, and severe hyponatraemia is defined as a serum sodium concentration less than 125 mmol/L, which may cause apnoea and convulsions. The causes of hyponatraemia are listed in Box 21.3. Care must be taken in the interpretation of serum sodium, as red cell haemolysis in blood samples obtained by squeezing may lower the apparent serum level.

In the assessment of infants with hyponatraemia, serum potassium, creatinine and osmolality should be measured as well as urinary sodium and osmolality (or specific gravity). A careful fluid input and output chart should be kept for these infants.

CLINICAL TIP: Sodium is essential for normal growth. If a preterm baby has poor growth despite adequate calories check the serum sodium. If the sodium level is less than 133 mmol/L, supplementation will be required. If the sodium level is in the lower end of the normal range (133–135 mmol/L), check the urinary sodium excretion. If this is also low, consider adding sodium supplements to improve growth.

$$\text{Na required (mmol)} = 135 - \text{actual Na} \times \text{weight (kg)} \times 0.5$$

where 0.5 represents the 'Na space', which may vary between 0.3 and 0.7 depending on birth weight, gestation and postnatal age.

If hyponatraemia is severe (<118) there is danger of water intoxication and rapid correction (up to 128 mmol/L) using 3% normal saline is needed followed by slow correction with normal saline infusions.

Hypernatraemia

Hypernatraemia is defined as a serum sodium concentration greater than 150 mmol/L. Newborn infants, particularly those born preterm, rapidly become dehydrated and hypernatraemic if fluid intake is reduced or abnormal losses occur where water loss exceeds sodium loss. There are two main causes of hypernatraemia:
- **Reduced renal excretion.** The newborn kidney is less efficient at excreting excess salt than water, and so hypernatraemia is more likely in very immature infants than in older children.
- **Excessive water loss.** The lack of keratin in the skin of very tiny babies causes excessive transepidermal water loss. Phototherapy and radiant warmers aggravate this loss.

With hypernatraemia the serum osmolality is high and this may be associated with intracerebral haemorrhage. The causes of hypernatraemia are:
- mismanaged intravenous fluids
- dehydration; delay in establishing oral feeds
- vomiting and diarrhoea
- bowel obstruction: necrotizing enterocolitis (NEC)
- osmotic diuresis: hyperglycaemia
- excessive use of sodium bicarbonate
- congenital hyperaldosteronism
- faulty technique in making up formula feeds.

Box 21.3 Causes of neonatal hyponatraemia

- Maternal hyponatraemia following excessive administration of 5% dextrose or oxytocin in labour
- Inadequate sodium intake
- Vomiting and diarrhoea
- Inappropriate excess of intravenous fluids
- Inappropriate antidiuretic hormone secretion
- Congestive cardiac failure (e.g. patent ductus arteriosus)
- Diuretic treatment
- Indometacin or Ibrufen for treatment of PDA (due to increased intravascular volume)
- Renal failure
- Sepsis
- Cystic fibrosis
- Bowel obstruction
- Congenital adrenal hyperplasia (salt-losing variety)

Treatment

Treatment of hyponatraemia depends on the cause. If it is due to haemodilution (inappropriate antidiuretic hormone secretion or excessive intravenous water) then water restriction is the first line of treatment. If it is due to sodium loss, then careful replacement with hypertonic saline according to the equation:

Treatment

The serum sodium is reduced by slow infusion of dextrose solution. Too rapid a reduction in hypernatraemia may be deleterious, resulting in cerebral fluid shifts and convulsions.

Potassium metabolism

Hyperkalaemia

This is defined as a serum potassium concentration greater than 6.5 mmol/L, and it may cause life-threatening ventricular dysrhythmias if levels exceed 7.5 mmol/L. Spurious hyperkalaemia occurring with haemolysis during blood sampling should not be confused with true hyperkalaemia.

Pathological causes include renal failure, acidosis, shock, hypoxia and blood transfusion. It is particularly likely to occur spontaneously in very ill, premature infants within 72 h of birth.

Treatment

First-line treatment should consist of stopping all potassium-containing fluids (e.g. parenteral nutrition) and maximizing renal output (e.g. consider furosemide administration). If this still does not work, insulin infusion may be required. One needs to be careful with use of calcium resonium in preterms with poor gut function.

Salbutamol infusion has been shown to reduce serum potassium by 1 mmol/L in the first hour after starting the infusion.

Hypokalaemia

This is defined as a serum potassium concentration less than 2.5 mmol/L (depending on laboratory standards). The causes are:
- diuretic treatment
- alkalosis
- inadequate intake of potassium
- vomiting and diarrhoea
- congenital adrenal hyperplasia.

Treatment

If the hypokalaemia is due to dietary potassium deficiency, it can be replaced orally by adding it to the milk. The normal requirements are 2–3 mmol/kg per day.

Intravenous potassium replacement must only be given in the presence of known and adequate renal function, according to the formula:

$$K \text{ required (mmol)} = (3.5 - \text{actual K})$$
$$\times \text{weight (kg)} \times 0.3$$

This is given by slow intravenous infusion up to a maximum of 0.5 mmol/kg/hour under ECG control.

Endocrine gland disorders

Disorders of thyroid function

Hypothyroidism

Untreated hypothyroidism is associated with severe intellectual impairment and as such is an important cause of subsequent disability. Because early recognition and effective treatment offer an excellent outcome in the majority of cases, the early detection of congenital hypothyroidism is essential.

The incidence of congenital hypothyroidism in the UK and Australia is approximately 1/3500 live-born infants. Causes of hypothyroidism can be subdivided as shown in Table 21.3.

Screening tests

The aim of screening is to detect all infants with clinically significant congenital hypothyroidism at an early stage in order to effect appropriate treatment to avoid brain damage. Screening is performed on heel-prick blood obtained at the same time as the Guthrie test. In the UK and Australia, thyroid-stimulating hormone (TSH) is assayed. Deficiency of circulating thyroid hormone causes the pituitary to release more TSH to stimulate the thyroid. TSH assay is more sensitive in screening for hypothyroidism than thyroxine assay, but fails to detect the rare cases due to pituitary/hypothalamic failure. It does not detect deficiency of thyroid-binding globulin. If TSH levels are high (>40 mU/L), the infant is urgently referred for definitive investigations of thyroid function. A borderline assay (15–40 mU/L) requires a repeat Guthrie card screen at 28 days of life.

Clinical features

Most infants detected by a screening programme will be clinically normal. The classic signs of severe or untreated hypothyroidism include poor feeding, constipation, abdominal distension, umbilical hernia, mottled skin, coarse puffy facies with a large protruding tongue, hypotonia, hypothermia, failure

Table 21.3 Causes of hypothyroidism in the neonate	
Primary, affecting the thyroid gland (90%)	
Dysgenesis (75%)	Ectopic thyroid (30%)
	Absent thyroid (30%)
	Hypoplastic thyroid (15%)
Dyshormonogenesis (20%)	Multiple causes involving biochemical defects in thyroid gland function. These are usually associated with a goitre at birth and are autosomal recessive in inheritance
Isoimmune (5%)	Occurs as the result of transplacental antibodies and may cause permanent or transient hypothyroidism
Secondary, affecting the pituitary or hypothalamus (10%)	
Transient neonatal hypothyroidism	This is the cause of 10–20% of all positive screening tests
Excessive use of iodine containing solutions for skin cleansing	Hence not used these days

to thrive, persistent jaundice and both growth and developmental delay.

Transient hypothyroidism

This refers to babies who have a positive screening test but whose thyroid function subsequently normalizes without treatment. Prenatally acquired causes include maternal thyroid deficiency, antithyroid drugs and thyroid antibodies acquired transplacentally. In the neonatal period the most common transient abnormality is due to topically applied iodine-containing antiseptics. Elevated TSH levels are related to the surface area swabbed and the frequency of skin swabbing.

Investigations

Once a positive screening test has been notified, the following investigations are required:
- Serum thyroxine and TSH.
- Thyroid autoantibodies in mother and baby.
- Radioisotope scan to localize the position of an ectopic or hypoplastic thyroid.
- Ultrasound scan of the thyroid gland.
- Radiography for bone age – this is delayed in hypothyroidism.
- Enzyme assays may be required in the investigation of inborn errors of thyroid metabolism.

Treatment

Treatment consists of L-thyroxine initially. Monitoring of the dose will be by growth assessment, bone age, physical appearance and thyroid function tests. Treatment is lifelong in all but transient cases.

Prognosis

The outcome for congenital hypothyroidism depends on the severity of intrauterine hypothyroidism and the delay in establishing effective treatment after birth. The pretreatment venous thyroxine level is the best predictor of eventual IQ; in those with high levels, even with effective treatment after birth, mild educational, motor and behavioural problems are likely at 10 years.

If diagnosis and treatment are delayed until 3–6 months of age, only 50% of treated children achieve an IQ greater than 90. If diagnosis and treatment are commenced by 3 months, 75% will achieve an IQ greater than 90.

Neonatal hyperthyroidism

This is a rare condition that occurs in about 1–10% of infants born to women with Graves' disease. Women suffering from thyrotoxicosis (or who have been treated with subtotal thyroidectomy) may have circulating TSH-receptor-stimulating antibodies that cross the placenta. Neonatal hyperthyroidism secondary to maternal antibodies usually remits after 2–5 months when the maternal antibodies have disappeared.

Clinical features

The infant is usually growth restricted and often has a small goitre at birth and develops irritability and diarrhoea, with failure to gain weight despite feeding well. The most important feature is tachycardia, which may not be present at birth but develops rapidly within 48 h. This may be severe enough to precipitate cardiac failure. In some cases symptoms can be delayed for up to 6 weeks after birth.

Management

All infants born to thyrotoxic women should be carefully monitored for tachycardia for the first 48 h of life. If symptoms develop, propranolol (2 mg/kg per day) is the treatment of choice. The condition is self-limiting and it should be possible to stop treatment by 2–3 months.

Abnormalities of the adrenal gland

Neonatal adrenal disorders fall into the categories of hyperplasia and hypoplasia.

Congenital adrenal hyperplasia

Congenital adrenal hyperplasia (CAH) is a rare but important autosomal recessive disorder of adrenal function with an incidence of 1/10,000; 95% of cases are due to 21-hydroxylase deficiency. Figure 21.4 shows the metabolic pathway for adrenal hormones. An enzyme block causes failure of cortisol production, which results in central overstimulation of the adrenal by adrenocorticotropic hormone (ACTH). This leads to the overproduction of adrenal hormones produced downstream of the enzyme block, and it is the effect of this overproduction that produces the clinical features of CAH.

Clinical presentation

Deficiency of 21-hydroxylase presents in one of two ways:
• **Virilization.** This is usually obvious in male infants, who may be born with hypertrophic, pigmented genitalia. Female virilization may be missed, as on cursory examination the virilized clitoris may be mistaken for a penis.
• **Salt-losing.** This is due to an excessive aldosterone effect on the renal tubules and occurs in 75% of cases. Hyponatraemia does not usually become obvious until the second week of life, and is associ-

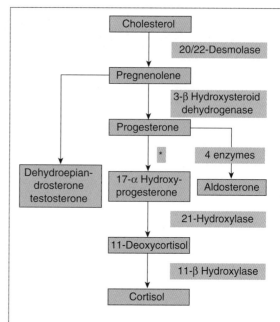

Figure 21.4 A simplified diagram to illustrate the synthesis of adrenal hormones. The asterisk represents the enzyme 17-α-hydroxydehydrogenase.

ated with a high serum potassium. Symptoms of vomiting and poor feeding precede shock in these babies.

The other forms of CAH are extremely rare but may present with poor virilization and hypertension (Table 21.4).

Investigations

Plasma 17-α-hydroxyprogesterone is markedly raised in the common 21-hydroxylase deficiency type of CAH. Biochemical abnormalities for the other enzyme defects are shown in Table 21.4. Countries with a high incidence of this condition may screen the entire population of newborn babies.

Treatment

• **Emergency.** Intravenous fluid replacement, electrolyte correction and mineralocorticoids (fludrocortisone) and hydrocortisone (three times a day).
• **Long term.** Medical management consists of replacement therapy with fludrocortisone and other corticosteroids, usually under the supervision of a paediatric endocrinologist. Surgical treatment may

Table 21.4 Clinical and biochemical features of enzymatic defects in congenital adrenal hyperplasia

Enzyme defect	Virilization	Under-virilization	Salt loss	Hypertension	Urinary 17-ketosteroids	Plasma 17-OH progesterone
20/22-Desmolase	–	+	++	–	↓	↓
3-β OH steroid dehydrogenase	+	+	+	–	←	Normal or ↑
17-α OH steroid dehydrogenase	–	+	–	+	↓	↓
21-Hydroxylase	+	–	+ –	–	←	← ++
11-β-Hydroxylase	+	–	–	+	←	←

+ = present – = absent arrow = equivocal.

be required for the enlarged clitoris in virilized females.

Prenatal therapy

It is now possible to determine whether a fetus is affected by 21-hydroxylase deficiency where there is a family history of this condition. Diagnosis may be made by identifying the gene mutation on tissue obtained at chorionic villus biopsy, or by assay of hormones in amniotic fluid. Dexamethasone given to the mother from 10 weeks of gestation inhibits ACTH overstimulation and reduces the extent of fetal virilization.

Adrenal hypoplasia

This is a rare condition and may arise as primary adrenal failure or secondary to pituitary hypoplasia (as occurs in anencephaly), but may occur in infants with an otherwise normal brain. Adrenal hypoplasia is most often suspected by unrecordable oestriol estimation performed during pregnancy. The infant of any such pregnancy should have adrenal function carefully assessed postnatally. There are also X-linked and autosomal recessive forms of adrenal hypoplasia.

At birth the infant may show hyperpigmentation and hypoglycaemia. Alternatively, symptoms may be delayed until later in infancy. Severe metabolic collapse with profound hypotension may be the first feature of this condition. Adrenal hypoplasia may be confused with CAH, but virilization is not seen and salt loss rarely occurs.

Infants with a family history or low oestriols during pregnancy should have short and long Synacthen tests to investigate the cortisol response to stimulation. Treatment involves lifelong replacement with cortisol and possibly aldosterone.

Ambiguous genitalia

The subject of ambiguous genitalia is complex and one where the neonatologist, the paediatric endocrinologist and the paediatric surgeon must work together to achieve the optimal physical and psychological result for the child and family.

The neonate with ambiguous genitalia may represent a medical emergency. Assessment and subsequent gender assignment must consider the future physical and sexual development of the child.

Parents are informed of the medical concern and the baby is examined in their presence. Terms such as 'underdeveloped' or 'overdeveloped' should be used, and 'intersex' and 'pseudohermaphrodite' avoided. The naming of the baby should be delayed until the definitive sex of rearing has been determined.

Clinical assessment

The following are useful guidelines that should be followed.

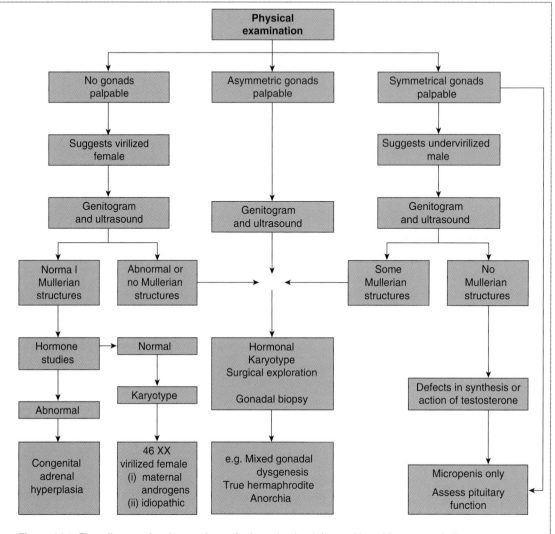

Figure 21.5 Flow diagram showing a scheme for investigating infants with ambiguous genitalia.

- Is the baby a female who has been virilized?
- Is the baby a male who is undervirilized?
- Are gonads palpable in the inguinogenital region? If palpable gonads are present, it is almost certain that they are testes.

A diagnostic flow chart can be based on these observations (Fig. 21.5).

Discussion of the various conditions and their individual treatment is beyond the scope of this text. CAH has been discussed above.

Inborn errors of metabolism

The term 'inborn error of metabolism' was introduced by Garrod in 1896 to describe a group of genetically determined biochemical disorders caused by specific defects in the structure or function of protein molecules. Some of these have no clinical manifestation, such as histidinaemia, whereas others have major clinical sequelae, for example phenylketonuria (PKU). The majority are inherited as auto-

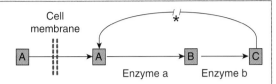

Figure 21.6 Representation of metabolic pathways with a negative feedback loop.

somal recessive disorders but some are sex linked, including Hunter's syndrome, Lesch–Nyhan disease, Menkes' syndrome and ornithine transcarbamylase deficiency.

Metabolic disorders may be understood if the hypothetical biochemical reaction shown in Fig. 21.6 is considered. This reaction may be interfered with at the following sites:
• Failure of substance A to cross into cells, e.g. Hartnup's disease (failure of tryptophan to enter cell).
• Deficiency of enzyme a. This may cause disease by the accumulation of precursor A, as happens in galactosaemia with the build-up of galactose-1-phosphate.
• Alternatively, a deficiency of enzyme a may be associated with the build-up of alternative metabolic products derived from the metabolites of high levels of precursors of A. An example of this is phenylketonuria, with the production of high levels of phenylketones.
• Deficiency of end-metabolic products (C in Fig 21.6) as occurs in albinism, where there is failure to produce melanin.
• Failure of positive feedback control. This occurs when the end product of metabolism is required to switch off a hormone-controlled loop system. CAH is an example of this condition. Failure of cortisol production by an enzyme block results in failure to inhibit ACTH, with consequent adrenal hyperplasia. This is represented by the asterisk in Fig. 21.6.

The inborn errors of metabolism may be diagnosed clinically, in either an asymptomatic phase or an acute early symptomatic phase. Preferably they are diagnosed by screening programmes for the newborn.

Newborn screening

There are many important principles inherent in newborn screening. The following criteria should be satisfied:
• The disease is a significant health problem.
• The disease has a latent or asymptomatic phase.
• There is a commonly accepted and successful therapy.
• The natural history of the disease is understood.
• The test is suitably sensitive (few false negatives) and specific (few false positives).
• The screening programme is cost effective.
• The test sample is acceptable to the patient and easily obtained.
• Adequate facilities for diagnosis and therapy exist.
• There is a commitment to careful follow-up.

The incidences of diseases that have been considered for newborn screening are given in Table 21.5. Screening programmes that have been adopted in parts of Europe, Australia and the USA include
• **Phenylketonuria**.
• **Hypothyroidism**.
• **Galactosaemia**.
• **CAH**.
• **MCAD**.
• **Cystic fibrosis**. Neonatal screening by elevated immunoreactive trypsin on a dried blood spot detects 90% of cases with severe disease. Positive

Table 21.5 Incidence of diseases considered for newborn screening

Specific metabolic disease	Approximate incidence
Cystic fibrosis	1/2500
Hypothyroidism	1/3500
Phenylketonuria	1/15,000
MCAD deficiency	1/15,000
Hartnup's disease	1/18,000
Histidinaemia	1/18,000
Galactosaemia	1/30,000
Homocystinuria	1/150,000
Maple syrup urine disease	1/250,000

cases can then be screened by analysis for the ∆F508 mutation, which accounts for 80% of cases of cystic fibrosis. Widespread screening for this condition is now available in the UK and Australia. Evidence shows that those babies with the disease do better if the diagnosis was made early by screening rather than presenting later in life.
• **Medium-chain acyl-CoA dehydrogenase (MCAD) deficiency.** This condition is as common as phenylketonuria and presents with collapse (implicated in some cases of sudden infant death syndrome, SIDS) and severe hypoglycaemia. If the condition is recognized, hypoglycaemia can be avoided by careful attention to carbohydrate intake, and the prognosis is excellent. Screening using a dried blood spot from a newborn infant is possible using a tandem mass spectrometer. The availability of tandem mass spectrometry in many countries has expanded the range of metabolic disorders that can be screened on the day 3–5 blood spot.

Presentation of inborn errors of metabolism in an acutely ill child

Inborn errors of metabolism as a group are very rare and may present in a number of different ways. In the newborn, presentation is usually dramatic and the infant is very ill. Inborn errors of metabolism must always be considered in the differential diagnosis of an acutely ill infant when there is no obvious alternative diagnosis.

In considering infants with possible inborn errors of metabolism, particular attention should be paid to the following:
• **Family history.** Most such conditions are inherited as an autosomal recessive disorder, hence consanguinity should be asked about. A family history of unexplained stillbirths or neonatal deaths is important.
• **Onset of illness related to feeds.** Some of the disorders only become manifest when the infant ingests milk (e.g. galactosaemia).
• **Is there a characteristic smell?** Infants with isovaleric acidaemia smell of sweaty feet, and in maple syrup urine disease the baby smells of curry.
• **Dysmorphic features.** Peroxisomal disorders (e.g. Zellweger's syndrome) show characteristic facial features. Cataracts are features of galactosaemia.

Diagnosis

Affected infants present in a variety of ways, but the most frequent are:
• **Encephalopathy.** Symptoms include convulsions, apathy, coma and profound hypotonia. Early onset of severe seizures suggests pyridoxine deficiency and non-ketotic hyperglycinaemia.
• **Hypoglycaemia.** This is seen particularly in the organic acidaemias and type I glycogen storage disease. Ketonuria in the absence of hypoglycaemia suggests an organic acidaemia.
• **Acid–base disturbance.** This is seen frequently in any sick baby and is usually not related to inborn errors of metabolism. Calculation of the anion gap may be helpful:

$$\text{Anion gap} = \text{serum } (Na^+ + K^+) \text{ mmol/L} - \text{serum } (Cl^- + HCO_3^-) \text{ mmol/L}$$

If the anion gap is greater than 25 mmol/L then the patient is likely to have a specific organic acidaemia.
• **Hepatic failure.** Rapidly progressive liver disease with rising levels of conjugated bilirubin suggests galactosaemia, α_1-antitrypsin deficiency or tyrosinaemia.

If an inborn error of metabolism is suspected, the following investigations should be undertaken as a matter of urgency:
• Amino acid concentrations in blood and urine (freeze all additional urine specimens for more detailed subsequent examination).
• Organic acid analysis.
• Plasma ammonia.
• Serum lactic acid level.
• Urine for ketone estimate.

Management

Definitive treatment depends on the precise underlying condition. While awaiting a diagnosis the following management points are important:
• Stop all milk feeds.
• Treat metabolic acidosis with infusions of sodium bicarbonate.
• Prevent catabolism by giving 10–15% dextrose infusions, together with insulin if necessary.

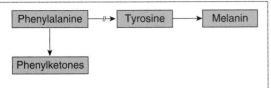

Figure 21.7 Metabolism of phenylalanine. The broken arrow represents the enzyme defect in phenylketonuria.

• Remove toxic waste products by peritoneal dialysis (see Chapter 18).
• If there is hyperammonaemia ($>600\,\mu$mol/L), give sodium benzoate.

Phenylketonuria

PKU is an autosomal recessive condition and, in its classic form, is caused by a deficiency of the enzyme phenylalanine hydroxylase, which converts phenylalanine to tyrosine. Absence of the enzyme results in the accumulation of phenylalanine and its metabolites (Fig. 21.7). In untreated patients the accumulation of phenylalanine and phenylketones produces a clinical picture of neonatal convulsions, later mental impairment, epilepsy and eczema. Affected children usually have fair hair and skin with blue eyes, owing to a relative lack of melanin, which is metabolized downstream from tyrosine.

Malignant hyperphenylalaninaemia has recently been described and is due to a deficiency of biopterin in the liver. This is required as a cofactor for the enzyme phenylalanine hydroxylase.

Diagnosis

This may be suspected from screening tests and confirmed by definitive investigations.

Screening

Screening for PKU was formerly based on the Guthrie test, which is a bacterial inhibition assay on blood absorbed on to blotting paper from a heel-prick sample. The infant needs to be on an adequate milk diet for 48 h before testing. This is particularly important in preterm and ill infants. Antibiotic treatment of the infant may inhibit the bacteria

that produce the Guthrie reaction. Most screening laboratories now use a radioimmunoassay for phenylalanine.

Definitive diagnosis

This involves recalling the infant for definitive biochemical investigations of blood phenylalanine and tyrosine levels, together with urinary phenylketones.

Treatment

This consists of a diet low in phenylalanine and tryptophan instituted within 20 days of age.

With early treatment the prognosis is good, provided careful control is maintained. The diet should probably be lifelong, but sustained at least into the early adolescent years. In the rare cases of malignant hyperphenylalaninaemia, treatment with biopterin will be necessary.

Such conditions are best managed in specialized metabolic clinics.

Maternal phenylketonuria

Undiagnosed maternal PKU may cause the infant to be brain damaged owing to the passage of toxic phenylpyruvate products across the placenta. All women with seizures or low IQ should be tested at booking in the antenatal clinic for urinary phenylketones by means of a simple stick test (Phenistix, Ames Ltd). Women known to have PKU should be well controlled on their diet before conception in order to prevent neurological compromise of the fetus.

Galactosaemia

This rare autosomal recessive condition has many variants, but only classic galactosaemia presents early in the neonatal period. Classic galactosaemia is due to a deficiency of the enzyme galactose-1-phosphate uridyl transferase. It presents with severe illness in the first week of life, with vomiting, encephalopathy, jaundice, failure to thrive, cataracts, hepatomegaly and a coagulation disorder. If treatment is not started the infant will die.

Diagnosis

If galactosaemia is suspected clinically, the urine should be tested for reducing substances. If the urine is positive on Clinitest tablet testing, but negative for glucose on a glucose oxidase stick test, then assay of galactose-1-phosphate uridyl transferase should be performed. A proportion of children with galactosaemia do not show reducing substances in their urine, and an enzyme assay should be performed if the condition is suspected.

Treatment

This consists of careful dietary control using galactose-free milk (see Chapter 9).

Prognosis

Unlike other inborn errors of metabolism early diagnosis does not appear significantly to improve the outcome of galactosaemia, as the fetus has been damaged before birth. Most have significant developmental delay despite adequate dietary management.

Screening

Outcome is not markedly improved by early diagnosis, which weakens the argument for screening all newborns.

SUMMARY

Successful transition of a fetus from *in utero* to *ex utero* life requires a number of adaptations including establishment of a normal glucose homeostasis and metabolic processes. Most of the time such adaptations take place without any difficulty, but on occasions this process does not happen as usual, resulting in increased mortality and morbidity. An understanding of the normal physiologic processes controlling these individual adaptations, both *in utero* and after birth, is necessary to be able to provide a framework for further assessment if needed.

Prompt recognition and early treatment is necessary in all affected babies and this requires a coordinated approach from paediatrician and other professionals, such as specialists in metabolic and endocrine diseases, because of the complexities of such problems. Considering that the harmful effects of many of these conditions can be either prevented or at least ameliorated, many countries have introduced neonatal screening programme for certain conditions specially if their prevalence is high and they are amenable to treatment.

 Now visit **www.essentialneonatalmed.com** to test yourself on this chapter.

CHAPTER 22
Neurological disorders

Key topics

Introduction

Development of the brain is not only a complex but a continuous process starting from very early fetal life, right through gestation and continuing through the first few years of life. The milestones of central nervous system (CNS) development include formation of neural tube and hemispheres, neuronal proliferation, migration and wiring of the brain, synaptogenesis and mylenation. The developing brain is also an extremely vulnerable organ and is subject to a wide range of insults, both in nature and timing, that may alter its structure and function. Advances in diagnostic techniques such as neuroimaging and molecular biology have improved our understanding of the mechanism of perinatal brain injury and this in turn should help to predict long-term neurodevelopmental outcomes.

Brain development

Development of the brain is a continuous process starting from very early fetal life, right through gestation and until the end of the first decade of life. The pattern of brain growth and development is illustrated in Fig. 22.1.

Neuronogenesis

The first neural tissue appears at about 18 days with the neural crest, from which the neural tube develops. There is a phase of rapid neuronogenesis occurring from 4 to about 18 weeks of gestation.

Essential Neonatal Medicine, Fifth Edition. Sunil Sinha, Lawrence Miall, Luke Jardine.
© 2012 John Wiley & Sons, Ltd. Published 2012 by John Wiley & Sons, Ltd.

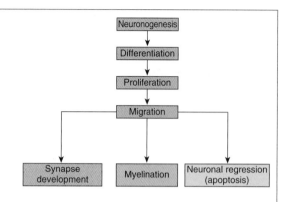

Figure 22.1 The sequence of brain development.

Differentiation

The primitive neural cells differentiate into the different populations of cells, both neurons and glia, that make up the mature brain. This process occurs mainly from weeks 4 to 18.

Proliferation

There is a vast increase in the number of neuronal cells up to about 18 weeks of gestational life, most of which die as part of the neuronal regression process (see below).

Neuronal migration

Neurons are produced deep in the brain and migrate to the cortex and other sites. Final migration of neurons has been achieved by 25 weeks of gestation.

Neuronal regression

The process of apoptosis ensures that only neurons that have achieved a functional capacity within the nervous system survive. Most neurons, during the course of migration, do not acquire this function and regress as part of normal brain development.

Synapse development

Full function in the brain depends on the dendrites of each neuron developing and making many connections (on average each neuron is in contact with 10,000 other neurons). These connections are called synapses. Establishing new synaptic contacts is part of the process of development and learning.

Myelination

Glial cells are associated with the process of myelination and there is rapid growth of these cells from 24 weeks as they migrate to their final sites. Myelination is not complete until the age of about 12 years.

Factors adversely influencing brain growth and development may operate at different times. Community-based studies of disabled children, relating the timing of the brain insult to either prenatal, perinatal or postnatal events, show that prenatal insults account for more disability than perinatal and postnatal causes together. The approximate proportions for neurological handicap in a community are shown in Table 22.1. Table 22.2 lists the relatively common insults that may cause prenatal, perinatal or postnatally acquired disability.

Table 22.1 Estimated timing of events that cause neurological handicap in a community

Prenatal	70–75%
Perinatal	20%
Premature	60%
Full-term	40%
Postnatal	5–10%

The brain is not a homogeneous organ. Specific areas of the brain grow at different times and rates. Thus, growth restriction at any one time (e.g. due to malnutrition) distorts the general growth of the brain and may selectively affect a particular area. Unlike general body growth, the brain has only one opportunity to develop properly and thus interference with growth at a particular time in development may be irreversible.

Malformations of the central nervous system

Abnormalities of the brain can be classified as **malformations** (a developmental defect in which the

Table 22.2 Causes of neurological disability related to the timing of onset of the insult		
Prenatal	**Perinatal**	**Postnatal**
Down's syndrome	Birth asphyxia	Hypothyroidism
Neural tube defects	Intracranial haemorrhage	Meningitis
Other chromosomal disorders	Periventricular leukomalacia	Inborn errors of metabolism
Viral infection	Ototoxic drugs	Trauma
Intrauterine growth restriction	Kernicterus	
Toxins and drugs	Hypoglycaemia	

brain was never normal) and **deformations**, where an external insult has affected normal brain development causing an abnormality in subsequent structure.

Malformations of the CNS apparent at birth result from abnormalities in CNS development. These can be divided into two groups: disorders of dorsal induction and disorders of ventral induction.

• **Dorsal induction** refers to the formation and migration of the neural tube, with subsequent development of the anterior tube into the primitive brain structures. These processes occur during the third and fourth weeks of gestation. Disorders occurring at this time include anencephaly, encephalocoele, myelomeningocoele and meningocoele. These are collectively known as **neural tube defects** (NTDs), and the incidence of babies born with these disorders has fallen markedly over the last 15 years.

• **Ventral induction** refers to development at the ventral end of the neural tube, and particularly cleavage into bilateral hemispheres and ventricles, with thalamic and hypothalamic growth. These processes occur mainly in the fifth and sixth weeks of gestation. The commonest disorder occurring at this time is **holoprosencephaly**, which

may be associated with abnormalities in facial development.

Neural tube disorders (NTD)

NTDs in general, and spina bifida in particular, have become much less common in recent years. There are two main reasons for this: periconceptual folate supplementation and antenatal fetal screening. In some women the risk of a baby with NTDs is increased. This includes families with a history of an affected child, or where the mother herself has the condition. A number of anticonvulsant drugs administered to the mother (particularly sodium valproate) are associated with a considerably increased risk.

It is now known that folic acid is an important substrate for normal early neural tube development, and periconceptual supplementation of at-risk women with folic acid reduces the incidence of NTDs by approximately 75%. As it is not possible to know which women are at increased risk until their first baby is born with spina bifida, it is now recommended that all women intending to become pregnant take regular folate for 3 months before conception.

The second factor in the falling incidence of NTDs is early fetal ultrasound to detect congenital spine or brain abnormalities. In many developed countries virtually all pregnant women are screened at about 18 weeks of gestation. The detection of a seriously abnormal fetus offers the opportunity for the parents to consider terminating the pregnancy.

Anencephaly

In this condition the forebrain is absent; it occurs as the result of an insult before 24 days' gestation. With routine fetal scanning and termination of pregnancy this condition is now rarely seen at birth. Anencephaly is incompatible with life and results in stillbirth or neonatal death.

Encephalocoele

In this condition there has been failure of midline closure of the skull, usually with herniation of the brain. Up to 80% of cases occur in the occipital

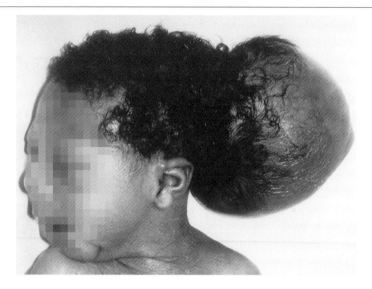

Figure 22.2 Occipital encephalocoele. This infant was operated on. Although he has severe visual impairment, at 2 years he was otherwise normal.

region (Fig. 22.2). This lesion occurs about 28 days after conception. The prognosis depends on the amount of brain in the sac. If the infant is microcephalic with a large encephalocoele, the prognosis is very poor. Neurosurgery is necessary to close the defect.

Spina bifida

This is a developmental failure of fusion of the vertebral column, often with an external protrusion of the meninges and cord. A meningeal sac of cerebrospinal fluid (CSF) with normal underlying spinal cord is referred to as a **meningocoele**, and if there is associated abnormality of the cord it is a **myelomeningocoele**. The abnormalities produced may be classified according to their severity.

Spina bifida occulta

In this condition the vertebrae are bifid but there is no meningocoele or myelomeningocoele sac (Fig. 22.3). This abnormality is seen in 10% of the population and is usually of no clinical significance. In a small proportion the spinal cord may be tethered and with growth becomes stretched, causing irreversible neurological signs in the lower limbs and

bladder. This condition should be suspected if there are lesions over the midline of the lower back. Such lesions include:
- a deep sinus
- a naevus
- a tuft of hair
- a soft fatty swelling referred to as a lipomyelomeningocoele – this is particularly likely to be associated with later neurological signs.

All newborn infants with any of these clinical features should be investigated with real-time ultrasound and, if spinal cord tethering is suspected, referred to a neurosurgeon. The prognosis is much better with early repair before the onset of neurological symptoms.

Spina bifida cystica

This includes meningocoeles and meningomyelocoele (Fig. 22.3). The incidence of this lesion in liveborn infants is now about 1/1000 births, but is considerably higher in some parts of the world.

Meningocoele

These account for 20% of spina bifida cystica lesions. In this condition there is no herniation of nervous tissue, and consequently no neurological

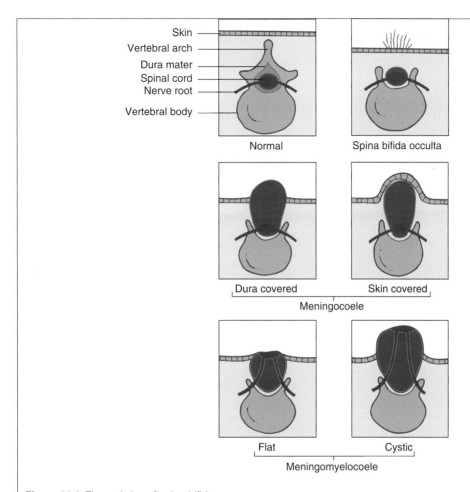

Figure 22.3 The varieties of spina bifida.

deficit. There is a risk of meningitis if the sac leaks CSF.

Myelomeningocoele

These account for 80% of spina bifida cystica lesions. They are associated with herniation of nervous tissue and permanent neurological deficit (Fig. 22.4). The clinical feature are listed in Box 22.1

Investigations

The neural arches of the vertebrae are poorly mineralized at birth, and spinal radiography is of little value except for the assessment of scoliosis. Ultra-sound examination of the spine in the newborn period allows visualization of the spinal cord: if it does not move with respiration, this suggests that there may be tethering.

Management

A careful assessment of the newborn infant by appropriate specialists is necessary before a definite treatment plan can be formulated. Treatment is always discussed with the parents, whose wishes should be considered. Many centres use Lorber's criteria for conservative treatment. Lorber followed a large number of babies with meningomyelocoele, and identified the following bad prognostic criteria:

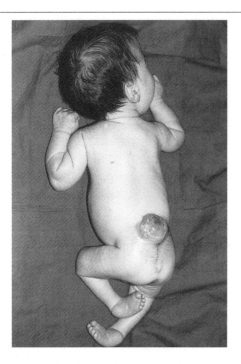

Figure 22.4 Lumbosacral meningomyelocoele.

- total paralysis of the legs
- thoracolumbar or thoracolumbosacral lesions
- severe kyphoscoliosis
- hydrocephalus at birth
- other major congenital malformations

If one or more of these features are present at birth, he recommended conservative management. This consists of nursing care only, but does not rule out subsequent reappraisal of the need for neuro-surgery. Some centres close the skin lesion routinely even if opting for palliative care.

If active treatment is indicated, the following approach would be adopted:

- **Early neurosurgery.** Closure of the sac within 24 h of birth, with ongoing assessment for hydro-cephalus and insertion of a ventriculoperitoneal shunt, if indicated.
- **Orthopaedic assessment and treatment** as necessary.
- **General surgical treatment.** Urinary incontinence is a major problem, and girls usually require an ileal conduit, whereas boys may be managed at

Box 22.1 Clinical features of myelomeningocoele

The spinal abnormality is obvious at birth; clinical examination should assess the following features:

- **Site of lesion.** About 70% are lumbosacral
- **Covering of sac.** Usually meninges, but occasionally the sac is ruptured, leading to CSF leakage and consequent risk of meningitis
- **Neurological examination**:
  motor loss – this is generally lower motor neuron in type and the extent depends on the site of the lesion
  sensory loss – this depends on the position of the lesion, and the level is often asymmetrical
  neurogenic bladder – the patient usually dribbles urine constantly and has a distended expressible bladder
  patulous anal tone
- **Hydrocephalus.** Ninety percent of infants with meningomyelocoeles have an associated abnormality of the brain and skull base, referred to as the Arnold–Chiari type II malformation. This includes prolapse of the medulla, cerebellum and fourth ventricle through an abnormal foramen magnum into the cervical canal. Not all infants develop hydrocephalus, but most have ventricular dilatation on ultrasound scans. Progressive enlargement of the head may occur with advancing age
- **Orthopaedic abnormalities.** These are common and include talipes (see Figure 22.4), dislocated hips, kyphosis, scoliosis and contractures of the lower limbs
- **Miscellaneous abnormalities.** These include renal, cardiac and visceral defects and chromosome disorders

least initially with a penile collecting system or intermittent catheterization. The aim of treating faecal incontinence is to produce a firm stool to prevent soiling and faecal impaction.

- **Supportive care.** Pressure sores need to be prevented by careful positioning and skin care. Psychological and social problems are common and parents need careful support and counselling.

• **Genetic counselling.** This will be necessary for future pregnancies.

Screening for neural tube defects

There are two main aspects of screening for NTDs:

• **Alpha-fetoprotein (AFP).** Blood is taken from the mother at 14–18 weeks' gestation and the level of AFP is measured. AFP in the first trimester normally increases with gestational age, and an accurate assessment of the duration of pregnancy is essential in assessing the significance of the AFP level. Those women with high serum levels should have repeat samples taken 1 week later. Only 10% of pregnancies complicated by a high serum AFP level are associated with NTDs. Multiple pregnancies, exomphalos and other abnormalities may cause high levels. AFP is raised in 90% of cases of anencephaly, and in most cases of open myelomeningocoele. A skin-covered lesion will not have raised levels.

• **Ultrasound screening.** Various abnormalities are assessed, including careful examination of the lower spine for a skin defect and examination of the skull base for the 'banana' sign (a feature of the Arnold–Chiari malformation) or a 'lemon' sign involving the frontal bones.

Disorders of ventral induction

Holoprosencephaly

This is a rare condition where there is a failure of midline fusion of the CNS. There may also be midline defects of the eyes, lips and palate. Half of these lesions are associated with abnormal chromosomal patterns, most often trisomy 13 or 18. The prognosis for normal development is hopeless.

Holoprosencephaly may present as complete alobar forms or as partial forms, referred to as lobar or semilobar, and the diagnosis is made on ultrasound or CT/MRI examination. The appearances of agenesis of the corpus callosum and septo-optic dysplasia may be confused with holoprosencephaly if care is not taken. If septo-optic dysplasia is suspected, assessment of the baby's vision and hypothalamic/pituitary function should be made.

Disorders of head size and shape

Microcephaly

This is defined as an occipitofrontal head circumference more than two standard deviations below the mean for the infant's gestational age. The child may show microcephaly in proportion to weight and length (symmetrical growth restriction) or, more ominously, have a small head but a normally grown body. Microcephaly may be primary or secondary. Primary microcephaly results from disorders of neuronal proliferation (lissencephaly) or cellular migration (such as in Zellweger's syndrome). Secondary microcephaly implies normal growth up to a point when a major insult has occurred, after which brain growth fails. Table 22.3 lists various causes of microcephaly. The prognosis depends on the underlying cause and is generally poor except for familial cases.

Craniostenosis (craniosynostosis)

In this condition the skull sutures fuse prematurely resulting in distortion of head shape (Fig. 22.5).

Table 22.3 Causes of primary and secondary microcephaly

Primary	Secondary
Familial	Intrauterine growth retardation
Autosomal recessive	Meningitis
X-linked recessive	Hypoglycaemia
Chromosomal	Asphyxia
Trisomy 13	Periventricular leukomalacia
Trisomy 18	
TORCH infections	
Maternal phenylketonuria	
Lissencephaly	
Fetal alcohol syndrome	

The underlying cause should be diagnosed and treated wherever possible. The prognosis is usually poor and treatment is supportive.

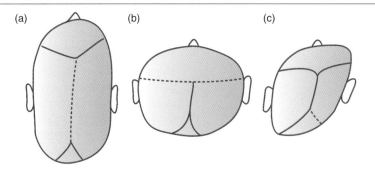

Figure 22.5 Premature suture closure leading to craniostenosis. (a) Scaphocephaly (sagittal suture); (b) turricephaly (coronal suture); and (c) plagiocephaly (single lambdoid suture).

The most common form of craniostenosis is premature closure of the sagittal suture, giving a scaphocephalic head shape (boat shaped, see Chapter 6). Premature closure of the coronal suture leads to a turricephalic head (towering head), and closure of one lambdoid suture results in plagiocephaly (oblique head). Positional plagiocephaly also results from the baby lying on one side of the head with resultant distortion in shape. Autosomal dominantly inherited craniofacial deformities which are associated with some other abnormalities include:
- Apert's syndrome (acrocephalosyndactyly)
- Crouzon's syndrome (craniofacial dysostosis)
- Carpenter's syndrome (acrocephalopolysyndactyly).

Management

Skull radiographs may confirm the clinical suspicion but CT scan provides better assessment of the state of the cranial sutures. Surgery is indicated if premature fusion of the sutures causes raised intracranial pressure. Surgery for purely cosmetic reasons is not indicated except in very select cases.

Macrocephaly (large head)

Macrocephaly is the term used to describe a large head where head circumference is more than two standard deviations above the mean. It can result from a variety of causes which can be broadly subdivided into

- enlargement of the skull bones
- enlargement of brain itself (megacephaly)
- enlargement of CSF spaces (hydrocephalus)
- enlargement of other structures (such as brain neoplasm or intracranial haematoma).

A large head can be an isolated finding and familial or associated with disorders of growth (Soto's syndrome). There are a number of genetic conditions which are also known to be associated with macrocephaly, for example Beckwith–Wiedemann syndrome, neurofibromatosis type 1 and fragile X syndrome.

Hydrocephalus

Hydrocephalus is caused by an imbalance between the production and the absorption of CSF, with resultant dilatation of the cerebral ventricles. This can also result from obstruction to CSF circulation. The term macrocephaly or megalencephaly should not be confused with term hydrocephalus.

Classification

Non-obstructive hydrocephalus
In this type there is no interference with CSF flow. The excessive production of CSF is usually due to a papilloma of the choroid plexus.

Obstructive hydrocephalus
See Fig. 22.6 for site of obstruction. Obstructive hydrocephalus can be divided into non-communicating and communicating.

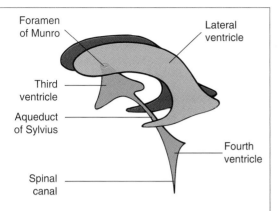

Figure 22.6 Diagram to show intracerebral drainage of cerebrospinal fluid. Reproduced from Levene 1987, with permission of Churchill Livingstone.

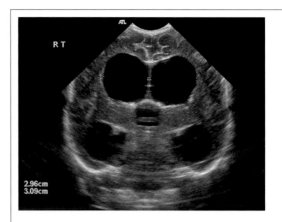

Figure 22.7 Coronal ultrasound scan showing massive dilatation of both lateral and third ventricles.

Non-communicating

There is little or no communication between the ventricles and the subarachnoid space. There are three common sites of obstruction:

- Aqueduct of Sylvius (due to stenosis or atresia).
- Occlusion of the foramina of Luschka and Magendie as a result of basal adhesions. This is the commonest site of blockage and is usually due to intraventricular haemorrhage.
- Arnold–Chiari type II malformation secondary to spina bifida cystica.

Communicating

CSF can escape from the intracranial system via the foramina of Luschka and Magendie, but cannot be absorbed at the arachnoid granulations situated over the surface of the brain. This is usually due to arachnoiditis following either meningitis or intraventricular haemorrhage (IVH).

Clinical features

Hydrocephalus due to congenital abnormalities may be present at birth or diagnosed *in utero* by ultrasound examination. Follow-up studies have shown that about 50% of babies born with apparently isolated fetal ventriculomegaly (no other congenital malformation detected) are normal. The prognosis is poor if the ventriculomegaly is associated with spina bifida or brain abnormality.

Ventricular dilatation occurring after IVH can be detected by serial cranial ultrasound examinations (Fig. 22.7). Ventriculomegaly may be quite advanced before abnormal head growth is noted. A 'sunset' appearance of the eyes is a late sign in neonatal hydrocephalus and may be seen in infants without dilated ventricles.

Investigations

It is recommended that all infants with IVH have weekly ultrasound scans to detect ventricular dilatation. Accurate measurement of the occipito-frontal circumference at weekly intervals is essential in all infants, especially those with intracranial pathology.

Management

This depends on the underlying cause and the degree of ventriculomegaly.

If treatment of the general condition is thought to be appropriate, then ventriculoperitoneal shunting is the treatment of choice. If the infant is unfit for surgery, then temporizing management is necessary by intermittent or continuous drainage of CSF from the ventricles.

Research into the management of posthaemorrhagic hydrocephalus has not suggested that early or aggressive therapy is advantageous to the baby.

The use of acetazolamide and furosemide (furosemide) treatment in established posthaemorrhagic hydrocephalus is associated with a worse prognosis than babies not treated with these drugs. In the last 5 years, evaluation of the direct instillation of thrombolytic agents into the ventricles of babies with early posthaemorrhagic hydrocephalus has not been promising for the safe treatment of this condition.

The important factors in the management of posthaemorrhagic ventricular dilatation (PHVD) are probably the extent of the initial haemorrhage and the intraventricular pressure.

The following management protocol can be followed:
• Twice weekly ultrasound measurement of ventricular size.
• If there is progressive ventricular dilatation, then careful measurement of occipitofrontal head circumference should be performed on alternate days.
• Measurement of CSF pressure if:
  • there is a progressive increase in ventricular size on ultrasound to a point 4 mm above the 97th centile for ventricular index (Fig. 22.8)
  • there is a progressive increase in occipitofrontal head circumference above the 97th centile
  • there are symptoms of raised intracranial pressure (apnoea, poor feeding, irritability, etc.).

CSF pressure can most safely be measured by lumbar puncture. Pressure is measured either by a fluid manometer or measuring the height of a column of CSF in cmH_2O. Two important criteria must be applied to these measurements:
• There is free flow of CSF. If less than 5 mL of fluid is obtained, it suggests that the obstruction is non-communicating and that the pressure can only be measured by ventricular tap.
• The infant is lying quietly when the pressure measurement is made. If the infant is agitated or crying, the measurement is unreliable. Sometimes it will be necessary to sedate the infant to obtain accurate measurements.

In infants with non-communicating ventricular dilatation, or those who are very unstable and in whom the handling involved in lumbar puncture is unacceptable, ventricular tap is the alternative (see Chapter 29).

If the pressure is elevated (>10 cm H_2O, >7.5 mmHg), then further treatment is warranted. If the CSF protein is less than 1 g/L, then a ventriculoperitoneal shunt should be inserted. If the protein is in excess of 1 g/L, a ventricular reservoir or access device will be necessary to prevent the maintenance of raised intracranial pressure. This can later be converted to a shunt. Drug treatment for posthaemorrhagic hydrocephalus should be avoided.

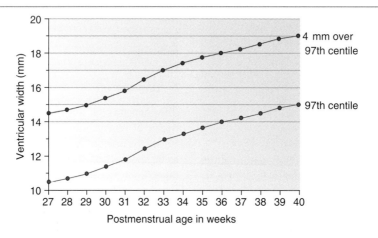

Figure 22.8 Indication for intervention for significant ventriculomegaly. The lower line is the 97th centile for normal ventricular size. The upper line defines ventricular dilatation severe enough to require treatment.

Prognosis

Complications of surgery include shunt obstruction, infection (ventriculitis) and the need for shunt revision. The long-term outlook depends on the cause and severity of the hydrocephalus, presence of any associated brain parenchymal abnormality seen on scans and any subsequent complications.

Hydranencephaly

In this condition there has been almost total loss of brain substance (encephalomalacia) owing to an early massive insult *in utero* such as a vascular insult, infection or trauma. There is usually sparing of the cerebellum and basal ganglia. There is no treatment and the prognosis is hopeless.

Porencephaly

Porencephaly is a non-specific term given to describe any cystic cavities in the brain, which may or may not communicate with the lateral ventricles. They can be congenital or acquired following meningitis, intracerebral haemorrhage (ICH) or cerebral atrophy. The commonest cause is extension of an IVH into brain parenchyma (an intraparenchymal haemorrhage; see Fig. 22.10).

Diagnosis is made by ultrasound or MRI examination.

Lissencephaly

This is an abnormality of neuronal migration and may be due to an intrauterine viral infection, or vascular or asphyxial insult that occurs in the first half of pregnancy. The brain appears smooth and is often microcephalic. Lissencephaly is usually associated with dysmorphic features and neonatal convulsions that are very difficult to control. It may also be due to a genetic disorder, including Miller–Dieker syndrome and Walker–Warburg syndrome.

Intracranial haemorrhage

ICH in the newborn is a common finding at autopsy, and 70% of infants who die have evidence of some degree of ICH. Subdural haemorrhage,

which 50 years ago was the most common type of ICH, is now rare, and intraventricular haemorrhage (IVH) has replaced it as the commonest ICH seen in the newborn infant. There are five important types of neonatal ICH:
- subarachnoid (SAH)
- subdural
- intraventricular (IVH)
- intracerebral (ICH)
- intracerebellar.

Subarachnoid haemorrhage

Blood in the subarachnoid space is most commonly secondary to IVH, which tracks through the ventricular system.

Primary SAH is a common and usually benign condition and is seen in both premature and full-term infants. It occurs as a response to hypoxia or trauma, and is usually seen as a discrete area over the convexity of the brain.

Clinical features

SAH is usually asymptomatic, but when symptoms do occur seizures and apnoea are most commonly seen in full-term infants on the second day of life. Between seizures the infant is usually neurologically normal.

Diagnosis

Ultrasound is very unreliable in detecting SAH, and CT or MRI is much more sensitive for this diagnosis. The CSF is usually heavily blood-stained and does not clear in successive tubes.

Prognosis

A good prognosis can be given if there are minimal neurological signs in the neonatal period and if the predisposing traumatic or hypoxic injury is mild.

In approximately 90% of cases infants with seizures as the primary manifestation of the haemorrhage are normal on follow-up. Rarely the patient dies or is left with serious neurological sequelae, such as hydrocephalus, which presents weeks to months after the initial insult.

Treatment

There is no specific treatment. Bleeding disorders should be excluded and, if present, treated appropriately (see Chapter 20). Shunting for posthaemorrhagic hydrocephalus may rarely be required.

Subdural haemorrhage

Subdural haematoma was formerly relatively common but now rare because of reduced incidence of birth trauma. It is classically due to rapid changes in head shape during labour and delivery. More frequent use of brain imaging has shown that clinically insignificant, relatively small subdural haemorrhages are a common feature of babies born by vacuum extraction.

Pathogenesis

There are three basic origins of subdural haemorrhage:
• Tentorial laceration with rupture of the straight sinus, resulting in an infratentorial haematoma.
• Falx cerebri laceration and rupture of the inferior sagittal sinus, giving rise to a haematoma of the longitudinal cerebral fissure.
• Rupture of superficial cerebral veins with a subdural haematoma over the temporal lobe – usually unilateral and accompanied by subarachnoid blood.
    Several predisposing factors have been established (see Box 22.2).

Clinical features

Subdural haematomas may present as a recognizable symptom complex including tense fontanelle,

---

Box 22.2 Predisposing factors for subdural haemorrhage

• Rigid birth canal – primipara, elderly multipara, small pelvis
• Infant with large head
• Labour – precipitous or prolonged
• Presentation – breech, foot, face or brow
• Delivery – difficult forceps, difficult rotation
• Vacuum extraction

---

hypotonia, lethargy and facial palsy. If the haemorrhage involves the posterior fossa, then apnoea, irregular sighing respiration, fixed bradycardia, opisthotonus and skew deviation of the eyes may occur. If there is only a minor haemorrhage, the baby may be asymptomatic. Signs of hydrocephalus may develop. Asymptomatic subdural haemorrhage is increasingly recognized by increased use of MRI.

Investigations

Subdural haemorrhage over the brain convexity or associated with tentorial tears may be seen on ultrasound, particularly if large. A midline shift may be the only clue to a convexity subdural collection. A CT/MRI scan is more sensitive for diagnosis than ultrasound.

Treatment

In convexity subdural haemorrhage, subdural taps through the anterior fontanelle under strict aseptic conditions are necessary. Repeated taps may be required. Neurosurgical evacuation of thrombus is rarely required.

Intraventricular haemorrhage (IVH)

IVH is usually assumed to have arisen from the rupture of capillaries within the germinal matrix of the caudate nucleus. The condition occurs in premature infants. In some infants the bleeding may be massive, with involvement of the cerebral parenchyma (Fig. 22.9). The initial bleeding occurs into the germinal matrix (also called the subependymal plate), which lies over the head of the caudate nucleus. The germinal matrix is present between 24 and 34 weeks of gestation and rapidly involutes after this time. Rupture into the ventricles (hence the term IVH) occurs in 80% of cases of germinal matrix haemorrhage. Rarely IVH is seen in full-term infants. Changes in cerebral blood flow probably precipitate the bleeding, and infants with respiratory distress syndrome (RDS) are most likely to have an unstable cerebral circulation. Conditions are recognized to be important risk factors associated with onset of IVH are listed in Box 22.3.

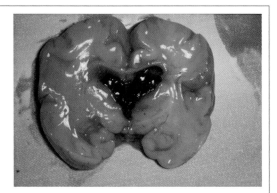

Figure 22.9 Post mortem specimen showing bilateral intraventricular haemorrhage with ventricular dilatation.

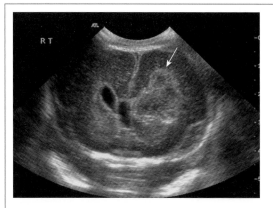

Figure 22.10 Coronal ultrasound scan showing massive left sided IVH with venous infarction of the left parietal lobe with porenchephalic cyst developing (arrow).

Box 22.3 Risk factors associated with onset of intraventricular haemorrhage

- Prematurity
- RDS and pneumothorax
- Intermittent positive-pressure ventilation
- Hypercapnia (high $PaCO_2$)
- Metabolic acidosis
- Coagulation disorder

Clinical features

- **Minimal signs**. Approximately 60% of infants with IVH have no major clinical symptoms. Neurological examination reveals subtle changes in tone, including a tight popliteal angle, and roving eye movements (slow nystagmus) for some weeks after the haemorrhage has occurred.
- **Intermittent deterioration** over a period of days, with increasing signs of apnoea, bradycardia, metabolic acidosis and seizures.
- **Massive collapse** with neurological signs (seizures, coma), shock and anaemia.

Diagnosis

Real-time ultrasound is the method of choice. There is no generally agreed method for grading the sever-

ity of IVH. The two most commonly used schemes are outlined below:
- **Grade 1**: subependymal and/or minimal IVH
- **Grade 2**: intraventricular clot within the lateral ventricle
- **Grade 3**: intraparenchymal involvement. This is usually unilateral and occurs as a result of venous infarction (Fig. 22.10).

The second scheme is called the Papile classification:
- **Grade 1**: subependymal germinal matrix haemorrhage;
- **Grade 2**: IVH with no ventricular dilatation;
- **Grade 3**: IVH with ventricle distended by blood;
- **Grade 4**: intraparenchymal haemorrhage.

Complications

There are two main complications of IVH: post-haemorrhagic ventricular dilatation, leading to hydrocephalus, and porencephaly (see above).

Treatment

There is no specific treatment once IVH has occurred. Careful attention to respiratory management, coagulation disturbances and blood pressure is important in ill infants in an attempt to reduce the likelihood of IVH.

A variety of drugs have been evaluated to assess their effectiveness in preventing IVH when given shortly after birth (vitamin E, indometacin and ethamsylate) but there is no convincing evidence that these drugs reduce adverse outcome in survivors and hence they should not be routinely administered to very premature babies. A more pragmatic approach is to avoid those clinical risk factors (see above) which are known to predispose IVH.

Intracerebral haemorrhage

This is due to venous infarction secondary to IVH or to rebleeding into periventricular ischaemic areas of the brain. Other causes of primary ICH include:
- coagulation disturbances
- cerebral artery occlusion
- TORCH infection
- thalamic haemorrhage
- arteriovenous malformation (very rare)
- tumour (very rare).

Diagnosis is made by ultrasound examination or CT/MRI.

Intracerebellar haemorrhage

This type of haemorrhage occurs in about 5% of preterm infants. It may be due to hypoxic insults, a traumatic breech delivery or head compression. No treatment is available and cerebellar hypoplasia may develop in surviving infants.

Periventricular leukomalacia

Periventricular leukomalacia (PVL) literally means softening of the white matter around the ventricles, and if severe is a major risk factor for the subsequent development of cerebral palsy. It is due to damage to the developing oligodendroglial cells inhabiting the periventricular white matter during the vulnerable period between 26 and 34 weeks of gestation.

Causes

It used to be thought that cerebral underperfusion of the periventricular white matter, as occurs in neonatal hypotension, was the cause of PVL because of the potential vascular watershed at an immature

gestation, but more modern studies have shown this proposal to be unlikely. A number of associated factors are correlated with the development of PVL and these include:
- **Twin-to-twin transfusion syndrome**.
- **Maternal chorioamnionitis**. Infection of the fetal membranes or the fetoplacental unit releases inflammatory proteins called cytokines, which are neurotoxic to the immature brain.
- **Severe fetal asphyxia** (e.g. massive placental abruption, cord prolapse).
- **Complications of severe neonatal lung disease** such as tension pneumothorax.
- **Hypocarbia**. Severe and prolonged hypocarbia (low $P\text{CO}_2$ <4 kPa) is often associated with the development of PVL and should be avoided by appropriate blood gas monitoring in babies receiving mechanical ventilation.
- **Necrotizing enterocolitis** (this may be due to cytokine release).
- **Postnatal dexamethasone administration** for chronic lung disease if given in the first 96 h of life.

Diagnosis

Diagnosis is made by real-time ultrasound, which initially shows areas of echodensity in the white matter; these may resolve spontaneously or progress to cystic degeneration (Fig. 22.11) The prognosis for babies who show persistent echodensity without cystic changes ('flare') is uncertain. More subtle white matter oedema may be detected on MRI, and this may not be evident on ultrasound, but the clinical significance of these lesions is probably negligible.

Neonatal stroke

This is a cardiovascular event occurring around the time of birth with pathological or radiological evidence of focal arterial infarction. Stroke is the second commonest cause of neonatal seizures and results in cerebral palsy and neurodevelopmental delay, mainly affecting the speech. Its exact incidence is difficult to determine, as often the affected babies remain asymptomatic during the newborn period, but is estimated to occur in 1 in 4000 deliveries. The aetiology is multifactorial and summarized in Box 22.4.

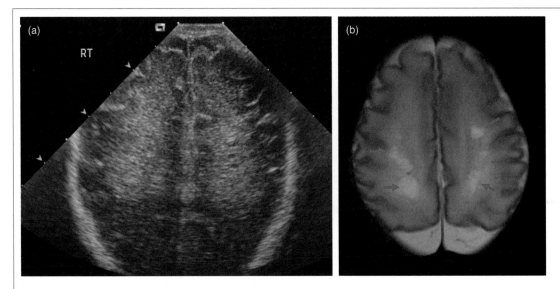

Figure 22.11 Cystic periventricular leukomalacia (PVL): (a) Cerebral ultrasound showing PVL; there is bilateral periventricular 'flare' with cysts on the left side (arrowed) which appeared at 14 days of life. (b) T2-weighted MRI scan on the same patient 6 days later shows extensive bilateral cystic PVL (arrows).

Box 22.4 Risk factors for neonatal stroke

- Cardiac disorders
- Haematological disorders characterized by hypercoagulable state thrombo-embolism (factor V Leiden mutation, protein S and protein C deficiency)
- Infection
- Maternal disorders (autoimmune and coagulation disorders)
- Vasculopathy

Diagnosis relies mainly on neuroimaging. MRI provides a better delineation of the lesion (Fig. 22.12). The commonest vessel to be affected is middle cerebral artery. It is mostly unilateral but can be bilateral.

Treatment is supportive using anticonvulsants, maintenance of adequate perfusion, and use of thrombolytics such as low molecular weight heparin or warfarin. Affected babies require long-term neurodevelopmental surveillance because of high risk of developmental delay. Screening of families for prothrombotic disorders can be helpful for counselling.

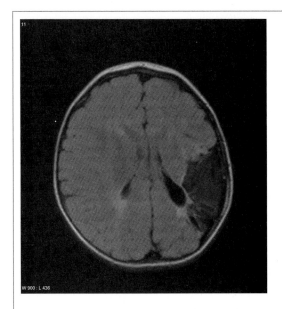

Figure 22.12 Neonatal stroke. MRI scan showing ischaemic infarction of the brain (dark) in the territory of left middle cerebral artery.

Hypoxic–ischaemic encephalopathy

Clinical features

Asphyxia is the simultaneous combination of hypoxia and ischaemia, and the clinical neurological syndrome associated with this is referred to as hypoxic-ischaemic encephalopathy (HIE).

After the initial resuscitation, the infant may be flaccid, hypotonic and unresponsive. The clinical signs characteristically progress over the first 12–24 h, and then gradually improve in all but the most severe cases.

The severity of the HIE syndrome is ascribed retrospectively to one of three grades: mild, moderate or severe (Table 22.4):

• **Grade I** includes increasing irritability with some degree of hypotonia, together with poor sucking, which recovers by 3 days of age. These infants often appear to be 'hyperalert', a state in which they seem hungry but feed poorly and respond vigorously to minimal stimuli. Other causes of irritability, such as hypoglycaemia and infection, must be excluded.

• **Grade II** includes more marked abnormalities of tone, with marked lethargy and usually a lack of interest in feeding. Seizures often develop between 12 and 24 h after the insult but are not severe. These infants classically show a differential increase in tone, in the neck extensors more than in the neck flexors, and leg tone is greater than that in the arms. Improvement in these symptoms over the first week of life is essential before allocation to this group.

• **Grade III** describes the most severely affected infants. They may initially breathe normally but rapidly become comatose, requiring ventilatory support. At this time they are profoundly hypotonic and often have multiple seizures, which are frequent and difficult to control. They are often areflexic. Fatalities occur predominantly in this group, and there may be no improvement prior to death.

Management of encephalopathy

Treatment is largely directed towards complications. General measures include

• adequate tissue oxygenation
• maintenance of optimal environmental temperature
• treatment of possible infection
• correction of coagulation disturbances
• correction of electrolyte imbalance
• avoidance of hypoglycaemia.

Specific complications include:

• intracranial haemorrhage
• hypotension
• seizures
• cerebral oedema.

Hypotension may lead to further cerebral hypoperfusion, and low systemic blood pressure must be rapidly recognized and effectively treated with volume and/or inotropic support. The latter may be guided by echocardiographic assessment. Continuous intravascular blood pressure monitoring is the most reliable measurement method.

Seizures are common and may be subtle, at least in their early stages. Their recognition and treatment are of paramount interest.

Treatment aimed at minimizing cerebral oedema, including fluid restriction (less than usual requirement) is traditional in birth asphyxia, but there is very little data to prove its beneficial effects.

Cerebral neuroprotection

It is now recognized that the immature brain is remarkably resistant to the effects of acute brain

Table 22.4 A scheme for the clinical severity of hypoxic–ischaemic encephalopathy

Grade I (mild)	Grade II (moderate)	Grade III (severe)
Irritability	Lethargy	Coma
Hyperalert	Seizures	Prolonged seizures
Mild hypotonia	Marked abnormalities of tone	Severe hypotonia
Poor sucking	Requirement for tube feeding	Failure to maintain spontaneous respiration

injury such as hypoxic–ischaemic insult (asphyxia). The acute asphyxial insult may cause some initial neuronal injury, but sets in a train of process of abnormal biochemical events that leads to delayed neuronal death, which may occur over days rather than hours. There is no one single route to neuronal death, but rather a whole series of pathways, which may be interconnected. These involve damage to the cerebral vasculature (in part mediated by macrophages), free radical generation, excessive calcium entry due to glutamate neurotransmitter overstimulation, and apoptosis. Apoptosis is 'programmed cell death', a normal function of any cell that does not receive survival signs from adjacent cells. This process is energy requiring and is different from neuronal necrosis. Apoptosis is a normal process in the developing brain, but insults such as asphyxia may exacerbate the process, leading to delayed neuronal loss. Table 22.5 summarizes mechanisms of neural loss to assist the reader in understanding the background to the potential therapies.

Therapeutic Hypothermia

Hypothermia is the most promising technique to protect the mature brain following severe perinatal asphyxia. Recent randomized control trials and their metanalysis have shown benefit from cooling the baby's brain within 6 h of delivery to 33.5 °C for a total of 72 h compared with a normothermic control group. Hypothermia also appears to be a relatively safe technique and is now the standard of care.

It is recommended that: active cooling is used only in larger NICUs, that significant cerebral corti-cal suppression is confirmed with cerebral function monitoring (CFM) trace and that all babies are logged into a national or international database for follow-up purposes. Many centres now recommend passively cooling babies with apparent perinatal asphyxia, pending transfer to a cooling centre. It is very important that this is done with continuous rectal temperature monitoring to avoid excessive hypothermia.

Known complications include mild coagulopathy, and rarely, subcutaneous fat necrosis. Rewarming should be undertaken slowly to avoid hypotension. There is some evidence that cooling can offer a window of opportunity to use other agents to prevent secondary neuronal loss. Currently there is promising research evidence that cooling with coadministration of inhaled xenon gas shows even greater neuroprotection.

Prognosis

The severity of HIE is the best clinical guide to prognosis. Babies with mild (Grade 1) encephalopathy have an excellent prognosis; those with moderate encephalopathy have a 25% risk of serious sequelae, including cerebral palsy and mental retardation. Severe (Grade 111) encephalopathy has a poor prognosis, with 80% of infants dying or surviving to be severely handicapped, but about 20% of such infants may survive without significant disability. These data are before cooling adds further benefit.

As well as cerebral palsy, mental retardation, epilepsy, deafness, blindness, microcephaly or

Table 22.5 Mechanism of neural loss			
	Primary intracellular insult	**Reactive reperfusion**	**Secondary delayed response**
Na/H_2O flux/neural instability	+++	–	–
Calcium influx	+++	+	+
Glutamate receptor	+++	–	+
Free radical	++	–	++
Macrophage	++	++	+
Apoptosis	–	–	+++

Categories of a EEG

- Normal amplitude
  - Upper margin of band >10 μV
  - Lower margin >5 μV

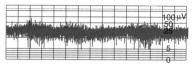

- Moderately abnormal amplitude
  - Upper margin >10 μV
  - Lower margin ≤5 μV

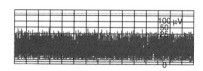

- Suppressed amplitude
  - Upper margin <10 μV
  - Lower margin <5 μV

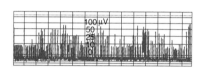

Figure 22.13 The prognostic values of different forms of aEEG tracings in babies with hypoxic-ischaemic encephalopathy. Whilst the top and middle tracings are mostly indicative of good prognosis, the suppressed amplitude with continuous low voltage with seizure activity (burst suppression) as seen in the bottom panel is invariably associated with worst prognosis in terms of death and neurodisability.

hydrocephaly may all occur as sequelae to perinatal asphyxia. Minor handicaps such as specific learning difficulties, behavioural problems and clumsiness may not manifest until many years after birth. The best investigations to predict outcome following perinatal asphyxia are:

- **Electroencephalography (EEG) or CFM.** Very abnormal EEG/CFM traces 6 h after birth indicate a 70% risk of adverse outcome (death or severe disability). The most abnormal traces in mature babies include an isoelectric or very low voltage signal and burst suppression (Fig. 22.13). Complete normalization of the CFM, with a normal voltage and sleep wake cycle by 24 h, offers a good prognosis.
- **Doppler assessment of cerebral haemodynamics.** Doppler assessment of the anterior or middle cerebral arteries has also been found to be a good predictor of a bad outcome, but is only reliable at 24 h after birth. A Pourcelot resistance index (PRI) of <0.55 on Doppler assessment accurately predicts adverse outcome.
- **MRI.** The change that best predicts a bad outcome is abnormality in signal intensity in the posterior limb of the internal capsule (PLIC) and basal ganglia (Fig. 22.14) with 90% sensitivity and

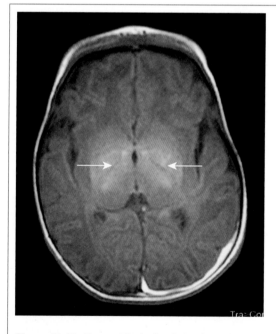

Figure 22.14 Abnormality in the thalamic nuclei (arrows) in a term baby indicating a poor prognosis following acute intrapartum asphyxia.

100% specificity; and positive predictive value of 100%.

Neonatal convulsions

The terms 'convulsion', 'fit' and 'seizure' are used interchangeably to describe clinically evident, episodic events occurring in the neonatal period and arising from a brain disorder. The incidence of neonatal seizures is 5–8/1000 liveborn infants. It may be difficult to decide whether movements made by the sick neonate are abnormal or not. In addition, jitteriness must be distinguished from the infant having convulsions (Table 22.6).

Seizure type

The five basic descriptive types of convulsions in the newborn are subtle, tonic, multifocal clonic, focal clonic and myoclonic. The preterm infant with a less well-organized immature CNS is more likely to show subtle convulsions.

Subtle

These may be difficult to distinguish from jitteriness. There are a number of recognized types:
• horizontal deviation of the eyes with or without jerking

• chewing or sucking movements
• bicycling movements
• rhythmic or dancing movements of the eyes
• apnoea, which may be the only feature of seizures.

Tonic

Tonic convulsions are characterized by extensor spasms of the trunk and limbs with opisthotonic posturing. They may occur predominantly in preterm infants.

Multifocal clonic

These involve a non-ordered progression of clonic movements of the limbs. They occur predominantly in term infants.

Focal clonic

Well-localized clonic jerking of a limb or jaw is seen with the focal clonic type. They are sometimes associated with a convexity haemorrhage (e.g. subdural).

Myoclonic jerks

Occasional myoclonic jerks may be normal in the newborn but multiple myoclonic jerks are usually pathological. They may be difficult to distinguish from jitteriness.

Electroconvulsive dissociation

With the introduction of more clinical cotside continuous monitoring of brain electrical function, referred to as 'cerebral function monitoring' (CFM) or 'amplitude integrated EEG' (aEEG), it has become apparent that the correlation between abnormal clinical movements and electrical abnormalities is often poor. This is referred to as electroconvulsive dissociation (ECD). ECD becomes more apparent after treatment with antiepileptic drugs (see below). CFM or aEEG is increasingly used in neonatal units to determine whether apparently abnormal movements are due to cortical seizure activity. Figure 22.15 shows an example of ECD. Whether all electroconvulsive seizures require drug treatment is controversial and is discussed below.

Table 22.6 Important features in distinguishing the jittery infant from one who is having convulsions

	Jitteriness	Convulsions
Stimulus provoked	Yes	No
Predominant movement	Rapid, oscillatory	Clonic, tonic
Movements cease when limb is held	Yes	No
Conscious state	Awake or asleep	Altered
Eye deviation	No	Yes

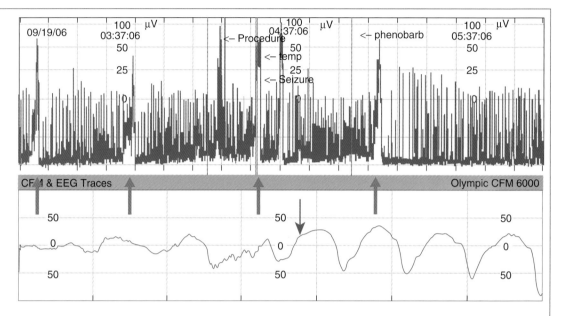

Figure 22.15 Trace from a cerebral function monitor. There are frequent electroconvulsive seizures (red arrows). The clinically evident seizures are marked in the upper panel with black arrows showing electroconvulsive dissociation. The blue arrow indicates the onset of seizure activity on the raw EEG panel.

Aetiology

The major causes of neonatal convulsions depend on the time of onset and whether the infant is term or preterm. Table 22.7 lists the more common causes of neonatal seizures and indicates their time of onset.

Perinatal asphyxia

This is the commonest cause of neonatal seizures. Such seizures usually present on the first day of life as subtle in type, progressing to multifocal clonic and tonic seizures. They usually improve and cease within 4–5 days. Status epilepticus may occur with severe hypoxic–ischaemic encephalopathy.

Intracranial haemorrhage

All types of ICH may present with fits. The infant who convulses as a result of SAH usually appears to be neurologically normal between fits. Seizures secondary to cerebral contusion, especially a convexity subdural or subarachnoid collection, may exhibit predominantly focal features. All full-term infants with convulsions should have an ultrasound scan or MRI scan to exclude this as the cause.

Infections

Intracranial bacterial and non-bacterial infections account for a significant number of neonatal convulsions. The most common infecting organisms are the Gram-negative bacilli, group B β-haemolytic streptococcus and the TORCH group.

Neonatal abstinence syndrome

Over 65% of the babies of opioid-dependent women will show withdrawal symptoms in the first 3–5 days after birth. Symptoms of the neonatal abstinence syndrome include irritability, hypertonia, tremors and hyperactivity in over 70% of affected infants. Convulsions occur in less than 10% of cases. Other common symptoms include yawning, snuffliness, sweating, sneezing, diarrhoea, vomiting and poor feeding.

Management of the neonatal abstinence syndrome is discussed in Chapter 4.

Table 22.7 Causes of neonatal convulsions indicating whether they occur early or late. The overall frequency of convulsions is indicated by the number of '+' signs shown

	Time of onset and relative frequency	
	0–2 days	2–10 days
Asphyxia	+++	–
Neonatal/perinatal stroke	+++	+
Intracranial haemorrhage	++	+
Hypocalcaemia	++	+
Hypoglycaemia	++	+
Infection	+	++
Developmental abnormalities	+	+
Drug withdrawal	+	
Inborn errors of metabolism	+	+
Pyridoxine deficiency	++	

Crack cocaine is a commonly abused drug in pregnancy. It may cause fetal cerebral artery infarction, with resultant neonatal convulsions.

Metabolic

Derangements of electrolytes such as hypocalcaemia, hypomagnesaemia, hyponatraemia and hypernatraemia as well as hypoglycaemia and hyperbilirubinaemia may cause convulsions.

Inborn errors of metabolism

These are individually very rare and include maple syrup urine disease, urea cycle defects, organic acidaemias and galactosaemia. They often present once the baby is on full milk feeds and there may be a family history. Screening investigations when inborn errors of metabolism are suspected include urinary amino acids and organic acids, serum lactate and ammonia. See Chapter 21 for further details.

Box 22.5 Diagnostic evaluation of an infant with seizures

- **History.** Family history of neonatal convulsions, maternal drug ingestion, antenatal and intrapartum infections, perinatal asphyxia, birth trauma
- **Examination.** Developmental anomalies, signs of sepsis
- **Metabolic.** Test for hypoglycaemia. Blood is obtained for assay of calcium, magnesium, phosphate and sodium
- **Lumbar puncture.** Meningitis, haemorrhage
- **Septic work-up and TORCH serology.** Meningitis, encephalitis
- **Cranial ultrasound followed by CT or MRI as indicated.** Intracranial haemorrhage, developmental anomalies of the brain

Pyridoxine deficiency

This is very rare but must be considered where there is a history of very early convulsions and where the convulsions are resistant to standard anticonvulsant medication. This condition can now be diagnosed by measuring pipecolic acid in urine as a diagnostic marker.

Newborn infants with convulsions need a diagnostic evaluation (Box 22.5), consisting of a careful history and examination and laboratory investigations. It is unusual not to find a cause for the convulsions as idiopathic epilepsy rarely, if ever, commences in the newborn period.

Additional investigations include:
- urinary and serum amino acids
- urine for organic acids
- serum lactate
- serum ammonia
- galactose-1-phosphate uridyl transferase activity.

Treatment

Specific treatment

The underlying cause of the convulsion is treated if possible.

Hypoglycaemia

If the infant is hypoglycaemic, 10% dextrose should be given as an intravenous bolus followed by an infusion.

Hypocalcaemia

If serum calcium is less than 1.5 mmol/L, the baby is given calcium gluconate intravenously with ECG monitoring. If convulsions are recalcitrant to calcium and the serum magnesium level is low, magnesium sulphate heptahydrate should be administered by slow intravenous infusion under ECG control.

Asphyxia

This is discussed fully above.

Infection

The management of meningitis is discussed in Chapter 10.

Inborn errors of metabolism

Exchange transfusion may be helpful in some cases, and megavitamin therapy is also recommended.

Anticonvulsant drug treatment

Before considering drug treatment it is necessary to ask whether convulsions are just a marker of existing brain damage or whether the seizures in their own right cause additional neuronal injury. Recent animal studies support the notion that short but frequent seizures do cause both additional structural and functional brain damage. This swings the pendulum towards more aggressive management with antiepileptic drugs.

First-line anticonvulsant therapy is with intravenous phenobarbitone loading dose with a further half loading dose for persistent seizures. If the baby continues to have seizures then phenytoin should be given by slow intravenous infusion. Third-line anticonvulsant management is with a midazolam infusion. Lidocaine (lignocaine) by continuous infusion is becoming more widely used for resistant seizures but must not be used if phenytoin has been given previously because of the possibility of cardiotoxic effects.

A number of newer anticonvulsants such as levetiracetam (Keppra) and topiramate are now considered for use in newborns.

Stopping anticonvulsant drugs

Only about 10% of babies with neonatal seizures will have convulsions in the first year of life after discharge from the hospital. It is therefore advisable to stop all anticonvulsant medication in the newborn, provided the baby is showing no abnormal neurological signs.

Prognosis

The prognosis for infants who have had neonatal convulsions depends on the underlying cause. A summary of the outcome following neonatal convulsions is given in Table 22.8.

Neonatal hypotonia ('floppy infant')

There are a large number of causes of neonatal hypotonia. Hypotonia is a very significant symptom

Table 22.8 The chance of normal outcome depending on the cause of the neonatal seizure

Cause of seizures	Chance of normal development (%)
Hypoxic–ischaemic encephalopathy	50
Subarachnoid haemorrhage	90
Other intracranial haemorrhage	50
Hypoglycaemia	50
Hypocalcaemia	90
Bacterial meningitis	20–50
Developmental, structural CNS abnormality	0
Idiopathic	75

and should never be ignored. Generalized floppiness may be due to abnormalities in a variety of anatomical sites:
- brain (asphyxia)
- spinal cord (trauma)
- anterior horn cell (spinal muscular atrophy)
- nerve root (brachial plexus injury) – this causes hypotonia only of the affected limb
- peripheral nerve (trauma)
- neuromuscular junction (myasthenia gravis)
- muscle (congenital dystrophy).

Clinical features

These infants are lethargic, show little movement and lie in the classic 'frog' posture with the hips abducted and external rotation of the limbs (Fig. 22.16). This posture must be differ-

entiated from the normal posture of a preterm infant.

There are two main groups of infants in this category:
- **Non-paralytic.** Weak infant with hypotonia and normal muscles, e.g. cerebral hypoxia. Tendon reflexes are preserved (upper motor neurone disease). This form may progress to cerebral palsy with increased tone.
- **Paralytic.** Weak infant with hypotonia and muscular disease, e.g. spinal muscular atrophy (Werdnig–Hoffmann disease) with absent tendon reflexes (lower motor neurone disease).

The two groups can also be distinguished by the ability of the infant to move his/her limbs against gravity, either spontaneously or following a stimulus. The paralytic infant is unable to maintain the posture of an elevated limb, and has a poverty of spontaneous movement.

Causes

Table 22.9 lists causes of paralytic and non-paralytic hypotonia.

Spinal muscular atrophy (Werdnig–Hoffmann disease)

This is caused by an abnormality of the anterior horn cells in the spinal cord and is an autosomal

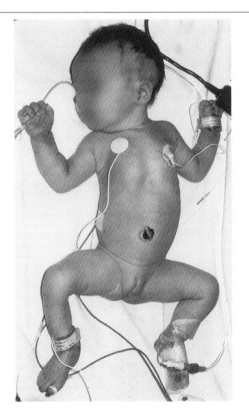

Figure 22.16 An infant with severe hypotonia showing the characteristic 'frog' posture.

Table 22.9 Causes of hypotonia in the newborn	
Paralytic	**Non-paralytic**
Spinal muscular atrophy (Werdnig–Hoffmann)	Birth asphyxia
Congenital muscular dystrophy	Down's syndrome
Congenital myopathy	Prader–Willi syndrome
Congenital myotonic dystrophy	Skeletal and connective tissue disorders
Myasthenia gravis	Drugs Benign congenital hypotonia

recessive disorder. The infant presents with profound weakness and hypotonia, although the face is usually striking by its expressiveness because the facial muscles are not involved. Congenital contractures are sometimes present. Diagnosis used to be based on muscle biopsy but new genetic testing is now available which can be done on a blood sample. There is no treatment and the infant dies in the neonatal period or soon after.

Myasthenia gravis

Ninety per cent of cases of myasthenia gravis occur as a result of maternal disease (specific IgG passing through placenta) but are transient and last 6–12 weeks, with complete recovery. Rarely a congenital form occurs without maternal disease. Infants show intermittent hypotonia responsive to edrophonium (Tensilon) or neostigmine.

Congenital muscular dystrophy

A condition of unknown cause but inherited as an autosomal recessive disorder, this may present in the newborn period with generalized hypotonia; the infant is often born with severe contractures. The prognosis may be reasonably good, as improvement in the weakness may occur. Diagnosis is by muscle biopsy.

Congenital myotonic dystrophy

This is a genetic disorder due to chromosomal triplet repeat expansion, but the mother is the affected parent in 90% of cases of neonatal disease. The mothers of all floppy infants should be screened for clinical evidence of myotonia or weakness (inability to close the eyelids tightly and bury the eyelashes, or inability to release grips after clenching the hand). A specific DNA test is now available to diagnose this condition which can be performed on a blood sample. Severely affected infants require ventilatory support and have severe feeding difficulties.

Benign congenital hypotonia

This is a diagnosis of exclusion and cannot be made in the neonatal period. Prader–Willi syndrome needs to be excluded.

Investigations

In all infants with significant weakness or hypotonia the following investigations should be performed:
- **Creatinine phosphokinase (CPK)**. This is often high in the first week of life in normal children. Only in blood taken after 2 weeks of life are high levels of CPK of clinical significance.
- **Chromosomal analysis and specific DNA testing** where available.
- **Electromyography**.
- **Motor nerve conduction velocities**.
- **Muscle biopsy**, if the pathology department has adequate facilities for sophisticated histochemical staining techniques.

Prognosis

This depends on the underlying cause of the hypotonia. In many cases the prognosis is poor and for this reason establishing a reliable histological diagnosis is very important.

SUMMARY

- Congenital malformation of the CNS accounts for a major proportion of infants born with congenital anomalies but their incidence has declined significantly because of preventative measures (such as folic acid supplementation for spina bifida), better antenatal diagnosis and availability of parental choice to terminate pregnancy.
- Improvements in neuroimaging techniques such as MRI and Doppler techniques along with neurophysiological tests such as aEEG or CFM have enhanced the diagnosis and prognostication of CNS lesions.
- A number of brain protective strategies such as head or total body cooling (therapeutic hypothermia) and pharmacological agents seem to show beneficial results, both short term and long term, such as reduced mortality and better neurodevelopment outcomes.

CHAPTER 23

Neurodevelopmental follow-up and assessment of hearing and vision

Key topics

Introduction

Although advances in neonatal–perinatal care have dramatically improved the survival of very premature babies, they remain at high risk for adverse neurodevelopmental outcomes and therefore a carefully planned follow-up of these babies has now become an essential part of the neonatal care service provision with an aim to help in:

- **Early identification** of major problems such as cerebral palsy, developmental delay, major hearing or visual impairment. This in turn should facilitate further diagnostic test, assessment, and involvement of other relevant professionals and agencies.
- **Screening** for other problems (e.g. squint, speech delay, growth failure) and implementation of early remedial measures.
- **Maintenance of optimal health** in order to achieve the utmost potential for growth and development.
- **Support to parents/caregivers** regarding the child's problems, prognosis and the need for consultation with other specialists (such as ophthalmologists, paediatric surgeon, orthopaedic surgeon, neurosurgeon, neurologist, psychologist and clinical geneticist) and therapists (such as physiotherapists, speech and language therapists and occupational therapists).

Essential Neonatal Medicine, Fifth Edition. Sunil Sinha, Lawrence Miall, Luke Jardine.
© 2012 John Wiley & Sons, Ltd. Published 2012 by John Wiley & Sons, Ltd.

Neurodevelopmental outcome

A high proportion of at-risk infants develop **transient** neurologic abnormalities including abnormalities of muscle tone such as hypotonia or hypertonia, hyperexcitability, poor postural control, feeding difficulties and persistence of primitive reflexes. Although most of these transient abnormalities may resolve by the second year of life, it might also be an indicator of later neurological dysfunction and such babies require close and longer-term neurodevelopmental surveillance. Further problems could emerge during the school age years, such as specific learning difficulties, behavioural problems and attention deficit hyperactivity disorder (ADHD), even in presence of normal intelligence.

Major neurologic disabilities include the following:
- moderate to severe cerebral palsy
- blindness in both eyes (registered blind)
- severe deafness (requiring hearing aid)
- significant delay in cognitive development
- intractable seizures (epilepsy).

Cerebral palsy

The term cerebral palsy (CP) refers to a loop of non-progressive, but often changing, motor impairment syndromes secondary to lesions of the developing brain and includes three components:
- abnormalities of tone, reflexes, coordination, and movements
- delay in motor milestones
- aberration in primitive reflexes (retention> 6 months).

CP is classified by the number of limbs involved and the severity of the condition (see Box 23.1).

Another way to classify CP is to describe it as 'non-disabling' or 'disabling'. A functional measure, the Gross Motor Function Classification System (GMFCS) has been developed to systematically evaluate functional skill in different motor activities such as sitting, walking, jumping and running, and this seems to provide a more stable measure of functional ability over time.

CP occurs more frequently among babies with extremely low birthweight (LBW) as compared to

---

Box 23.1 Classification of cerebral palsy

- All four limbs= quadriplegia
- Two limbs (usually the legs) = diplegia
- Both limbs on the same side = hemiplegia
- One limb = monoplegia

Severity of CP may be classified as:

- **Mild**: impairment interferes with but does not prevent age-appropriate function
- **Moderate**: walks with assistive device or does not walk, sits independently or with support
- **Severe**: no ambulation ,no sitting even with support

---

controls with normal birthweight. Recognized risk factors include abnormal cranial ultrasound findings, particularly large intraventricular/periventricular haemorrhage (PV-IVH) and periventricular leukomalacia (PVL), severe respiratory distress requiring prolonged ventilation, refractory hypotension, postnatal corticosteroid therapy and multiple births. In contrast, among term infants, in many cases no cause can be found despite extensive investigation.

As in most infants, neurological impairment may be transient; the diagnosis of CP should be delayed until a time when motor development has been established, which is usually 3–5 years of age unless the abnormalities are severe and obvious. Similarly, assessment of cognitive function may not be accurate until 3 years of age.

Clinical risk factors for adverse neurodevelopmental outcomes

Certain perinatal and neonatal conditions which are recognized risk factors for adverse neurodevelopmental outcome, are listed in Box 23.2 and Box 23.3.

Structured plan for follow-up assessment

- Listening to the parents/caregivers' concerns.
- Regular anthropometric measurements: weight, length, and head circumference.

Box 23.2 Usual risk factors for adverse neurodevelopmental outcomes in very preterm and LBW babies

- Birthweight <750g or <25 weeks' gestation
- Perinatal brain injury:
  Severe grades of intraventricular periventricular haemorrhage
  Periventricular cystic leucomalacia
  Persistent ventriculomegaly due to cerebral atrophy
  Posthaemorrhagic hydrocephalus requiring shunt
- Neonatal seizures
- Bronchopulmonary dysplasia
- Neonatal meningitis
- Congenital malformation affecting brain
- Chromosomal abnormality

Box 23.3 Common clinical risk factors for adverse neurodevelopmental outcome in term infants

- Hypoxic–ischaemic encephalopathy (HIE)
- Meningitis/encephalitis
- Neonatal seizures
- Neonatal stroke
- Severe intrauterine growth retardation
- Congenital malformation of brain
- Persistent severe hypoglycaemia
- Bilirubin encephalopathy

- Review of systems particularly for any health problem including feeding.
- Assessment of vision and hearing.
- Neurological/neurodevelopmental assessment:
  Assessment of posture, tone, reflexes, and presence of primitive reflexes
  Assessment of gait and detailed neurological examination in older children
  Achievement of developmental milestones after correcting for prematurity (especially for chil-

dren less than 24 months chronological age in those born extremely preterm)
- Structured developmental assessment, such as the Bayley Scale of Infant Development (BSID-II or III) and Griffiths Mental Developmental Scales.

Most studies these days use BSID-III, which includes a Mental Developmental Index (MDI), a Psychomotor Development Index (PDI), and a Behaviour Rating Scale (BRS) to assess developmental outcomes of high-risk infants in the first 3 years of life with high reliability. Bayley scores of 100 represent the mean ± standard deviation of population of normal infants born at term. A score of less than 70 (two standard deviations below the mean) is used as evidence of significant developmental delay.

Hearing impairment (deafness)

The importance of early diagnosis in hearing-impaired children is obvious, as appropriate sound amplification and the provision of specialized educational facilities will enable the deaf child to realize his/her maximal potential. Speech in deaf children is much better if hearing aids are fitted in the first 6 months of life.

Hearing impairment takes one of the following forms:
- **Conductive.** This involves abnormalities of the external auditory meatus, the tympanic membrane or the ossicles within the middle ear. This can rarely be congenital if the meatus has not yet canalized; much more commonly it is due to infection or serous exudate within the middle ear.
- **Sensorineural.** Abnormalities or damage to the cochlea or brainstem nuclei cause 'nerve' deafness.
- **Mixed.** Not uncommonly children with sensorineural deafness may also develop infection, which may further impair hearing as a result of conductive loss.

Screening for hearing in the neonatal period

Two methods for screening are used: the otoacoustic emissions (OAE) and auditory brainstem response (ABR) tests. All newborns in the UK have OAE testing and those at high risk will go on to have an automated ABR test.

Otoacoustic emissions

The OAE technology detects the physiological response from the outer hair cells within the cochlea, which are present in 98% of normally hearing babies. As sensorineural hearing impairment is associated with abnormal function of the outer hair cells this is a very sensitive and accurate test for hearing impairment. An automated OAE test is used for routine screening of all newborn infants.

Auditory brainstem responses

The ABR technique measures evoked electrical signals detected by surface electrodes from within the hearing pathways of the brain in response to sounds at predetermined frequencies and loudness. ABR tests the whole auditory pathway rather than just the cochlea and is more valuable in screening high-risk babies, particularly those who have been subject to neonatal intensive care, as they are at more risk of developing retrocochlear hearing impairment (auditory neuropathy).

It is important to be able to refer babies with abnormal responses to neonatal hearing tests for rapid assessment and treatment with hearing aids if deafness is confirmed. Part of the screening protocol requires appropriate response, follow-up and treatment.

Incidence

Deafness remains a common cause of disability, with approximately 2–3/1000 children requiring hearing aids and a considerably larger number having a permanent mild bilateral impairment or significant unilateral deafness.

The prevalence of severe congenital or early hearing impairment is 1.5–2/1000 live births, and in 90% this is due to sensorineural causes. Deafness is, however, much more common in infants who have received intensive care, reaching an incidence of about 30/1000, a marked increase compared to the general population.

Although conductive deafness is an uncommon cause of permanent hearing loss, it is a common

> ### Box 23.4 Indications for routine auditory assessment
>
> - Family history of hearing impairment
> - Congenital perinatal infection, particularly rubella, CMV, syphilis
> - Anatomical malformations:
>   Cleft palate
>   Ear anomalies
>   Syndromes (e.g. Down's, Treacher–Collins)
> - Hyperbilirubinaemia:
>   >340 μmol/L (20 mg) for full-term infants
>   >240 μmol/L for infants <1500 g
> - Bacterial meningitis
> - Severe perinatal asphyxia
> - High aminoglycoside serum levels

condition. In a study of infants receiving intensive care, up to 25% were found to have evidence of otitis media while on the neonatal unit. Babies intubated and receiving ventilatory support are most at risk of otitis media. If this condition is recognized and adequately treated, it is unlikely to lead to long-term hearing impairment.

Aetiology

There are a large number of causes of sensorineural hearing loss affecting the newborn. Many high-risk babies can be recognized on history taking and physical examination (Box 23.4). The most important are detailed below.

Genetic causes

With the reduction in incidence of rubella embryopathy, inherited causes now account for 50% of all cases of severe sensorineural hearing impairment: 80% are due to single gene autosomal recessive disorders and 15% to autosomal dominant disorders. Deafness due to chromosomal abnormalities or syndromic causes is rare. Genetic disorders often present late and are frequently progressive. The age of onset of hearing loss is not useful in distinguishing environmental from genetic loss.

Syndromic causes

The main syndromes causing hearing impairment are:
• **Branchio-oto-renal syndrome**. Although this is a rare dominant disorder (1:40,000) it is the commonest syndromic cause of deafness. There are branchial clefts, ear abnormalities and renal anomalies.
• **Pendred's syndrome** (autosomal recessive). Goitre and profound deafness.
• **Waardenburg's syndrome** (autosomal dominant). White forelock, different-coloured eyes and deafness.
• **Usher's syndrome** (autosomal recessive). Retinitis pigmentosa leading to blindness and deafness.

Congenital infection

A variety of prenatally acquired viruses can cause permanent deafness.

Rubella

The full-blown syndrome (now very rarely seen) includes microcephaly and cataracts in addition to deafness, but hearing impairment may be the only abnormality. Active infection may continue well after birth, and deafness that is not apparent in the newborn period may develop later in childhood.

Cytomegalovirus

In infants with evidence of cytomegalovirus (CMV) infection at birth, 30% will have hearing impairment, and in those with asymptomatic infection almost 20% will subsequently develop hearing loss. As hearing loss is usually progressive, repeat screening might be indicated, and targeted testing at 9–12 months is recommended.

Meningitis

Deafness is an important complication of neonatal meningitis, and the organisms *E. coli*, group B β-haemolytic streptococcus and listeria are particularly liable to cause deafness. The infection causes direct inflammatory involvement of inner ear structures leading to permanent hearing loss. It has been suggested that dexamethasone may reduce the chances of deafness in neonatal meningitis, but as

this has not been consistently shown it cannot be recommended as part of meningitis treatment.

Bilirubin toxicity

Sensorineural deafness is part of the clinical spectrum of kernicterus (bilirubin encephalopathy). indeed, deafness may be the only neurological manifestation. Neonates whose cochlear nuclei are damaged by hyperbilirubinaemia may pass an OAE screening test, but will be picked up on an abnormal ABR.

Drugs

Aminoglycoside antibiotics (gentamicin, amikacin, netilmicin, tobramycin and kanamycin) are potentially ototoxic but the risk of deafness in neonates treated with these drugs is probably overestimated. Provided that the appropriate dosages and intervals between doses are used together with measurements of trough levels, these drugs are unlikely to contribute significantly to the numbers of deaf neonates. Trough levels (immediately before the next dose) are used to calculate the drug regimen. High peak levels indicate too high a dosage, and high troughs indicate that the interval between dosages should be lengthened. Recent studies have suggested that combined use of aminoglycosides and furosemide increases the risk of sensorineural hearing loss in LBW infants. It is now known that ototoxicity related to high gentamicin level only occurs in presence of a specific mitochondrial RNA mutation which can be tested.

Incubator noise

It has been suggested that noisy incubators are an important cause of neonatal deafness, but there are few data to support this in the present era of relatively quiet incubators. Unnecessary environmental noise should always be avoided in the neonatal nursery (see Chapter 24).

Management

Now that routine neonatal screening for deafness is widely used and high-risk babies are screened by ABR, more rapid diagnosis of deafness is made with more effective intervention. Fitting of hearing aids from a young age is important, and a cochlear implant later in childhood has been shown to be effective for certain children. Because of increased risk for bacterial meningitis, all children with cochlear implants should be monitored and vaccinated specifically against *Streptococcus pneumoniae*.

Visual impairment

Visual impairment as a result of prematurity is relatively common, although usually not severe; however, approximately 2% of babies born extremely preterm are registered blind. The most important cause of blindness is retinopathy of prematurity (ROP), but severe brain damage occurring during neonatal/perinatal period can also be associated with **cortical visual impairment** along with other disabilities.

Retinopathy of prematurity

ROP, formerly known as retrolental fibroplasia, is a relatively common condition affecting the most immature infants. Studies in the 1950s proved a direct association between oxygen dosage and the development of retinal abnormalities, and the controlled use of oxygen reduced the incidence of this condition. More recently, it has been noted that the relationship between oxygen and ROP is more complex, particularly in preterm babies.

The key to the pathophysiology of ROP is abnormality in the expression of the vascular endothelial growth factor (VEGF), which is normally stimulated by relative hypoxia as occurs in the fetus. Hyperoxia after birth causes VEGF to be downregulated with consequent vaso-obliteration and cessation in the growth of new blood vessels within the retina. This in turn leads to hypoxia of the non-perfused retina with secondary local upregulation of VEGF leading to neovascularization and in the most severe cases the development of retinal fibrosis and detachment.

Classification of retinopathy of prematurity

The diagnosis of ROP is made clinically by means of indirect ophthalmoscopy after prior pupillary

Box 23.5 Severity of retinopathy of prematurity

- **Stage 1 (demarcation line).** A thin white line of demarcation in the periphery of the retina separating the avascular retina anteriorly from the vascularized retina posteriorly.
- **Stage 2 (ridge).** The line is more extensive and forms a ridge.
- **Stage 3 (proliferation).** Ridge with vascular proliferation immediately posterior to it (Figure 23.1).
- **Stage 4.** Retinal detachment – subtotal.
- **Stage 5.** Retinal detachment – total.

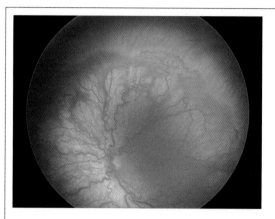

Figure 23.1 Stage 3 retinopathy of prematurity (ridging and vascular proliferation) with plus disease (tortuosity of posterior retinal vessels).

dilatation with 0.5% cyclopentalate eyedrops. The examination is performed by a trained paediatric ophthalmologist, as considerable expertise is required. The description of severity of ROP given in Box 23.5 follows the recommendations of the international classification of the staging of ROP.

Mild ROP never progresses beyond stage 2 and does not require treatment. Stage 3 or worse is severe and requires treatment.

Location by zone

The location of ROP is described by the zone involved. The zones are centred on the optic disc.

- **Zone 1.** Extends from the optic disc to twice the disc–foveal distance.
- **Zone 2.** From the periphery of the nasal retina in a circle around the anatomical equator.
- **Zone 3.** This is anterior to zone 2 and is present temporally, inferiorly and superiorly, but not in the nasal retina.

Extent

The extent is recorded in 'clock hours' 1–12 around the retinal circumference.

'Plus' disease

'Plus' is added to any stage of ROP if the following signs of activity are seen:
- tortuosity and engorgement of retinal vessels
- vascular engorgement and rigidity of the iris
- vitreous haze
- pupil rigidity.

Threshold disease

A further concept is 'threshold' disease. This refers to the presence of a combination of five continuous clock hours or eight cumulative hours of stage 3 ROP in zones 1 and 2 together with 'plus' disease.

More recently it has been recognized that the most immature infants may develop a more virulent form of ROP referred to as 'pre-plus disease' and aggressive posterior ROP. These babies may need treatment earlier than more mature infants (see below).

Incidence

ROP is common in very premature infants; the incidence is 65–70% in babies of birthweight less than 1251 g, but only about 5% of these require treatment and 1–2% are blind as a result of severe ROP. In Western countries ROP accounts for only 6% of children with severe visual impairment, usually in the most immature infants. By contrast, in developing countries ROP is the cause of visual impairment in about 40% of children, and often affects larger babies of 1.5–2.0 kg. More severe forms of ROP (stage 3 or worse) occur in about 50% of babies with birthweight 750 g, 30% of babies 750–999 g and in only 18% of babies 1000–1250 g.

Screening

Screening for ROP with indirect opthalmoscopy or a retinal camera is recommended in all babies weighing less than 15001 g or less than 31 weeks' gestation at birth. In the event of sight-threatening disease developing (such as prethreshold, threshold plus disease or stage 3), it will only occur at or after the baby is 31 weeks of postmenstrual age (where PMA = gestational age + postnatal age) and after 4 weeks from birth. No new sight-threatening ROP occurs after 46 weeks PMA. Therefore in order to detect all cases of acute ROP in a timely manner, babies should be screened for signs of potentially severe disease starting at 30 weeks if born <27 weeks or in 4–5th week if born 27–31[+6] weeks. PMA and thereafter weekly. If significant disease is not present by 36 weeks PMA, screening can be stopped.

Prevention

The P_{O_2} of at-risk infants should be maintained at 6–10 kPa (50–80 mmHg). There has been much speculation as to what should be the ideal range for maintaining oxygen saturation target which will save life without causing more ROP. On the basis of risk/benefit analysis of data from recent studies such as SUPPORT and BOOST trials, it seems that a saturation target of 90–95% should provide a safe target limit without increasing the risk of adverse clinical and visual outcomes.

Treatment

Instead of cryotherapy, which was used in the past, laser therapy has now become more widely used to treat acute ROP. Treatment should be confined to centres with special expertise in its use.

Criteria for laser therapy for ROP include:
- Zone II 'plus' disease with stage 2 or 3 ROP
- Zone I 'plus' disease with stage 1 or 2 ROP
- Zone I stage 3 ROP.

Cerebral visual impairment

This refers to an abnormality of the brain that renders the child functionally blind or with a major visual disability where the child finds it difficult to make visual sense of the world. These children often have major disability acquired in the perinatal period, including CP (see Chapter 22).

Causes of cerebral visual impairment include:

- brain malformations
- PVL
- hypoxic–ischaemic brain injury
- hydrocephalus
- meningitis and encephalitis.

Cataracts

Cataracts account for blindness in 20% of children with severe visual handicap. Box 23.6 details the causes of cataracts seen in the neonatal period.

Diagnosis

Cataracts should always be sought at the routine neonatal examination. Normally, on shining a light directly into the infant's eye, a 'red reflex' is seen. Loss of this red reflex suggests cataract, although retinoblastoma will give a similar appearance. If there is any doubt, careful ophthalmic examination should be performed by an experienced person.

Treatment

Urgent referral to an ophthalmologist is essential. Unless most of the pupil is occluded by the cataract, it can be left and observed. If surgical treatment is necessary, the lens is removed and contact lenses are placed.

Box 23.6 Causes of cataracts seen in the neonatal period

- Congenital rubella syndrome (see Chapter 10)
- Other prenatal infections (CMV and toxoplasma) less commonly
- Prematurity: cataracts may be due to trauma rather than prematurity *per se,* and are usually transient requiring no treatment
- Galactosaemia (see Chapter 21)
- Hypocalcaemia
- Lowe's syndrome (oculocerebrorenal syndrome): an X-linked condition
- Down's syndrome: 5–10% of these children have cataracts at birth
- Inherited: usually as an autosomal dominant condition
- Idiopathic: accounts for up to 50% of cases

Glaucoma (buphthalmos)

Congenital glaucoma occurs in 1/10,000 births and is usually bilateral. It may be a familial condition or associated with vascular malformation affecting the face, e.g. Sturge–Weber syndrome. The eye appears large (buphthalmos) in only one-quarter of infants with congenital glaucoma. The commonest presentation is the observation of a cloudy cornea. The treatment is surgical.

SUMMARY

Advances in neonatal perinatal medicine has led to significant improvement in survival of very low birthweight (VLBW) babies but a significant proportion of these babies develop complications which can result in lifelong neurologic morbidities, including CP, blindness and deafness. Not surprisingly, long-term follow-up of these at-risk babies has now become a standard of clinical care and a marker for quality control of the service provided. There are already many reports of neurodevelopmental abnormalities in ex-VLBW infants in early childhood, but increasing evidence is accumulating of adverse outcomes and special health care needs at school age and in young adults.

Profound hearing and visual impairments are also major causes of severe disability arising from the neonatal period. Assessment of both hearing and vision in infants is usually possible before the child leaves the neonatal unit, and early diagnosis is essential for optimal management of any deficiencies.

There are already some established protocols for screening certain complications which leads to their early identification and it is hoped that early intervention will prevent or at least ameliorate their severity.

CHAPTER 24

Developmental care and the neonatal environment

Key topics

Introduction

Human newborn babies, especially preterm newborns, are exquisitely vulnerable to the environment around them. They are born at a relatively more immature stage than many mammals and are dependent on immediate warmth and nutrition being provided by their mother. When this is not possible, for example in the context of a sick infant admitted to the neonatal intensive care unit (NICU), it is vital that the environment around the baby is controlled to provide the optimum care and nurture and to avoid causing any harm. The importance of early parental involvement, good positioning, noise reduction and avoiding painful stimuli in facilitating normal development is increasingly being understood. This chapter explores the key issues.

Thermoregulation

Normal physiology

Full-term infants are able to regulate their own body temperature but less effectively thanolder children or adults. The small for gestational age (SGA) infant, and particularly the preterm infant, has greater problems in maintaining body temperature. After birth, the core and skin temperature of the term newborn can drop at a rate of approximately 0.1 °C and 0.3 °C per minute respectively, unless immediate precautions are taken.

Essential Neonatal Medicine, Fifth Edition. Sunil Sinha, Lawrence Miall, Luke Jardine.
© 2012 John Wiley & Sons, Ltd. Published 2012 by John Wiley & Sons, Ltd.

The temperature of an infant will depend on the site at which it is measured. Normal core temperature ranges between 36.7°C and 37.3°C, and can be measured by a rectal thermometer; however, this is not routine practice and should usually be avoided. Axillary temperature approximates to core temperature and is the preferred site for recording temperature in newborn babies. Skin temperature is lower than core temperature and is recorded by taping a thermistor to the abdomen. Normal abdominal temperature is 35.5–36.5°C in a term infant and 36.2–37.2°C in small premature infants. If the difference between abdominal and peripheral (e.g. toe) temperature is large, then the infant is vasoconstricted to conserve heat (or because he/she is infected or shocked). If the difference is small, the infant may be vasodilated and attempting to lose heat. The World Health Organization classifies a core body temperature for newborns of 36–36.4°C as mild hypothermia, 32–35.9°C as moderate and less than 32°C as severe hypothermia. At these temperatures a special low-reading thermometer will be required to obtain an accurate reading.

Mechanisms of heat loss

Heat is lost from the body to the environment in four different ways: conduction, convection, evaporation and radiation. These mechanisms are illustrated in Fig. 24.1 and the ways to minimize their effects in the nursery are described in Table 24.1.

Physiological mechanisms to conserve heat

When exposed to cold the normal baby tries to conserve heat by a variety of means:

- Peripheral vasoconstriction.
- Increased heat production through increased basal metabolic rate, increased voluntary muscular activity, involuntary muscular activity – shivering. Shivering is virtually non-existent in preterm infants and their ability to increase muscular activity is limited.
- Non-shivering thermogenesis. Full-term infants are born with a layer of brown fat, mainly around the neck, between the scapulae and along the aorta. Brown fat can be rapidly metabolized to generate heat. This is under the control of the sympathetic nervous system.

Why is the newborn prone to heat loss?

The newborn is particularly susceptible to heat loss for a number of reasons: see Box 24.1

Box 24.1 Reason why heat loss is a particular problem for newborn babies

- Babies have (like all small mammals) a relatively large body surface area to weight ratio. A preterm infant's limited ability to flex limbs and trunk increases the exposed surface area for heat loss
- Babies have a limited ability to shiver
- Babies (especially preterm and SGA babies) have a lack of subcutaneous fat
- Babies (especially preterm and IUGR babies) have a deficiency of brown fat and reduced glycogen stores
- Babies are born wet (liquor, meconium, blood), predisposing to evaporation

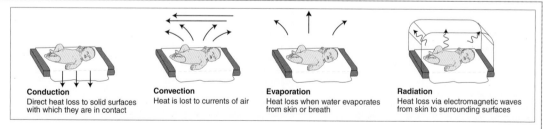

| **Conduction** Direct heat loss to solid surfaces with which they are in contact | **Convection** Heat is lost to currents of air | **Evaporation** Heat loss when water evaporates from skin or breath | **Radiation** Heat loss via electromagnetic waves from skin to surrounding surfaces |

Figure 24.1 Heat loss: (a) by conduction, (b) by convection, (c) by radiation, (d) by evaporation. From Warren, I. Nursing the Neonate, 2nd Ed. 2010. Wiley Blackwell.

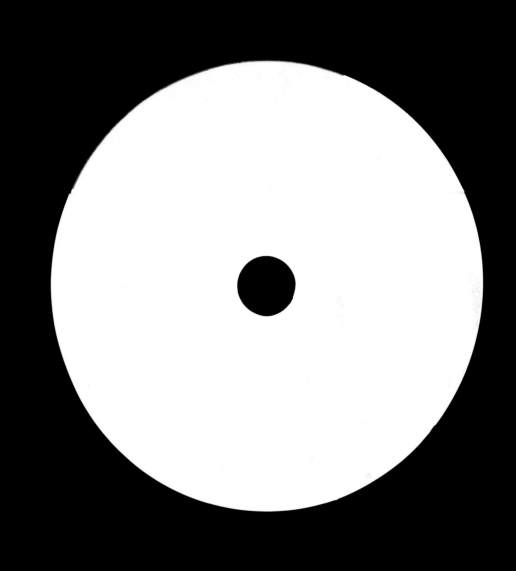

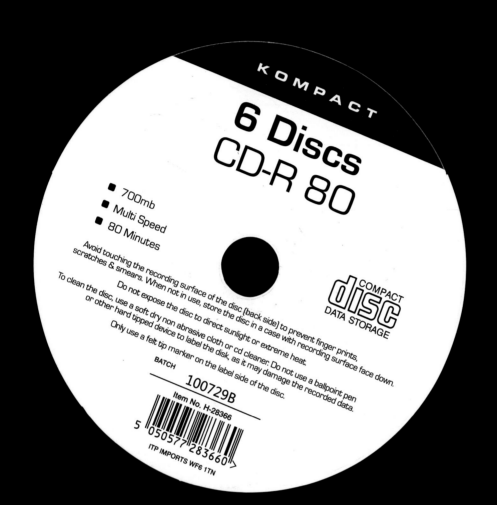

KOMPACT

6 Discs
CD-R 80

- 700mb
- Multi Speed
- 80 Minutes

COMPACT
disc
DATA STORAGE

Avoid touching the recording surface of the disc (back side) to prevent finger prints, scratches & smears. When not in use, store the disc in a case with recording surface face down.

Do not expose the disc to direct sunlight or extreme heat.

To clean the disc, use a soft dry non abrasive cloth or cd cleaner. Do not use a ballpoint pen or other hard tipped device to label the disk, as it may damage the recorded data.

Only use a felt tip marker on the label side of the disc.

BATCH
100729B

Item No. H-28366

5 050577 283660 7

ITP IMPORTS WF6 1TN

Table 24.1 Mechanisms of heat loss and prevention

Mechanism	Example	Prevention
Conduction	Heat loss into a cold surface directly under the baby. Heat loss into cold(er) equipment	Warm the Resuscitaire towels prior to delivery Discard wet towels Prewarm the incubator Do not place cold radiography plates directly in contact with the baby's skin Warm hands and stethoscope before examining the baby Kangaroo care – placing baby directly against a parent's chest
Convection	Heat loss directly into currents of air	Place newborn preterm infants in a plastic bag or wrap Do not place the baby near open windows or air vents Use closed incubators rather than open platforms if possible Close the doors to the nursery Close the incubator doors after a procedure
Evaporation	Heat lost when water evaporates from the baby's skin as water vapour Evaporation of water (and therefore heat loss) from the lungs during expiration	Place newborn preterm infants in a plastic bag or wrap Dry newborn term infants immediately with warm, dry towels Humidify the environment (e.g. the incubator) Humidify and warm ventilation gases Cover open tissue (e.g. skin burns or gastroschisis)
Radiation	Heat loss (via infrared radiation) to another surface, which is not in contact with the baby or down a concentration gradient via surrounding air	Maintain the whole nursery at a warm temperature Use double-walled incubators Do not come between the baby and an overhead heater Cover the baby's head (large surface area) with a hat

Prevention of excessive heat loss

The ways in which heat loss can be prevented in general are described in Table 24.1. Specific issues are described below.

Labour ward

The provision of warmth and prevention of heat loss is the first essential step in stabilization of the newborn. It comes before airway and breathing in all resuscitation algorithms. The baby must either be dried completely with a prewarmed, clean towels or (if preterm <32 weeks) be placed, still wet, into a large plastic bag which provides a 'mini-incubator' around the baby and prevents evaporative and convective heat loss. The bag must clearly not cover the baby's head, which should be covered with a hat. Radiant warmers or heated mattresses are used. Heating gel packs can be used for extreme preterm babies.

CLINICAL TIP: An 'emergency preterm delivery box' containing hats, plastic bags/wraps, heating gel pads and preterm intubation equipment should be kept on the labour ward so that wherever a preterm baby is delivered, the neonatal team can institute thermal care immediately.

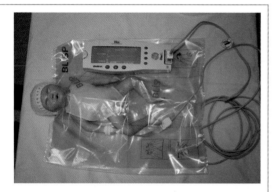

Figure 24.2 Demonstration of the use of a plastic wrap and hat to aid thermoregulation in the newborn preterm infant. With thanks to Dr Fiona Wood.

For a healthy term newborn skin-to-skin contact immediately after birth is recommended. The infant is thoroughly dried and placed on the mother's chest and abdomen with a light blanket around them. This reduces radiant and conductive heat loss, promotes temperature stabilization and improve bonding and lactation.

Nursery

Very low birthweight (VLBW) infants do not have a superficial layer of keratin, and consequently water and heat are lost through the permeable skin. Adequate ambient humidity in the incubator prevents this. Infants should be dressed, including a hat, to reduce radiant and convective heat loss whenever possible. Modern incubators provide a thermoneutral humidified environment and have warm air 'curtains' that minimize convection currents when doors are opened for procedures.

Closed versus open incubators

Babies are generally provided with a thermoneutral environment by nursing them in either a closed incubator (with doors and ports to allow access) or on a servo-controlled heated platform, with an overhead radiant heater or heated mattress. The thermoneutral temperature is that at which the baby expends least additional energy maintaining body temperature. The thermoneutral range is much narrower in preterm infants than in older children (Fig. 24.3).

Closed incubator (see Fig. 24.4a)

These reduce heat loss, allow good humidification and to some extent muffle external noise. In modern incubators temperature can be set to either 'air' or 'baby' mode. In **air mode** a thermistor measures the environmental temperature and regulates the heater to maintain air at a constant preset temperature. The baby's temperature must be checked regularly. The air temperature required will vary depending on the baby's gestation, weight, postnatal age and whether they are dressed or naked (see Fig. 24.3) and may be as high as 35 °C. In **baby mode** a thermistor is attached to the baby, so the heater is servo-controlled to keep the infant's temperature constant. Overheating can occur if the thermistor becomes detached from the baby. Both systems require careful monitoring and alarm limits.

Humidification of the ambient air in the incubator is valuable in infants less than 30 weeks and less than 1000 g for the first 8–10 days to prevent excessive evaporative water and heat loss until maturation of the stratum corneum layer of the skin. All ELBW (extremely low birthweight) or hypothermic infants (temperature <35 °C) should be nursed in humidified incubators. However, such incubators carry the risk of bacterial contamination with *Pseudomonas aeruginosa* or serratia, which colonize the water reservoir and may lead to neonatal infection. This risk can be eliminated by changing the water every 24 h and using sterilized water.

Open incubator (platform with radiant warmer) (see Fig. 24.4c)

The infant lies on a mattress under a heating element which delivers radiant heat energy. It has a servo-controlled mechanism with a thermistor on the

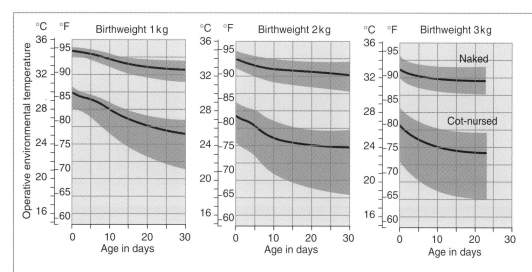

Figure 24.3 Thermoneutral temperature range for different birthweight infants. The upper graph represents infants nursed naked and the lower is for clothed babies. From Warren, I. Nursing the Neonate, 2nd Ed. 2010. Wiley Blackwell.

baby's abdominal wall, and the radiant heater is automatically switched on and off to maintain body temperature at a preset level (usually 36.5 °C).

The great advantage of this device is that in term infants it gives easy access to the infant for surgical or nursing procedures. It is also useful for rapidly warming cold babies (see below). Its disadvantages are obvious in that heat loss is large and transepidermal water loss considerable, particularly in the most immature babies. If very preterm babies have to be nursed on an open platform, a thin, clear plastic wrap can reduce insensible water loss and careful monitoring of fluid and electrolyte balance is essential. In general closed incubators are associated with fewer complications than open radiant incubators. There are now closed incubators which can convert quickly to overhead heated platforms at the push of a button (Fig. 24.4b).

 Link to *Nursing the Neonate*: Thermoregulation. Chapter 6.

Ventilator humidity

It is important to use adequate humidification and warming in all ventilator circuits as there can be high fluid and heat loss in babies being ventilated or on high-flow systems such as continuous positive airway pressure (CPAP) or high-flow oxygen therapy.

Neonatal cold injury

Prolonged exposure to a cold environment increases oxygen consumption and glucose utilization, and consequently the baby readily becomes hypoxic and hypoglycaemic. There is peripheral cyanosis with redness of the face, refusal to feed and lethargy, followed by oedema and sclerema (localized hardening of the subcutaneous tissue). Subcutaneous fat necrosis may develop. Cold-stressed babies may develop apnoeic spells, worsening of their respiratory distress syndrome, severe metabolic acidosis, hypoglycaemia, pulmonary haemorrhage and intracranial haemorrhage. There is a 60% increase in mortality if preterm babies become significantly hypothermic.

Hypoglycaemia and metabolic acidosis are most likely to occur on rewarming. Restoration of metabolic processes creates a demand for glucose and this should be anticipated. Regular tests for glucose must be performed. As blood pressure and perfusion improve the products of anaerobic metabolism are washed out into the circulation, causing a severe metabolic acidosis.

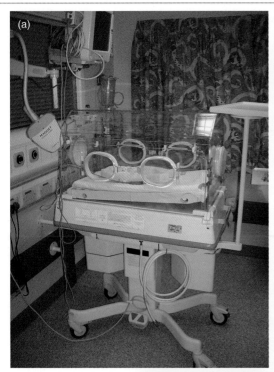
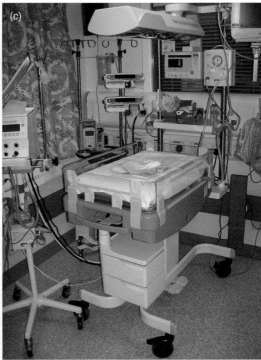
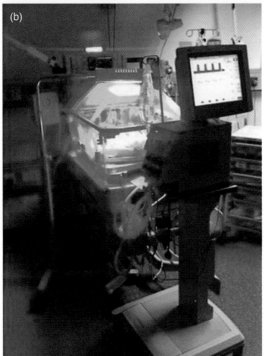

Figure 24.4 Three designs of intensive care incubator: (a) closed incubator; (b) hybrid; (c) open platform.

Therapeutic hypothermia

Controlled mild-to-moderate hypothermia (33–34 °C) has been proposed as treatment for potentially brain-injured near-term babies. This technique has been shown to be neuroprotective in babies born with moderate asphyxia. There is no evidence of benefit in preterm babies. The therapeutic value of hypothermia is discussed in more detail in Chapter 22.

Skin care on the neonatal intensive care unit

The skin of all newborns is relatively vulnerable, but in preterm babies the protective stratum corneum is not yet developed and there is little protective subcutaneous fat. This leads to massive transepidermal water loss in the first week of life before the keratin layers mature. Preterm skin is very vulnerable to bruising and extreme care should be taken when removing adhesive dressings as this may strip off the superficial layers of skin or in extreme cases lead to complete skin loss. Very adhesive tapes (e.g. Elastoplast or zinc oxide tape) should not be used to attach equipment or devices to the skin of very preterm babies.

The use of semipermeable non-adhesive dressings lowers the transepidermal water loss without any increased risk of colonization with bacteria, but by using modern well-humidified incubators this should not be necessary. Protecting the skin around stoma sites (e.g. around ileostomy sites, where loose stool cause dermatitis) is very important.

 Link to *Nursing the Neonate*: Stoma care. Chapter 20, p 353.

Emollients are considered to be effective in preventing water loss and protecting skin from cracking and fissuring. Their effect lasts only for about 3 h, necessitating repeated application. Some units encourage 'baby massage' with simple skin oils in more stable mature babies as part of a package of developmental care. Essential oils should not be used.

CLINICAL TIP: Regular application of moisturizing antiseptic skin washes can help reduce colonization with pathogenic strains of *Staphylococcus aureus*.

Optimizing the neonatal environment

The busy modern neonatal unit can be a noisy, stressful environment with equipment alarms, telephones ringing and bright artificial lighting – very different from the dark, muffled, secure environment of the womb. There is now increasing evidence that providing a nurturing peaceful environment and avoiding noxious stimuli (pain, excessive noise and interruption of the sleep cycle) can lead to improved developmental outcomes. Providing a calm, family friendly environment will also reduce parental stress and anxiety.

Link to *Nursing the Neonate*: The neonatal environment and care of families. Chapter 4.

Stimuli that may adversely affect the baby are listed in Table 24.2.

CLINICAL TIP: An automatic sound level monitor can make it easier to educate staff and visitors about maintaining a safe and comfortable noise level for babies in the nursery.

Procedural pain and analgesia

Sick newborn infants often require a number of investigations and practical procedures performing, many of which are undoubtedly painful (see Chapter 29). It is important that adequate analgesia is provided for these. Local anaesthetic, either topical (tetracaine or lidocaine/prilocaine) or injected (lidocaine), paracetamol and opioid analgesics should be considered. Non-pharmacological methods of analgesia are both important and have been shown to be remarkable effective: these include swaddling, skin-to-skin contact with mother, breastfeeding, and oral

Table 24.2 Adverse stimuli in the neonatal intensive care environment

Stimulus	Strategies to reduce harmful effects
Noise	Respond to alarms promptly and reduce volume to the minimum needed. Ensure doors and pedal-bin lids do not slam closed Close incubator doors carefully Keep conversations at a low volume (a wall-mounted sound monitor can help enforce this) CPAP circuits have been shown to be very noisy; the exhaust piping should vent outside the incubator Fit the baby with protective earmuffs during noisy MRI scans Keep background noise <45 dB and peak noise <65 dB
Light	Try to have periods during the day, and especially at night, when the lighting is dimmed Cover the baby's eyes when switching on an examination light to avoid startling Use protective eye shades when under intense phototherapy lights Some visible natural daylight is healthier for staff and parents
Pain	Prophylactic analgesia for procedural pain (see below) Discomfort from mechanical ventilation *may* require sedation Painful disorders (long bone fractures, osteomyeltitis, NEC) require adequate analgesia
Smell	Ensure incubators are cleaned regularly and water, clothes and bedding changed daily Avoid noxious chemicals (e.g. powerful cleaning agents) in the immediate vicinity of the baby
Thermoregulation	Ensure there are no draughts near the baby. Use incubators where appropriate. Close incubator doors Monitor temperature continuously if baby is in a servo-controlled environment (see above)
Overstimulation	Normal newborns sleep for most hours of the day. Sick infants and preterm infants must be allowed to rest and achieve a normal sleep–wake pattern Procedures, examinations and therapies should, wherever possible, be administered at times when the baby is awake. They should be clustered together. It is the role of the neonatal nurse to enforce this

sucrose. There is clear evidence that even very preterm infants feel pain. A variety of pain scores have been developed for neonatal practice and these can be used to guide therapy. A 'ladder' of escalating analgesia should be used until pain is adequately treated (pain score returns to normal). Preventing pain is much more effective than treating it once it occurs, but usually both are necessary. Examples of painful procedures and analgesic strategies are shown in Table 24.3.

Developmental care

'Developmental care' is a term used to describe the interventions that are used, especially in neonatal units, to promote healthy long-term development. It is often used to describe an overarching philosophy of humane, family-centred care that aims to promote healthy family attachment and reduce long-term stress and anxiety for the baby and reduce iatrogenic harm such as deformity and abnormal

Table 24.3 Procedural pain and analgesic strategies

Procedure	Analgesia	
	Before procedure	After procedure
Blood sampling	Venepuncture is less painful than heel-prick sampling. Choose the appropriate method: • topical anaesthetic (older neonates) • oral sucrose just before procedure	Usually not required
Venous or arterial cannulation (including PICC line)	Topical anaesthetic and/or oral sucrose	Not required if dressing applied to stabilize the cannula
Umbilical venous or arterial catheterization	None required. Ensure retaining stitches go through Wharton's jelly and not through skin	None
Tracheal intubation for mechanical ventilation	Premedication with short-acting opiate/sedative and short-acting muscle relaxant	Usually none. If on high pressures or agitated may need sedation with opiate infusion (see Chapter 29)
Lumbar puncture	Topical anaesthetic for 30 min	None
Chest drain insertion	Local anaesthetic (along tract)	None or opiate infusion depending on size/type of drain and condition of baby
RoP screening	Oral sucrose	None
RoP laser treatment	General anaesthetic or opiate infusion	Paracetamol or opiate infusion
Laparotomy or other surgery	General anaesthetic	Opiate infusion and or epidural anaesthesia
Immunization	Oral sucrose	Paracetamol (if required)

ROP, retinopathy of prematurity.

postural development that can arise from prolonged periods of time spent in the intensive care unit. It is important to remember that this often coincides with the period (24–37 weeks) when the brain is undergoing rapid development and neuronal organization, and so interventions that can promote normal neurological and behavioural development should be used where there is the evidence to support them (see Fig. 24.5).

Link to *Nursing the Neonate*: Chapter 18.

Kangaroo care

Holding and kangaroo care (where the baby is placed vertically against the mother's (or sometimes father's) naked chest, covered with a wrap (Fig. 24.6), was originally developed in Bogotá, Columbia, to maintain temperature regulation in preterm infants. Kangaroo care has been shown to provide a number of benefits to both parents and babies. A Cochrane Review details the benefits to mothers in terms of sense of competence and some short-term benefits, including a decrease in nosocomial infection and subsequent reduction in respiratory tract infection,

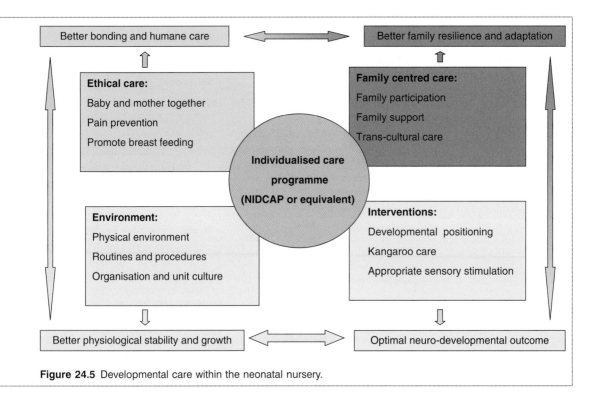

Figure 24.5 Developmental care within the neonatal nursery.

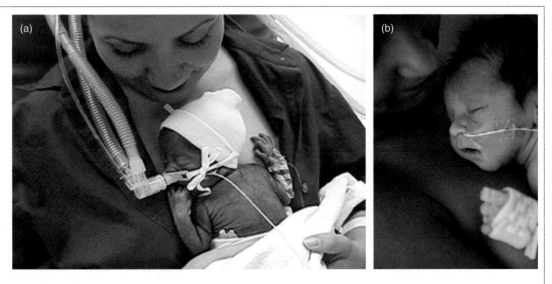

Figure 24.6 (a) Kangaroo care. Courtesy of Rady Children's Hospital – San Diego. (b) Skin-to-skin contact. With permission from Neama Firth.

and promotion of breastfeeding Allowing 24 h visiting and providing suitable areas to rest and make drinks on the neonatal nursery unit, and play areas and information for siblings, is important to promote good family dynamics and bonding.

Positioning

It is important that preterm infants or term infants who are very ill or who have neuromuscular problems are not just left sprawling in the position that gravity decides for them, but are instead 'nested' within a soft but supportive environment which keeps their body and limbs in a more physiological flexed position, provides them with boundaries and allows them to develop normally, including awareness of self (midline). In addition to this, gentle physiotherapy may be required to keep joint and limbs mobile. These assessments must be made on an individual basis, usually by skilled neonatal therapists.

Stimulation

It is clear that many preterm babies are overstimulated by the environment around them and the procedures carried out on them. Clustering care to certain times of the day and responding to behavioural clues is vital. 'Minimal handling' should be used by staff but should not discourage 'positive touch' by parents. When changing nappies or examining or turning babies they should not be startled, but carefully turned, with as much warning and preparation as possible, followed by gentle holding. This is time and labour intensive but important. Equally, mature babies, especially those still on the neonatal unit at several months of age, need an

individualized programme of sensory stimulation. Those with long-term artificial (nasogastric or gastrostomy) feeding may require an 'oral stimulation' programme to ensure they do not become orophobic and are able to develop normal oral feeding in the future.

> **CLINICAL TIP:** There is some evidence that toys or panels with contrasting colours or black and white stripes placed in the cot can help visual cortical development, but these should be used for short periods of time and changed frequently.

Newborn Individualized Developmental Care and Assessment Program

The Newborn Individualized Developmental Care and Assessment Program (NIDCAP) is a very individualized programme of developmental intervention based on repeated periods of observation. It is dynamic and changes with the needs of the baby and the family. It uses the concepts of 'approach' behaviours, which show the baby is receptive to intervention, and 'avoidance' behaviours. This programme was developed at the Boston Children's Hospital but is unfortunately unlikely to be practical in all health care systems as it is very resource intensive. However, as more evidence of the benefit of such programmes on long-term development emerges it is important that all units adopt a developmental care philosophy, whether it is based on NIDCAP or on those elements of the programme that can be delivered locally.

It is increasingly clear that newborn babies respond to and are affected by the environment around them. Compared with the womb, even the best-designed modern neonatal nursery is a hostile, noisy and dangerous environment which is challenging to the immature homeostatic mechanisms of a preterm baby. It is the duty of all neonatal practitioners to minimize the physical and psychological disturbance to the baby during a time of rapid neuronal migration and development and to support the whole family in adapting to their circumstances in order to promote the best long-term outcome.

SUMMARY

CHAPTER 25

Organization of perinatal services and neonatal transport

Key topics

Introduction

The majority of babies are born at or near term and are clinically well after birth. Specialist neonatal care is often provided in specific geographical locations where a critical mass of expertise can be placed. Ideally, pregnant mothers should deliver at a place that can provide the necessary care for their baby. For a variety of reasons, a number of babies will require emergency transport to a hospital that is capable of providing ongoing management. The care and transport of sick and premature infants requires specific skills, knowledge and resources.

Organization of perinatal services

Highly regionalized models for the delivery of perinatal services have developed over time. Perinatal services may provide:
- standard antenatal care
- antenatal care with maternal fetal medicine (MFM) services

- planned management of birth
- care and assessment of well newborn infants
- neonatal special care
- neonatal intensive care including care of extremely preterm and extremely low birthweight (ELBW) infants
- neonatal care of specific surgical and cardiac conditions

Essential Neonatal Medicine, Fifth Edition. Sunil Sinha, Lawrence Miall, Luke Jardine.
© 2012 John Wiley & Sons, Ltd. Published 2012 by John Wiley & Sons, Ltd.

- specialized transport services for infants requiring care at another facility
- follow-up and ongoing care after discharge from the neonatal service.

The goals of these perinatal services are to improve outcomes with high critical mass and provide cost-effective perinatal care.

Levels of perinatal care

Neonatal intensive care is a coordinated effort by health care providers in a defined geographical region to intervene in the reproductive process so as to make available to every neonate a level of medical care commensurate with the perceived risk of neonatal death or serious morbidity. The integration of neonatal and obstetric services into a perinatal programme offers the best opportunity for prevention and treatment.

A neonatal intensive care unit (NICU) should provide care for all babies born in a district or region, and babies requiring intensive care are referred to the intensive care nursery. Facilities for neonatal surgery and cardiology should be available in NICUs. When infants no longer require intensive care services they should be transferred back to the most appropriate service closest to their home.

Different countries have different ways of defining the levels of care (see Tables 25.1 and 25.2).

Tertiary perinatal services have a strong focus on quality improvement, evidence-based practice, risk reduction, clinical audit, ethics and research. The types of patients that should be cared for in NICUs are listed in Box 25.1 and the types of problems that can be admitted to a high-dependency unit are listed in Box 25.2. Level 1 special care is provided for all other babies who could not reasonably be expected to be looked after at home by their mother. Normal care is care given in a postnatal ward, usually by the mother under the supervision of a midwife or doctor but requiring minimal medical or nursing advice.

All maternity units must provide normal care for babies. A district general hospital with a consultant obstetric unit should provide special care facilities, and approximately 6% of infants will require this type of care.

Table 25.1 Levels of neonatal care in the UK	
Level 1 hospitals	Provide special care but do not aim to provide any continuing high-dependency or intensive care. This term includes units with or without resident medical staff. The requirement is for one nurse to every four babies
Level 2 hospitals	Provide high-dependency care and some short-term intensive care as agreed within the network. This requires one trained nurse to two babies
Level 3 hospitals	Provide the whole range of medical neonatal care but not necessarily all specialist services such as neonatal surgery. This requires one-to-one specialist nursing per cot

CLINICAL TIP: Regardless of the level of neonatal service provided, staff responsible for looking after babies need to be skilled in neonatal resuscitation, stabilization and examination.

The role of neonatal networks

Collaboration with a national neonatal network audits outcomes, provides benchmarking standards, develops clinical indicators, provides standardized guidelines and policies, allows consultation with the referring and receiving units, and facilitates research through critical mass.

Models of care

Ideally mother and baby should be kept together as much as possible so that models of care for babies with special needs, such as neonatal abstinence syndrome (NAS), infants of diabetic mothers, marginal prematurity (35–36 weeks), intravenous antibiotics and jaundice requiring intensive phototherapy, should be predominantly provided by parents.

Table 25.2 Levels of neonatal care in Australia and New Zealand	
Level 1 hospitals	(50–400 deliveries per annum). These provide services for uncomplicated maternity and newborn patients >36 weeks' gestation. The mature infant nursery provides basic life supports and receives back transfer from level 2 hospitals
Level 2 hospitals	(400–2000 deliveries per annum). These provide services for low- and medium-risk pregnancies and for babies >32 weeks' gestation. The special care nursery (SCN) is staffed by neonatal nurses and a paediatric registrar and consultant, and can provide stabilization of preterm and sick infants prior to neonatal retrieval
Level 3 hospitals	(usually >3000 births and >10,000 births in catchment area). These provide services for low-, medium- and high-risk obstetrics, have a maternal fetal medicine unit and a full range of ventilation options. The staff include neonatal nurses, neonatal registrars and a consultant, and there is access to a full range of paediatric subspecialties. These units may be located in obstetric hospitals, in general hospitals or in children's hospitals. There is a nurse:patient ratio of 1:2, or 1:1 for unstable infants
Level 4 hospitals	This is a term that is sometimes used to describe services provided to neonates requiring paediatric subspecialty care (e.g. those with complex metabolic and/or cardiac conditions, and surgical cases)

Box 25.1 Examples of problems that qualify for neonatal intensive care unit (level 3 in the UK and levels 3–4 in Australia and New Zealand)

- Any baby receiving any respiratory support via a tracheal tube and in the first 24 h after withdrawal of such support
- Any baby receiving nasal continuous positive airway pressure (NCPAP) for any part of the day and expected to require NCPAP for a prolonged period.
- Babies requiring >50% oxygen
- Any baby below 1000 g current weight
- Babies requiring major emergency surgery, for the preoperative period and postoperatively for 24 h
- Babies requiring complex clinical procedures:
  full exchange transfusion
  peritoneal dialysis
  infusion of an inotrope, pulmonary vasodilator or
    prostaglandin, and for 24 h afterwards
- Any other very unstable baby considered by the nurse in charge as needing one-to-one nursing

Box 25.2 Examples of problems that qualify for admission to a high dependency or level 2 unit/hospital

- Babies requiring short-term NCPAP and not fulfilling any of the criteria for intensive care
- Babies over 1000 g current weight and not fulfilling any of the criteria for intensive care
- Babies receiving total parenteral nutrition
- Babies having convulsions
- Babies receiving oxygen therapy and below 1500 g current weight
- Babies requiring treatment for neonatal abstinence syndrome
- Babies requiring specified procedures that do not fulfil any criteria for intensive care
  - care of an intra-arterial catheter or chest drain
  - partial exchange transfusion
  - tracheostomy care until supervised by a parent
- Babies requiring frequent stimulation for severe apnoea

Neonatal services should be developed to oversee a continuum of care between the different levels, hospitals and community-based primary health facilities.

Neonatal transport

In infants requiring neonatal intensive care, mortality is significantly lower if birth occurs in a hospital capable of providing that care rather than in a place that necessitates their transfer to another facility after birth. Therefore, if possible, the birth of a high-risk infant should occur in a hospital capable of providing the necessary care. If birth occurs in a place without the required facilities, the infant should be stabilized and transferred to an appropriate higher-level centre within the service network.

Transport *in utero*

The ideal time to transfer a potentially sick infant is *in utero*, if the problem can be anticipated. High-risk pregnancies should be transferred before delivery, and a high-risk fetus should be transferred *in utero* to a unit with perinatal intensive care facilities. In all cases there must be consultation with the receiving hospital before transfer. Unfortunately, not all neonatal problems can be recognized from an at-risk pregnancy, and some women are unwilling to be transported before delivery.

The rationale for transporting sick or low birthweight (LBW) neonates to special care or intensive care nurseries is based on the premise that specialized units reduce mortality and improve outcome, and that these advantages outweigh the risk of transport and physical or social disadvantages for the family. The incidence of intraventricular haemorrhage in infants born in a referring hospital after *in utero* transfer is significantly lower than in a similar group of outborn babies.

The decision to transfer a sick neonate will depend on the expertise of the intensive care nursery, the safety of travel and the facilities available at the hospital where the baby was born. Discussion with a neonatal paediatrician may obviate the need for transport or provide advice on the best methods of transfer. Personnel from the neonatal emergency

> ### Box 25.3 Possible indications for neonatal transfer
>
> - Gestational age <30 weeks
> - Respiratory distress of early onset or persisting more than 4–6 h
> - Oxygen requirement >50% or associated apnoea, meconium aspiration or suspected pneumonia
> - Apnoeic episodes
> - Convulsions
> - Hypoxic–ischaemic encephalopathy requiring hypothermia
> - Jaundiced infant in need of exchange transfusion
> - Bleeding
> - Surgical conditions
> - Congenital heart disease
> - Severe or multiple congenital abnormalities
> - Need for special diagnostic or therapeutic services
> - 'Unwell' infant with lethargy, poor perfusion, oliguria, etc.

transport service can assist with the decision on whether transfer is necessary.

Consideration should be given to the transfer of any infant if the facilities do not exist in the admitting hospital. Common indications for transfer are listed in Box 25.3.

Preparation for transport

The amount of stabilization required before departure depends on the baby's condition and the rate of progress of the disease. It is also influenced by the distance to be travelled, the duration of the journey and the mode of transport.

It is important not to waste time, power, oxygen or air. Always use the nursery or ambulance utilities where possible. Staff must be aware of the difficulties of detecting and correcting problems in transit, and must ensure appropriate stabilization before transport.

The infant should be resuscitated and his/her condition stabilized prior to transport. While awaiting transfer the referring hospital should provide the following care:

- The infant is kept warm (ideally servocontrolled to a skin temperature of 36.5 °C). Bubble plastic may help to reduce heat loss.
- The infant is given sufficient oxygen to maintain oxygen saturation in the normal range (91–95% for preterm infants and ≥94% for term infants).
- Adequate respiration is ensured (some babies will require additional respiratory support, e.g. nasal continuous positive airway pressure (NCPAP) or mechanical ventilation – see below).
- Insertion of intravenous access.
- Collection of a blood culture and commencement of intravenous antibiotics.
- Intravenous dextrose with maintenance of blood glucose above 2.5 mmol/L.
- Insertion of a nasogastric or orogastric tube. The baby is not fed during transport and the stomach is aspirated before leaving the referring hospital.
- Frequent observations of temperature, heart rate, respiratory rate, blood pressure and blood sugar by reagent stick.
- A photograph of the baby for the mother should be taken prior to transport.
- Other – specific conditions will require additional treatments on advice from the retrieving centre (e.g. prostaglandin E1 (PGE₁) infusion if possibility of duct-dependent cyanotic heart disease).

Before the transfer commences the referring hospital should also provide the following:

- completed perinatal data sheet
- signed parental consent for the infant's transfer and treatment
- copies of relevant records and results of tests, including radiographs
- if indicated, specimens should also be transferred with the baby (e.g. maternal blood, placenta, baby blood, etc.)

> **CLINICAL TIP:** In many instances venous access will be required for transfer, but do not attempt to put in an arterial line (peripheral or umbilical) before leaving. This is often best left to experienced operators at the receiving unit.

Important decisions to be made

Intubation

One of the most important decisions that needs to be made before transport is whether or not to intubate and ventilate the baby. This is influenced by factors relating to the particular baby, such as diagnosis, current condition and likely course, size and gestational age, and transport factors, such as the nature of the trip and operational conditions. If in doubt contact the receiving neonatologist. Once a baby is intubated, exogenous surfactant administration should occur where indicated. Before departure, it is essential to ensure the endotracheal tube is correctly positioned and safely secured.

Choice of vehicle

On the UK mainland infants are generally transferred by the road ambulance service. Occasionally, a fixed-wing aircraft (civil or military) is necessary for transportation overseas or over longer distances. In Australia there is usually a range of options, including road ambulance (up to 100–150 km), helicopter (up to 250 km) and fixed-wing aircraft (>200 km). The choice of vehicle depends on availability of vehicles and aircraft, distance, degree of urgency, weather conditions and other factors. Each transfer is considered individually on its merits.

Transport vehicles

Transport vehicles should be dedicated neonatal ambulance vehicles; these are desirable for large services where retrievals exceed 150 per annum. The vehicles must meet national passenger safety standards, and have adequate seating with safety restraints for staff. Adequate lighting and internal climate control are necessary. A fixed positive mounting system is required to restrain the transport system. Tolerable noise and vibration levels are an essential prerequisite. External communication should be available to allow the team to be directly connected to any telephone number at any stage of the transfer.

Aerial transport

Transfer by aeroplane or helicopter has several unique problems.

• Any air flight, even in a pressurized cabin, decreases ambient pressure with resultant expansion of gases in body cavities. This is particularly relevant in infants with pneumothorax, lung cysts or trapped gas in the bowel or the peritoneal cavity. Pain may occur as a result of expansion of air in the facial sinuses in larger infants.

• Inspired oxygen is decreased owing to the rarefied atmosphere.

• Noise and vibration may lead to loss of the gag reflex and promote vomiting, with resultant aspiration.

• Difficulty with illumination, observation and especially auscultation of the heart and lungs.

> **CLINICAL TIP:** When transporting a ventilated infant in a helicopter, auscultation of the infant becomes almost impossible because of the noise levels. Extubation or tube blockage can be particularly difficult to identify. In the event of an acute respiratory deterioration, a CO_2 detector can be used to confirm placement of the endotracheal tube. If no obvious cause is found for the deterioration, consider the possibility of pneumothorax and the need for emergency needle thoracotomy.

Who should accompany the baby?

A neonatal nurse experienced in transport should accompany term babies who are not critically ill. A neonatal doctor and nurse should escort any unwell or high-risk baby. It is desirable, but not always practicable, that the mother should be transported with her baby. If the mother is unwell then she should be transferred at a later stage as neonatal retrieval teams do not have the capability to look after an adult as well as the baby.

Transport equipment

There are a number of basic organizational requirements for providing and organizing neonatal transport equipment and these are listed in Table 25.3. Emergency equipment required is listed in Table 25.4.

The role of a neonatal transport service

An integral part of a successful neonatal transport programme is frequent communication with personnel in the referring nursery, and especially with the mother. The infant should be transferred back to the referring nursery at the earliest possible time.

A coordinated neonatal transport service organizes retrievals and return transfers of infants back to the base hospital, and is also involved with consultation services and education for outlying practitioners. It provides an active role in the coordination of all neonatal transport facilities, utilization of perinatal facilities and outreach education.

It plays a pivotal role in the coordination and utilization of perinatal facilities. The selection and standardization of transport facilities involves liaison with all transport providers. There is also a commitment to audit, research and quality assurance.

Care of parents

The transport team must be sensitive to the needs of the parents during this stressful period. They must introduce themselves to parents and explain the nature of the transport, treatment and likely prognosis. Parents are encouraged to touch their baby and are offered a photograph. An information booklet about the tertiary hospital is provided, and informed consent for transfer and care must be obtained.

Relationships with referring hospital and staff

The retrieval staff must be sensitive in relating to referral hospital personnel: they should never, either directly or by implication, criticize the referring doctor's management. Smooth communication and relationships between referring and receiving units are essential for effective regionalization of care.

Table 25.3 Basic requirements for neonatal transport

Quantity of equipment	A minimum of two sets of equipment are required for any one geographical area to allow for breakdown, maintenance, concurrent calls and twin transportation
Safety requirements	The equipment should satisfy all areas of safety regulation and other statutory requirements
Transport incubators	These must provide a neutral thermal environment under a wide range of external temperatures and environmental conditions There must be good lighting and visibility and easy access Incubators must be capable of operation from a variety of power sources including battery, mains, aircraft (24 V DC) and road vehicle (10–13 V DC) Most transport systems have an air compressor
Monitoring equipment	Monitoring of temperature, heart rate, inspired oxygen concentration and oxygen partial pressure and/or saturation is essential Blood pressure monitoring is desirable
Respiratory support	Independent supplies of oxygen and medical air are required to provide controlled inspired oxygen concentrations from 21% to 100%. Ideally, inspired gases should be heated and humidified Inhaled nitric oxide is now available for ventilators on transport incubator A mechanical ventilator able to provide intermittent positive pressure ventilation (IPPV) and continuous positive airway pressure (CPAP) is required A suitable hand-operated ventilator system, consisting of bag and mask with manometer, must be available as a back-up to mechanical ventilation
Suction	Suction equipment must have an independent power supply, and negative pressure must be controlled and adjustable Oral suction mucus traps must be available as back-up
Infusion pumps	Infusion by a constant-rate pump is required for intravenous and/or intra-arterial infusion Battery-operated syringe infusion pumps delivering a constant flow are used

Table 25.4 Essential equipment required for neonatal transport

Equipment for emergency intubation	Laryngoscope, endotracheal tubes with introducers, tape, CO_2 detectors
Equipment for emergency insertion of a chest tube	Intercostal catheters, Heimlich one-way flutter valve
Equipment for emergency insertion of an umbilical catheter	3.5 Fr and 5 Fr single-lumen and double-lumen catheters
Drugs for resuscitation	Adrenaline (epinephrine), normal saline, anticonvulsants, dopamine and dobutamine, bicarbonate, calcium gluconate, surfactant, and prostaglandin E_1 (Prostin)
Other miscellaneous items of equipment	Digital camera, paediatric stethoscopes, blood glucose meter and strips

Table 25.5 Specific conditions and managements for retrieval	
Diaphragmatic hernia	These babies should be intubated and ventilated Avoid bag-and-mask ventilation Be prepared for a possible pneumothorax The stomach must be frequently aspirated via a nasogastric tube Correct any acidosis before departure and consider paralysis if the baby is hypoxic
Oesophageal atresia with tracheo-oesophageal fistula	Replogle tube should be inserted into the upper pouch and placed on continuous suction Feeding is absolutely contraindicated Avoid intubation and mechanical ventilation if possible (as it can cause severe abdominal distension and further respiratory compromise in some cases) Nurse the infant prone with the body elevated to 30° from the horizontal
Exomphalos/gastroschisis/myelomeningocoele	The eviscerated lesions should be wrapped in a sterile plastic bag to prevent heat and fluid losses from evaporation and excessive cooling The infant is nursed on the surface opposite to the lesion Reposition the bowel if it appears to have impaired blood supply Assess perfusion and give fluid replacement if necessary
Bowel obstruction	Fluid and electrolyte disturbances should be corrected prior to transport and continuous nasogastric suction maintained throughout The infant should be nursed prone or lying on the right side with the head up An indwelling open nasogastric tube is placed in the stomach and aspirated intermittently An intravenous dextrose infusion is required
Pierre Robin sequence/choanal atresia	Ensure adequate airway, both while awake and when asleep The infant is nursed in the prone position and an oropharyngeal airway strapped in place. In some cases a long nasopharyngeal tube is positioned with tip just above the epiglottis Continuous observation of respiratory pattern, skin colour and oxygen saturation is required
Duct-dependent cyanotic congenital heart disease (e.g. pulmonary atresia, TGA with intact septum)	Infants who require a prostaglandin (Prostin, PGE) infusion to maintain the patency of their ductus arteriosus are at risk of apnoea If the baby is having apnoea or is at significant risk of apnoea, intubation and mechanical ventilation may be required prior to transfer

Staff should involve ambulance officers with equipment needs and educate them about the infant's condition. A debriefing with referring staff is an essential component of quality management improvement.

Special considerations

In certain conditions, a number of problems can be anticipated prior to transfer of the baby and these are listed in Table 25.5.

SUMMARY

Neonatal intensive care is now a highly specialized field of medicine. In order to provide a cost-effective critical mass, services are consolidated in specific geographical locations as part of a larger perinatal service. When problems are expected in a pregnancy, delivery should occur at a place that can provide the necessary care for that particular baby. The safest way for a baby to be transferred to another centre is *in utero*. If delivery occurs in a centre that is not capable of continuing the care of the baby, then emergency transport to another hospital will be required. The care and transport of sick and premature infants requires specific skills, knowledge and resources. Retrievals should be coordinated through a neonatal transport service that can provide the appropriate advice, staff, equipment and vehicles required.

 Now visit **www.essentialneonatalmed.com** to test yourself on this chapter.

CHAPTER 26

Discharge and follow-up of high-risk infants

Key topics

Introduction

Babies who have required neonatal intensive care are at high risk of long-term neurodevelopmental problems. Parents are often anxious around the time of discharge from hospital, particularly after a prolonged stay. Careful follow-up of these high-risk infants is essential to enable early identification of problems and the initiation of appropriate treatments. Specialized follow-up clinics play an important role in the long-term surveillance of these high-risk infants.

Discharge of high-risk infants

Before discharge the parents will need advice on feeding, sleeping, nutritional supplementation, introduction of complementary food and immunizations. They will need education about the preventable risk factors for sudden infant death syndrome (SIDS; see Chapter 14). An information booklet on these subjects may be issued to the parents. Some parents will also require training in basic resuscitation techniques, depending on the condition of the baby. In certain circumstances parents will require additional training before discharge (e.g. nasogastric feeding, gastrostomy care, tracheostomy care, etc.).

A full discharge summary should be sent to the infant's general practitioner and referring paediatrician/obstetrician at time of discharge. Parents should have a copy of the discharge summary. The summary should highlight ongoing care

Essential Neonatal Medicine, Fifth Edition. Sunil Sinha, Lawrence Miall, Luke Jardine.
© 2012 John Wiley & Sons, Ltd. Published 2012 by John Wiley & Sons, Ltd.

at discharge and need for follow-up. Parents should be advised about the role of the general practitioner in follow-up and the availability of other services such as a child health nurse or community clinics. Parents may also be provided with information on local support groups and other resources.

Rooming in

Ideally, the mother and father should 'room in' with their baby, or at least sleep in the hospital in close proximity to the baby for some days and nights before discharge, so that they can gain confidence and learn to care for their previously sick or preterm infant.

Feeding advice

Feeding of the low birthweight (LBW) infant is discussed in Chapter 9. The frequency of feeds depends on the maturity and neurological integrity of the infant, but 3–4 hourly feeds are usually necessary on discharge from the neonatal unit. The mother should be encouraged to demand-feed her baby, but feeds should not be more than 5 h apart during the day. Artificially fed infants are usually transferred from a preterm formula to a term formula before discharge although transitional formulas are now available and can be used in the interim. The maternal and child health clinic or the general practitioner should follow the growth of preterm and high-risk infants during the first year of life and plot length, weight and head circumference on appropriate percentile graphs.

Nutritional supplementation

Iron

Term infants receive sufficient iron from breast milk until about 6–9 months of age. Although the iron content in breast milk is low (0.5 mg/L), the absorption is excellent. The term infant being fed on iron-fortified formula receives sufficient iron until 6 months, at which time iron-containing foods such as cereals, vegetables, eggs and meat should be started. The preterm infant needs supplemental iron from 3 months of age, whether breastfed or not. In

some units iron therapy is commenced in hospital between days 14 and 28 with ferrous sulphate paediatric mixture, and is continued until solids are commenced.

Vitamins

Term infants probably receive adequate vitamins in their breast milk or vitamin-fortified breast-milk substitutes. However, preterm infants and other ill infants will require extra vitamins, especially D and C. Human milk fortifiers contain vitamins. Preterm infants with inadequate vitamin C intake often have an immaturity of the enzyme phenylalanine hydroxylase and may develop transient tyrosinaemia. In some units, a multivitamin preparation such as Dalivit, Pentavite or ABIDEC will be commenced in weeks 3–4 of life and continued until 6–12 months.

Fluoride

Fluoride drops are recommended in areas where the water supply is not fluoridated. It is important to adhere to recommended dosage schedules as excessive fluoride may cause tooth staining as a result of fluorosis. Fluoride drops should preferably be given in water rather than milk to permit better absorption.

Immunization

Details of the immunization schedules in the UK and Australia are shown in Tables 26.1 and 26.2. The current recommendations advise starting the immunization programme when the infant is 2 months of actual age, rather than age corrected for prematurity.

Contraindications to pertussis immunization

There are some circumstances in which pertussis immunization should be deferred or withheld.

• Immunization should be temporarily withheld if the child is suffering from any acute illness. Minor

Table 26.1 Immunization schedule in the UK

Age	Immunization (vaccine given)
Birth	hepatitis B and BCG to at risk groups
2 months	**DTaP/IPV(polio)/Hib** (diphtheria, tetanus, pertussis (whooping cough), polio, and *Haemophilus influenzae* type b) – all-in-one injection, plus: **PCV** (pneumococcal conjugate vaccine) – in a separate injection
3 months	**DTaP/IPV(polio)/Hib** (2nd dose), plus: **MenC** (meningitis C) – in a separate injection
4 months	**DTaP/IPV(polio)/Hib** (3rd dose), plus: **MenC** (2nd dose) – in a separate injection, plus: **PCV** (2nd dose) – in a separate injection
12–13 months	**Hib/MenC** (combined as one injection – 4th dose of **Hib** and 3rd dose of **MenC**) plus: **MMR** (measles, mumps and rubella – combined as one injection), plus: **PCV** (3rd dose) – in a separate injection
Around 3 years and 4 months	Pre-school booster of: **DTaP/IPV(polio)** (diphtheria, tetanus, pertussis (whooping cough) and polio), plus: **MMR** (second dose) – in a separate injection
Around 12–13 years (girls)	**HPV** (human papillomavirus) – three injections The second injection is given 1–2 months after the first one. The third is given about 6 months after the first one
Around 13–18 years	**Td/IPV(polio)** booster (a combined injection of tetanus, low-dose diphtheria, and polio)
Adults	**Influenza and PCV** if you are aged 65 or over or in a high-risk group **Td/IPV(polio)** – at any age if you were not fully immunized as a child

infections without fever or systemic upset are not reasons for withholding immunization.
• A history of severe local or general reaction to a previous dose.
• An evolving neurological abnormality or un-controlled epilepsy: immunization should be deferred until the child is assessed by a paediatric neurologist.

A family history of allergy is not a contraindication, nor is a perinatal or family history of fits, provided the child has not had an acute encephalopathic illness within 7 days. Children with evolving neurological conditions may be immunized when the condition has become stable. Pertussis vaccine in most countries is now acellular, with much lower complication rates than its cellular predecessor.

Special vaccine circumstances

BCG (bacille Calmette–Guérin)

In Britain and Australia, BCG is reserved for babies at risk for tuberculosis (TB) and is given by intra-dermal injection during the early neonatal period. Indications include:
• All infants living in areas of TB prevalence.
• Infants with parents or grandparents born in a country with a high TB prevalence.
• Babies born to previously unvaccinated recent immigrants from high-risk countries.

Table 26.2 Immunization schedule in Australia	
Age	**Immunization (vaccine given)**
Birth	Hepatitis B, tuberculosis only if high risk
2 months	**DTaP/IPV(polio)/Hib** (diphtheria, tetanus, pertussis, and polio, and *Haemophilus influenzae* type b) – all-in-one injection, plus: **PCV** (pneumococcal conjugate vaccine) - in a separate injection **Oral rotavirus**
4 months	**DTaP/IPV(polio)/Hib** (2nd dose) **PCV** (2nd dose) **Oral rotavirus** (2nd dose)
6 months	**DTaP/IPV(polio)/Hib** (3rd dose) **PCV** (3rd dose) **Oral rotavirus** (3rd dose)
12 months	**Hib/MenC** (combined as one injection – 4th dose of Hib and 3rd dose of MenC) plus: **MMR** (measles, mumps and rubella – combined as one injection), plus: Infant **Pneumococcal** if high risk
18 months	**Varicella** **Hepatitis A** if high risk
24 months	**Hepatitis A** (2nd dose) if high risk **Pneumococcal** if high risk
4 years	**DTaP/IPV(polio)** (diphtheria, tetanus, pertussis, and polio), plus: **MMR** (second dose) – in a separate injection
8 years	**Varicella** (2nd dose) **Hepatitis B** (2 doses) Girls only – **HPV** (human papillomavirus) – three injections The second injection is given 1–2 months after the first one. The third is given about 6 months after the first one
10 years	**DTaP** (diphtheria, tetanus, pertussis)
Adults	**Influenza** and **PCV** if you are aged 65 or over or in a high-risk group

• In Australia, Aboriginal neonates are considered to be high risk and BCG immunization is recommended.

Surveys in British children have shown that this vaccine is over 70% effective, with protection lasting at least 15 years.

Hepatitis B

Infants born to mothers who are hepatitis B surface antigen (HbsAg) positive should receive passive immunization with 100–200 IU of hepatitis B immunoglobulin and active immunization with hepatitis B vaccine as soon after birth as possible. The routine schedule for hepatitis B immunization in the UK and Australia are shown in Tables 26.1 and 26.2.

Modification to immunization schedule for preterm infants

Generally, preterm infants are immunized according to their actual postnatal age and not their corrected age. Some extremely preterm infants are still too unstable to receive diphtheria–pertussis–tetanus (DPT), Hib (*Haemophilus influenzae* type B) and polio at 2 months, and immunization needs to be deferred for some weeks.

CLINICAL TIP: Preterm infants require cardiorespiratory monitoring for 24–48 h after their first immunization because of the high risk of apnoea. They may need to recommence CPAP or even require a brief period of intubation and mechanical ventilation. Parents should be warned about these risks when consent for immunization is obtained.

Specialized follow-up clinics

In general it is very difficult to predict outcomes in the newborn period. The most useful predictor clinically remains gestation at birth (see Table 26.3). Other factors which help to predict outcome are listed in Box 26.1. Most preterm infants admitted to the neonatal unit grow and develop to be healthy, normal children. Some infants, however, develop significant disability (see Chapter 23). Categories of infant that should be considered for specialized follow-up are listed in Box 26.2.

Infants who are at high risk for adverse outcomes should be followed in specialized multidisciplinary clinics or at the very least, by a paediatrician. The follow-up of high-risk infants is a continuation of neonatal intensive care and an integral part of it. The benefits of following up high-risk infants in specialized clinics are listed in Box 26.3.

Box 26.1 Factors that increase the risk of adverse outcome in VLBW infants

- Periventricular leukomalacia
- Periventricular haemorrhage
- Posthaemorrhagic hydrocephalus
- Chronic neonatal lung disease
- Retinopathy of prematurity
- Intrauterine growth restriction
- Multiple birth
- Infection
- Encephalopathy and seizures
- Outborn baby
- Lack of antenatal steroids before delivery
- Male
- Significant hyperbilirubinaemia
- Hypotension

Table 26.3 Representative rates of disability in survivors analysed by gestational age

Gestation at birth (weeks)	Disability in survivors (%)	
	Major	Any
23	40	50
24	30	40
25–26	20	20
27–28	10	15
More than 28		10

Examples of major disability: blindness, deafness requiring hearing aids, inability to walk without assistance, or a low level of intellectual abilities.
Examples of less severe disability: short sightedness requiring correction with glasses, weakness on one side, clumsiness, learning difficulties, behavioural problems.

Data from Mater Mother's Hospital, South Brisbane.

Box 26.2 Categories of infants that should be considered for specialized follow-up

- Infants who were mechanically ventilated in the neonatal period including those infants treated with inhaled nitric oxide
- VLBW infants (<1500 g birthweight);
- Severe perinatal asphyxia including those requiring therapeutic hypothermia
- Infants with intracranial haemorrhage or periventricular leukomalacia
- Infants with neonatal convulsions
- Infants with meningitis or severe sepsis in the neonatal period
- Infants who have abnormal neurological examination at discharge
- Infants who had major surgery

Box 26.3 Benefits of specialized clinics in the follow-up of high-risk infants

- Early diagnosis of problems enables early intervention and perhaps a better long-term prognosis
- Evaluation of the perinatal factors that have an adverse effect on outcome, with subsequent modification of methods of delivery of perinatal intensive care
- Evaluation of the long-term prognosis of high-risk populations of infants
- Assessment of a cost-benefit analysis for perinatal intensive care

---

Most follow-up clinics will involve a multidisciplinary team containing a minimum of paediatricians, physiotherapists and psychologists. Other important members of the team may include speech pathologists, occupational therapists, dietitians, nurses, clinic staff, and research personnel.

Purposes of multidisciplinary follow-up clinics

Following high-risk children in a multidisciplinary follow-up clinic has several purposes including service, audit/quality assurance, research and education.

Service role

Follow-up is considered an integral part of assuming responsibility for high-risk infants and provides early identification of developmental disability, reassurance to parents, psychosocial support and referral for appropriate treatment. There is debate as to whether the multidisciplinary clinic personnel should provide treatment or merely have an evaluation role in follow-up of high-risk cohorts. The provision of health care by the clinic team gives greatest assurance of both a low attrition rate and an effective system of healthcare delivery.

Audit role

Multidisciplinary follow-up provides ongoing surveillance of morbidity, enabling evaluation of the impact of changes in obstetric and neonatal care on quality of survival of VLBW infants. Many advances in clinical practice have emanated from longitudinal cohort evaluation.

Research role

Follow-up programmes have a very important role in assessing the impact of perinatal care and monitoring the effect of new treatments. Almost all new treatments will require an assessment of the long-term developmental outcome before a decision is made as to their safety and efficacy. Ideally, staff should be blinded to the patient's history, so as to avoid biased assessments. Unfortunately, follow-up programmes are expensive, require patience and perseverance, take several years to complete before research findings are available, and run the risk of becoming outdated because current neonatal practice has changed.

Educational role

The clinic provides an excellent multidisciplinary resource for teaching allied health professionals and medical and nurse clinicians about child development and the needs of families of high-risk infants.

Follow-up of preterm infants

In preterm infants, growth and development should be assessed according to the corrected age:

$$\text{corrected age} = \text{postnatal age} - \text{number of weeks infant is preterm}$$

Data supporting this biological model suggest that, for infants of 28 weeks of gestation or less, correction should be continued for 4 years; in those 29–31 weeks for 2 years; those 32–34 weeks for 1 year; and in those 35 weeks and beyond no correction is made for gestational age.

Table 26.4 Complications in the first year of life in preterm infants

Medical	
Respiratory	Nasal congestion
	Exacerbation of bronchopulmonary dysplasia
	Recurrent wheezing
	SIDS
Cardiac	Patent ductus arteriosus
	Ventricular septal defect
Ophthalmic	Retinopathy of prematurity
	Strabismus
	Myopia
Auditory	Sensorineural hearing loss
	Conductive dysfunction
Surgical	Inguinal hernia, umbilical hernia, undescended testes, hydrocoele
Growth	Failure to achieve genetic growth potential
Gastrointestinal	Vomiting, gastro-oesophageal reflux, constipation, colic
Neurological deficits	
Major	Spastic diplegia/hemiplegia/quadriplegia
	Hypotonia, hydrocephalus, microcephaly, moderate to profound global delay
Minor	Ataxia, incoordination and clumsiness
Miscellaneous	Child abuse, neglect, deprivation, behavioural disturbances, emotional disturbances, failure to thrive

Problems encountered in follow-up

Common problems identified in preterm infants are shown in Table 26.4. Long-term outcomes are discussed in detail in Chapter 23.

Growth

The use of charts allows accurate assessment of these important parameters of physical growth. As a guide, term infants usually double their birthweight by 5 months and treble it by 1 year. The head circumference usually grows about 1 cm a month for the first 6 months, and then 0.5 cm a month for the next 6 months. Most babies increase their length by 20–30 cm (or 50%) in the first year of life.

The healthy preterm baby who is appropriate for gestational age (AGA) should grow at the same rate as a term infant, with the same growth patterns as low birthweight infants; that is, regaining birthweight at 2 weeks postnatal age and then accelerating, so that by the expected date of delivery the infant will be close to the expected weight of a term infant.

Growth failure often occurs in small for gestational age (SGA) and sick preterm infants, who receive inadequate nutrition and have higher metabolic requirements for the first 4–6 weeks after birth. In this latter group linear and head growth virtually cease, and even when adequate nutrition is established growth may remain suboptimal. The SGA infant usually loses little, if any, weight in the neonatal period and then rapidly gains weight to reach his/her potential growth percentile. This growth spurt may not be maintained, and a permanent deficit in somatic growth may persist into childhood.

CLINICAL TIP: Growth of head circumference is often difficult to interpret in preterm babies. This is partly due to the scaphocephalic head shape. For 3–4 weeks after birth, growth in head circumference is suboptimal at about 0.2 cm/week; then follows a period of rapid head growth (catch-up brain growth spurt) at about 1 cm/week for 1–2 months; the head then grows at the normal rate of 1 cm/month for the first 6 months and then 0.5 cm/month for the rest of the first year of life.

Postnatal development

A wide range of problems have been reported in graduates of the neonatal intensive care nursery. These are discussed in Chapter 23. Unfortunately no standard exists for the reporting of these outcomes and therefore it can be difficult to interpret published results. Issues to consider when interpreting published outcome studies on preterm infants are listed in Box 26.4.

There is great variability in infant development. The rate of progress is influenced by many factors, including gestational age, nutrition, intercurrent illness, environmental stimulation and emotional support. Milestones in development can be considered in four groups: social, speech and language, gross motor and fine motor. The ages for the acquisition of these skills and milestones are approximate and there are wide variations between normal babies. Table 26.5 summarizes some of these important milestones. If there is evidence of significant developmental delay or cerebral palsy, the child should be referred to a child development centre for more comprehensive assessment by a multidisciplinary team. The totality of handicapping conditions in VLBW infants relates to corrected postnatal age and is illustrated in Fig. 26.1.

Compared with their full-term peers, extremely preterm children tend to achieve lower levels of physical and intellectual performance. Some of the more commonly reported outcomes are listed in Table 26.6. These problems present at different ages and this is highlighted in Fig. 26.1. However, the

Box 26.4 Factors which need to be considered when interpreting published outcome data for neonates

- What is the denominator? Studies that include babies born alive in the labour ward compared with studies that report a denominator of only babies admitted alive to the neonatal unit may be associated with a 50% difference in outcome at the extremes of prematurity.
- Is data reported by gestational age or birthweight?
- What is the survival rate/approach to resuscitation at limit of viability?
- Is it a hospital-based or geographic population?
- What is the proportion of outborn babies? Outborn babies have higher rates of morbidity and mortality.
- Have they corrected for preterm birth?
- What is the attrition rate?
- What was the duration of follow up?
- What outcome measures have been used and how has disability been classified?
- How did they deal with untestable children?

majority of preterm infants rate their quality of life as high and they are less likely to participate in risk-taking behaviours such as heavy alcohol consumption and illicit drug use.

Definitions

Great care must be taken to use the terms 'handicap', 'impairment' and 'disability' correctly, so that comparisons can be made between different centres. The following are the internationally accepted World Health Organization (WHO) definitions.
- **Impairment**: any loss or abnormality of psychological or anatomical structure or function.
- **Disability**: any restriction or lack of ability (resulting from an impairment) in performing an activity in the manner or within the range considered to be normal.
- **Handicap**: a disadvantage for an individual arising from a disability that limits or prevents the fulfilment of a role that should be normal for that individual.

Table 26.5 Milestones in development. Note that ages are very approximate and there are wide variations between normal babies

Age	Social	Speech and language	Gross motor	Fine motor
1 month	Quietens when talked to	–	Holds head up momentarily	Fists clenched at rest
2 months	Smiling with good visual interest	Listens to bell	Chin off couch when prone	Hands largely open
3 months	Follows objects through 180°	Vocalizes when talked to	Weight on forearms when lying prone	Holds objects placed in hands
4 months	Laughs aloud	–	Pulling to sit: no head lag	Hands come together
6 months	Imitates	Localizes sound	Lying prone, pushes up on hands	Reaches for objects
7 months	Feeds him/herself with biscuit	Makes four different sounds	Sits unsupported	Transfers from hand to hand
9 months	Waves bye-bye	Says 'Mama'	Stands holding on	Pincer grasp
12 months	Plays 'pat-a-cake'	2–3 words	Walking unsupported	Gives objects
15 months	Drinks from a cup	4–5 words	Climbs up stairs	Tower of 2 cubes
18 months	Points to three parts of body	8–10 words	Gets up and down stairs	Tower 3–4 cubes
21 months	Dry (mostly) during day	2 word sentences	Runs	Scribbles circles
24 months	Puts on shoes	2–3 word sentences	Walks up and down stairs	Tower 6–7 cubes
$2\frac{1}{2}$ years	Recognizes colours	Knows full name		Copies with pencil
3 years	Dresses and undresses fully	Tells stories		Copies with pencil

Table 26.6 Adverse developmental outcomes in extremely preterm infants compared with controls

Intelligent quotient (IQ)	Studies consistently find mean IQs for ELBW infants are 0.7–1.0 SD less than term controls
Intellectual impairments	Subtle cognitive deficits include lower scores in maths, reading, spelling, visual short-term memory and executive function independent of IQ
School performance	ELBW infants are more likely to be in the lower half of performance in their grade and are twice as likely to repeat a grade versus term controls
Dyspraxia (clumsiness)	Dyspraxia is a common finding in ELBW infants. This is most obvious clinically when using ball skills (kicking and catching) and fine motor control
Attention deficit hyperactivity disorder and behaviour problems	Premature infants have approximately twice the rate of these problems compared to the general population

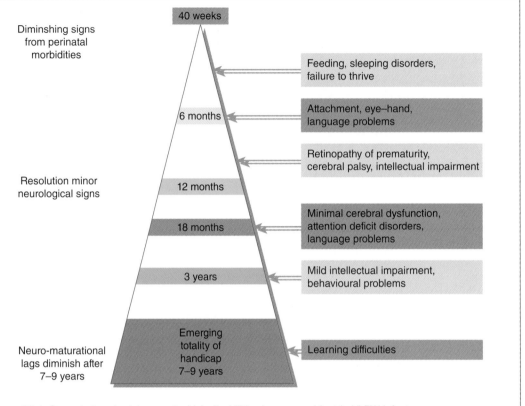

Figure 26.1 Corrected postnatal ages at which disabilities become evident in VLBW infants.

SUMMARY

The majority of infants who are discharged from the neonatal intensive care will have normal development and no major long-term problems. There is, however, a subgroup that are at particularly high risk and require ongoing surveillance. Parents will often need significant advice and support in preparation for discharge.

 Now visit **www.essentialneonatalmed.com** to test yourself on this chapter.

CHAPTER 27

Parent–infant attachment and support for parents of critically ill infants

Key topics

Introduction

Following important observations in the 1970s by Klaus and Kennell, it is now well accepted that a powerful parent–infant attachment ('bonding'), has usually been established especially in mothers, by the time of birth. At the same time, it also became very clear that little attention had been given to the possible effects on parents of the death of an infant who had had little or no opportunity for life. Since then there has been considerable literature on perinatal death, revealing that the care of recently bereaved parents leaves much to be desired. Thus, an understanding of the parent–infant bonding process can help the doctor and other health care providers to minimize the devastating effect of perinatal loss, and also to understand the effects of prematurity and congenital abnormality on a family.

For mothers a bond is formed quite early in pregnancy, stimulated by hormonal changes, psychological preparation and fantasies about the unborn child. 'Nesting' behaviour is manifested by the preparation of a nursery and the purchase of baby clothes. For the father the attachment process is less recognizable during the pregnancy but heightens with the birth, enhanced by an involvement with the delivery and handling of the baby. A sense of pride and hope for the future ensues.

Essential Neonatal Medicine, Fifth Edition. Sunil Sinha, Lawrence Miall, Luke Jardine.
© 2012 John Wiley & Sons, Ltd. Published 2012 by John Wiley & Sons, Ltd.

Parent–infant attachment (bonding)

Steps in attachment

The actual process by which attachment bonds are formed is unknown. There are thought to be critical stages essential to the establishment of attachment and these are listed in Box 27.1. The strength of the attachment during these stages may vary from one woman to another.

Most research, however, has concentrated on early contact in the immediate postnatal period. Extrapolation from animal research has proposed that there is a 'maternal-sensitive' or 'maternal-critical period', which is the optimal time for a bond of affection to develop between a mother and her infant. Although there is little doubt that the importance of this immediate postnatal period has been overemphasized in humans, this knowledge had major benefits such as early establishment of successful feeding and discharge from hospital. Some mothers are unable to achieve strong attachment without consistent contact. Failure to bond can result in rejection and resultant problems with child abuse, neglect and deprivation of nutrition, love and affection.

Parents learn to love their infant at varying times during the pregnancy and after birth. Parents are able to 'bond' to babies they have adopted, yet there has been no 'maternal-critical period'. It is apparent that humans differ from other animals in their patterns of bonding.

Box 27.1 Phases of parent–infant attachment (bonding)

- Planning the pregnancy
- Confirming the pregnancy
- Accepting the pregnancy
- Onset of fetal movements (quickening)
- Accepting the fetus as an individual
- The birth process
- Seeing the baby
- Touching the baby
- Taking care of the baby

Attachment after birth

After birth a mother initially demonstrates attachment to her baby in several ways.
- She is able to establish eye contact with the infant, who is in a state of arousal after birth.
- If she is left alone with her naked infant, she may touch each part of the body with her fingertips.
- A mother becomes overprotective of her infant in the first few days after delivery and becomes anxious about crying and minor difficulties. This anxiety may appear excessive to hospital staff and family around her.
- Babies may mimic the facial expressions of their parents, e.g. protrude their tongues.
- Breastfeeding may be used to comfort and pacify the infant.

Factors that promote attachment

- The parents together plan the pregnancy and attend antenatal educational and physiotherapy classes. The antenatal preparation of breasts and nipples will assist with subsequent breastfeeding.
- The father should support the mother during labour and witness the birth of the baby.
- Unless the baby is ill, the mother and baby should be permitted to respond to each other in their own time and manner. Unnecessary separation of infant and mother must be avoided.
- The infant should 'room in' with the mother for 24 h of the day and be taken out to the nursery at night only if the mother is ill, or if other mothers are being disturbed.
- Breastfeeding on demand, even at night, should be actively encouraged. However, if a mother fails in her attempts to breastfeed despite skilled help and advice, or does not wish to do so, she must not be made to feel inadequate or guilty. Successful bottle feeding is much better than unsuccessful breastfeeding.

Risk factors for failure to produce attachment

Mothers who plan their pregnancies have good expectations of the outcome, breastfeed their babies and rarely subsequently maltreat them. Some of the risk factors that may have an adverse effect on bonding and render the family 'at risk' for child safety concerns are listed below.

During pregnancy

- Unsupported pregnancies.
- Where the father was unfaithful or deserted the mother during pregnancy.
- Frequent pregnancies with excessive workload.
- Maternal depression during the pregnancy or a history of previous postnatal depression.
- Loss of an emotionally significant person in relation to the pregnancy, e.g. the maternal grandmother, grandfather, a loved sibling, a child of the mother or even a close friend, especially when the mother was somewhat isolated.
- Conception during a period of marital conflict.

During labour and delivery

- Being left alone and afraid in the labour ward, or when the mother perceived the staff as unconcerned.
- When the birth itself was more painful or prolonged than expected.
- When breastfeeding was thrust upon the mother by the staff.
- When the mother was unable to see the child after delivery, without explanation, or was told that the baby was damaged.
- When the mother herself was damaged as a result of the birth.
- When the father exhibited more interest in the infant than in his partner.

In the neonatal and postnatal period

- Prematurity.
- Congenital malformations.
- Critically ill infants requiring neonatal intensive care.
- Postnatal depression.
- There is a discrepancy between the idealized, perfect baby and the real baby: under these circumstances the parents require careful counselling and support.

Failure of bonding or attachment

When bonding fails there is non-acceptance or even rejection of the child. This may result in problems for both the child and the mother.

Long-term problems in the child

- **Child abuse.** Several studies have shown that preterm infants are overrepresented among abused children. Approximately 30% of physically abused children are premature, yet the overall incidence of prematurity is only 8%.
- **Non-organic failure to thrive.** Failure to thrive without organic cause is sometimes due to neglect or deprivation. Studies have revealed a fourfold increase among preterm infants and babies who require prolonged hospitalization in the newborn period.
- **Temper tantrums, infant colic, feeding problems, sleeplessness and vomiting.** Behavioural and feeding disorders are more common when an affectionate bond has not been formed.
- **Inadequate personality and poor interpersonal skills.** Infants who have been deprived of love and affection may subsequently have emotional and personality disturbances. They may become abusing or neglecting parents as adults, and so the cycle may repeat itself.

Problems in the mother

- Hesitant, clumsy handling of the baby.
- Anxiety states and depression.
- Mother states that 'the baby belongs to the hospital or nursing staff'.
- Feelings of inadequacy, disappointment, failure, deprivation and anger.
- Mother may complain that the baby does not bond with her.

Care of parents of critically ill infants

The modern intensive care nursery is a bewildering and frightening place for the parents of a recently delivered premature or sick infant. These parents often have feelings of extreme frustration, stress, guilt and helplessness and must be counselled sensitively. The total care of the high-risk neonate must include the parents. The approach to the parents is discussed in a chronological manner, from antenatal clinic through to discharge and follow-up.

Antenatal contact

Women with high-risk pregnancies or known fetal abnormality should be introduced, before delivery, to a 'baby doctor', whom they will probably meet after the baby is born. It is also helpful to the parents if they have the opportunity to visit the neonatal intensive care unit (NICU) before delivery, so that they are aware of the sights that will greet them when they first come to see their own baby. They might benefit from receiving an introductory book describing the nursery care and staff, and an introduction to a support group for parents of preterm babies or babies with a specific congenital anomaly.

Labour ward

When condition of the baby permits, the baby should be given to the mother for suckling and skin-to-skin contact for as long as possible immediately after delivery. The baby should be dried and warmed before being handled by the mother for skin-to-skin care. Even if the baby is critically ill, his/her condition should be explained and the mother should see the baby. The open visiting policy of the nursery should be explained to the parents.

Intensive care nursery

When the baby's condition is stable, the mother and father should come into the nursery to see and touch their baby. Careful explanations are given regarding abnormal signs (retractions, bruising, etc.) equipment (monitors, incubators, ventilators), and commonly performed procedures such as umbilical arterial/venous catheter, etc.).

There is every reason for the parents to be intimately involved with their critically ill infant from the outset. The premature infant has enough physiological problems already without adding attach-

ment problems to the list. The parents are informed that they may visit or ring the nursery 24 h a day, and that both parents will be kept informed of the baby's progress. Consideration should be given to providing a pamphlet explaining the intensive care nursery and encouraging the parents to become actively involved in their child's care. A digital photograph may help the mother to accept her baby for the day or two before she is able to visit the nursery.

Parents' first visit to the intensive care nursery

Parents should be greeted and welcomed to the nursery. Again, the equipment should be carefully explained. It is most important for the mother to be able to establish eye contact with her baby, and if appropriate the goggles used with phototherapy may be removed. Often the mother will have to look through the porthole to establish an *en face* position with her infant (i.e. align her head with her baby's). Some parents are very apprehensive of handling, and usually state that their baby is too fragile to touch.

The nursing staff must work through this anxiety with the parents and encourage them to touch, fondle and caress their baby. Once the parents realize that their baby can actually see them, respond to their voices and can be pacified by them, their attachment grows.

Parents' subsequent visits to the intensive care nursery

The parents should be encouraged to actively participate in their baby's care. They derive great satisfaction from holding the syringe through which milk is being fed, changing nappies and sponging the baby. Even though in an incubator, the baby can usually come out for a brief cuddle, or skin-to-skin ('kangaroo') care, provided care is taken to maintain body temperature and the patency of all attached tubes. This may even be possible when baby is receiving assisted ventilation.

Most mothers are only too happy to express their breast milk for their baby. It is remarkably well tolerated even in very preterm babies, considering the immaturity of the gastrointestinal tract at that gestational stage, and will decrease the incidence of necrotizing enterocolitis (NEC) and infection. The mother will need a great deal of empathy and support from staff members to continue breast expression for the 8–10 weeks before her infant will be able to suckle. The role of maternal milk in feeding the very low birthweight (VLBW) infant is discussed in Chapter 9. Breastfeeding (direct from the breast) should be encouraged while the mother is in hospital, so that the benefits of colostrum may be obtained.

Babies as individuals

Notes attached to the baby's bed should be encouraging to the parents, for example 'Mum is to feed me at 3 pm. I am looking forward to my first breastfeed. Love Billy'.

Parents are asked to provide the staff with the baby's name as soon as possible. The baby should be referred to by their first name, e.g. 'Billy' or 'Susie', where possible, and **never** as 'it'.

Appropriate decorations and mobiles, which may help parents adjust to a long hospital stay, can be attached to incubators. Parents are encouraged to use the pastoral care personnel of the hospital, or else to bring their own minister of religion to baptize or administer rites to the baby.

How is my baby doing?

The staff should answer this question in a realistic but optimistic way. Never should an unduly pessimistic attitude be conveyed, as this will only encourage detachment from the child. It has been shown that even if the baby dies, the parents gain from having attached to their child. Their grief is physiological and appropriate. Caution should be exercised when making predictions about outcome, and a problem-orientated approach to the baby should be avoided. It is easy for the parents to become involved with the intricacies of oxygen therapy and oxygen tension, rather than the baby as a whole.

The social worker

Social workers play an important role in the intensive care nursery. They can provide support, investigating the attitudes of parents towards the child, and at the same time may uncover social and financial problems. At times the social worker acts as the 'case manager' providing the continuum of care that can be difficult to achieve with nursing and medical rostering. Consideration should be given towards keeping a parental contact chart recording telephone enquiries, visits and the specific involvement of parents during these visits. This helps with communication, especially between nursing shifts.

Babies transferred from other hospitals

Parents of babies transferred from other hospitals into the intensive care nursery have unique problems. Prolonged parent–infant separation is common. If possible, the mother should be transferred along with the baby; but this may separate mother from her husband and other children. If the mother cannot be transferred, emailed digital photographs and daily progress reports should be provided. Whenever possible, the baby should be transferred back to the referring hospital for recovery care at earliest opportunity. Many tertiary perinatal hospitals have temporary accommodation facilities for 'out of town' families of high-risk infants.

Preparation for discharge

Early discharge for low birthweight (LBW) babies can safely be practised and may promote attachment. Babies can be discharged home even with birthweights as low as 1600 g, provided they are feeding well, the mother is handling competently, they are gaining weight steadily and there are no ongoing problems. These days, with outreach support, babies can go home while still having some tube feeds, if parents have been trained.

Caring for parents of an infant who dies

Birth and grief – a paradox

A birth is an event that is usually associated with joy and excitement. It is preceded by planning, expectations, dreams and hopes. For most people, having a baby brings with it changes in the family structure that affect each family member in a different way. The 9 months of the pregnancy are filled with adjustments in role for the mother, father and siblings, and with an awareness that a new life is growing within the mother. Grandparents and members of the extended family share in the preparations and hopes. In many families there may be ambivalent feelings perhaps because the pregnancy was unplanned or unwanted, or the siblings might be reluctant to share their parents with a new baby.

With these hopes and feelings, the news that the baby is dead comes as an unexpected catastrophe. For parents who have experienced miscarriage or a stillbirth, the fact that they have never known the baby can make their loss seem even more unreal and difficult to accept. When the baby survives for a short time, the parents have had an opportunity to experience their child as a living being.

Some of the common characteristics of normal grief are outlined in Box 27.2. The stages of grief are not necessarily in this order, and occupy a variable period of time. It has been suggested that a normal grief reaction lasts 6–9 months, although the most intensive phase lasts from 1 to 6 weeks. Grief reactions can also be delayed and often will reoccur on anniversaries.

Box 27.2 Stages of grief

- 'Shock'
- Emotional release
- Utter depression, loneliness and isolation
- Physical symptoms, e.g. choking, dyspnoea, empty feeling, weakness, fatigue, insomnia, loss of appetite
- Panic – about their own worth and the safety of other children
- Guilt
- Anger
- Inability to return to normal activities
- Overcoming grief
- Readjustment of life

Management of parents of critically ill babies

Parents of critically ill babies will all have their own special difficulties to overcome. However, guidelines which are known to decrease pathological grief and promoting normal reactions are given below

- The parents should be encouraged to visit the nursery and handle the baby.
- There should be frank discussions with the doctor regarding the chance and quality of survival of the infant.
- Where appropriate, parents of critically ill babies should be visited by the hospital priest or chaplain and asked if they would like to have their baby blessed according to their custom.
- Once death is imminent the parents are encouraged to cuddle the baby, who may die in their arms. In some instances the infant may be allowed home if suitable for palliative care. This is done in line with standard framework of clinical practice agreed locally in conjunction with national guidelines such as the one prepared by the British Association of Perinatal Medicine. Palliative care (supportive and end-of-life care) is an active and holistic approach to care throughout the infant's life, death and beyond. It embraces physical, emotional, social and spiritual elements and focuses on enhancement of quality of life.
- The parents should be permitted to express their emotions and feelings.
- If the mother is in the postnatal ward, she is offered the privacy of a single room and discharged early. Drugs to suppress lactation are sometimes appropriate.
- The staff should discuss death, autopsy and funeral arrangements with the parents at the earliest opportunity.
- A health visitor or social worker may visit the parents at their home if this is thought to be desirable.
- Preliminary autopsy results are discussed with parents as soon as they are available.
- A follow-up appointment is made 6–8 weeks after the death to discuss the autopsy findings and causes of death, and for counselling for further pregnancies.

In spite of these attempts to support the parents, the death of a newborn infant, whether sudden or expected, imposes a severe stress on the family. A longitudinal prospective study of bereaved parents has shown that parental distress, as manifested by anxiety and depression, is greatest at 6–8 weeks. Therefore, parents should be given an opportunity to re-book the appointments if that turns out to be more convenient for them.

> **CLINICAL TIP:** In the event of a baby's death, it is common courtesy to notify all medical staff who have been or are involved in the care of the baby and the family (e.g. obstetrician, visiting specialists, general practitioner, etc.).

Bereavement counsellors and perinatal loss support groups

Beneficial support, additional to that provided by doctors, nurses and social workers, can be provided by trained bereavement counsellors or by other parents who have experienced and recovered from perinatal loss, for example, in the UK the Stillbirth and Neonatal Death Support Group (SANDS). Invaluable support may also be provided by books and resource packages that help parents to understand the grieving process.

SUMMARY

All units involved with the care of sick infants should develop management strategies to promote the attachment of parents to their sick and preterm infants. A good parent–infant attachment has been shown to produce both short-term and long-term benefits in terms of physical and neurodevelopmental outcomes. Various forms of intervention are being implemented, either on individual basis such as NIDCAP and kangaroo care (see Chapter 24). As they involve a number of physiological processes, we do not know which individual item of intervention is most effective.

It should also be realized that bonding starts right at the stage of conception, runs through the entire pregnancy and extends well into the postnatal period. Therefore, the intensive care nursery should be designed to the needs of parents and babies, and staff should always encourage parental involvement in the care of their babies.

Babies who are ill or born preterm are already disadvantaged and likely to suffer more if their bonding with parents is not optimal. The compassionate care of parents who have suffered a perinatal loss involves a skilled multidisciplinary team approach.

 Now visit **www.essentialneonatalmed.com** to test yourself on this chapter.

CHAPTER 28

Ethical issues and decision-making process in the treatment of critically ill newborn infants

Key topics

Introduction

Ethics is the science of morals; the branch of philosophy concerned with human character and conduct. Ethical issues arise in the interactions of persons that involve the welfare or freedom of humans. They occur when one person or group of persons acts in ways that affect the welfare of another person or group of persons.

In the practice of medicine the best course of action is generally determined by humanist values (intrinsic value of human life). The very core of medicine is the respect for human life and the attempts to sustain and improve it. Life-sustaining treatment decisions for newborn infants are typically made in an environment of scarce resources and where the medical, ethical and personnel implications are complex and often ambiguous. Terminology such as 'sanctity of life', 'quality of life', and 'ordinary or extraordinary means' are unduly simplistic and usually unhelpful.

Essential Neonatal Medicine, Fifth Edition. Sunil Sinha, Lawrence Miall, Luke Jardine.
© 2012 John Wiley & Sons, Ltd. Published 2012 by John Wiley & Sons, Ltd.

Principles of ethical reasoning

Four major principles of ethical reasoning (described below) are particularly relevant to making decisions about newborn infants:

- beneficence
- non-malificence
- autonomy
- equity or distributive justice.

Beneficence (discontinuing futile treatment)

The traditional medical ethic is to act in ways that benefit the patient and do no harm. In many cases, however, the institution or continuation of treatment aimed at sustaining life is futile. Futile treatment is not likely to prevent death or serious compromise to the patient. There are difficulties in assessing futility, but medical determinations must be made so that treatments that offer no benefit, and only serve to prolong the dying process, should not be employed.

Non-malificence (burdensome treatment)

The primary ethical injunction for the doctor is 'first, do no harm' (*primum non nocere*). In making a decision to withhold or withdraw life-sustaining medical treatment the principle of non-malificence would require withholding treatment where it can be said that it harms the patient. This occurs when the treatment itself is an intolerable burden to the patient.

Autonomy

The patient has the legal right and ethical autonomy to refuse life-sustaining treatment and be allowed to die. The neonate has never been competent and therefore decision-making is based on the patient's 'best interests'. Generally the parents have the authority and responsibility to make decisions on behalf of their baby. The two rationales for giving the parents the responsibility are 'bearer of responsibility' and 'best advocate' grounds.

Equity or distributive justice

Doctors have an obligation to distribute benefits and burdens equally and, where differential treatment is given, to explain the reasons for this based on widely accepted criteria. This principle might mean that in some cases the patient's best interests should not or need not be the sole determining criterion.

Decision-making processes

Several approaches to decision-making process have been described.

'Wait until certainty' approach

In an aggressive treatment environment almost every infant who is thought to have any chance to survive has full treatment commenced and continued until it is clear that treatment should be withdrawn. The advantage of this approach is that it avoids the death of any infant who might have a good outcome, but at the cost of some infants for whom dying might be unnecessarily prolonged or who might survive with severe handicaps. This aggressive approach is understandable in societies where consumer rights, individualism and litigation are prevalent, such as in North American countries.

Statistical approach

This approach draws on the accumulated evidence in order to establish categories of patients for whom treatment should be withheld or withdrawn. This approach seeks to avoid 'creating' severely impaired children, even though this may be at the expense of the deaths of some infants who might have a good outcome. This approach has been widely adopted in the Netherlands and some Scandinavian countries.

Individualized approach (prognostic decision-making)

In this approach, treatment is initiated on any infant who has a chance of survival but the patient is continually assessed to determine whether this treatment is in the child's best interests. A determination to withdraw treatment is made earlier than in the 'wait until certainty' approach. For example, applying this approach to a 25 week, 750 g infant with respiratory distress syndrome (RDS) and refractory hypotension who develops a grade IV intraventricular haemorrhage (IVH) may enable the experienced physician to recommend withdrawal of treatment.

Antenatal diagnosis

A paradigm shift has occurred in the last two decades in ethical decision-making in perinatal medicine. In previous decades ethical decision-making usually occurred after the unexpected birth of an infant with a major congenital anomaly. However, most pregnant women now have biochemical and ultrasound screening (such as nuchal fold thickness) in the first trimester and almost all have ultrasound assessment at 17–19 weeks' gestation for congenital anomalies. In developed countries most major congenital anomalies are diagnosed antenatally before 20 weeks' gestation. Parents receive full multidisciplinary counselling and are supported in their decision-making process. A clinical care plan is developed and frequently a case manager supports the family.

The role of the Institutional Ethics Committee

Institutions and neonatal service providers usually have established general principles and a process for ethical decision-making. The Institutional Ethics Committee (IEC) may have a role to play in treatment decisions on 'imperilled' newborn infants. The IEC also has an important proactive role in ethical decision-making for obstetric and fetal patients but less so for commencing, continuing, withholding or withdrawing treatment in a neonate.

The roles of an IEC can be summarized as follows:
- Develop and ratify institutional guidelines.
- Act as an advisory and consultative body.
- Educate staff.
- Disseminate information.

- Absolve the attending physician from the decision-making process when necessary.
- Resolve differences of opinion.

There are no readily available algorithms that one can follow simply each time an ethical dilemma arises: rather, one must work through a complex series of moral, religious, cultural and legal issues to reach an acceptable conclusion.

Good ethics can only be exercised if the medicine practised is correct. Good ethics requires accurate medical facts; not even sound ethical reasoning will rescue a decision based on false assumptions. With the advances in medical technology has come a greater public awareness of neonatal intensive care.

Withholding and withdrawing life-sustaining treatment

Withholding life-sustaining medical treatment involves a choice to omit a form of treatment that is not considered beneficial, whereas withdrawal involves a choice to remove treatment that has not achieved its full beneficial intent.

Criteria for decision to withhold or withdraw life-sustaining medical treatment are usually based on:
- inevitability of death
- futility of treatment
- poor quality of life.

Whatever the reason, a structured decision-making process helps to ensure that appropriate views and preferences are made explicit. This includes:
- creating an optimal environment for discussion
- establishing the relevant facts
- developing consensus between parents and professionals
- exploring options and choose most appropriate action
- implementing decisions

Common neonatal ethical dilemmas

Most neonatal ethical dilemmas fall within the following four areas.

When not to resuscitate at birth

Unfortunately, junior physicians are often in the acute situation and may not have the relevant knowledge to make such a decision. Institutional guidelines are necessary to cover all situations. Mistakes can undoubtedly be made in those first few vital seconds, and if there is any doubt one must err on the conservative side of resuscitation. A decision can be reversed later on when full facts become available. Currently recommended indications for 'do not resuscitate' at birth includes only a few conditions such as:

• gestational age <24 weeks and/or birthweight <500 g
• severe central nervous system malformations
• absence of fetal/neonatal heartbeat for more than 10 min.

Infants with conditions such as suspected chromosomal anomalies (triploidy, trisomy 13 and trisomy 18), perinatal lethal renal disease and lethal skeletal disorders should probably be stabilised where possible and then fully assessed and investigated so that a rational decision can be made with all relevant information available. The approach to infants with a known major congenital anomaly is discussed below.

'How small is too small?': when not to resuscitate on gestational age or birthweight criteria

Human nature being what it is, we are straining to push back the frontiers of viability (technological imperative) to improve our statistics, and tend to accept death as failure.

Hospitals should develop guidelines based on their own survival and outcome data keeping in line with their regional and national trends. An approach could be to attempt resuscitation on all infants over 600 g and/or at least 24 weeks' gestation, and for selected infants between 500 and 600 g, depending on past obstetric history, the likelihood of infection, birth trauma and severity, initial asphyxia and parental wishes. Present indications suggest that infants less than 500 g and those less than 24 weeks' gestation have very poor outcome, even with intensive care treatment.

Saying that the neonatologist will attempt full resuscitation and subsequent intensive care for all infants of more than 24 weeks' gestation and/or birthweight greater than 600 g does not mean that the obstetrician must necessarily do everything possible for all these pregnancies, as they have two people to consider: not just the neonate but also the mother. At times there will be a dichotomy in the aggressiveness of care between obstetrician and neonatologist.

Major congenital malformations

The majority of malformations are now diagnosed antenatally, often before 20 weeks' gestation. Occasionally these may not become obvious until after birth.

Malformations can be considered under several categories.

• **Severe but not life-threatening abnormalities**. These babies should be given all appropriate medical and nursing care to promote survival and minimize later disability.
• **Potentially lethal conditions** that may be associated with severe handicap. Examples include:
   neural tube defects (myelomeningocoele, hydrocephalus, encephalocoele)
   birth asphyxia with evidence of severe hypoxic–ischaemic encephalopathy
   Parents are counselled so that they are fully aware of the clinical condition, including the sequelae and the management options available. If not diagnosed antenatally, life support measures may be instituted while the infant is fully assessed and all necessary information obtained.
• **Lethal abnormalities** (e.g. anencephaly, trisomy 13 and 18 encephalocoele). The majority of these will have been diagnosed antenatally. If the parents have decided to continue the pregnancy and the baby is born alive, he/she should receive comfort care only (warm, free from hunger and relieved of pain). No active means are taken to shorten life. At times these babies are discharged home under the parents' care sometimes in conjunction with a children's hospice. Parents and family receive ongoing counselling and support.

CLINICAL TIP: When a lethal abnormality has been diagnosed in utero and the parents have elected to continue the pregnancy, it is important that a clear birth plan is made before delivery. Things to consider include the mode of delivery (vaginal is normally recommended), resuscitation (what, if any, should be done), pain and symptom management, and discharge home. Introduction to the palliative care team before the birth may help to facilitate this.

Withdrawal of life supports

The situation regarding possible withdrawal of life supports arises in different circumstances.
• Clear-cut cases (e.g. confirmation of bilateral renal agenesis, trisomy 13 or 18, triploidy, irreversible cervical cord injury). To continue ventilation for these lethal conditions would be futile and under the circumstances would constitute 'extraordinary care'.
• Irreversible brain death following hypoxic–ischaemic injury.
• Preterm infant with progressive bronchopulmonary dysplasia, grade IV IVH with posthaemorrhagic hydrocephalus.
These cases may be clear cut when the infant can be recognized as dying despite maximal assistance, and death seems inevitable.

Selective withdrawal of neonatal intensive care

Reasons for considering re-orientation towards palliative care include:
• Prognosis extremely poor:
  short-term survival
  long-term outcome
• Therapy too burdensome.
The decision-making process involves:
  • Accurate and complete medical facts:
    subspecialist consultation
    scientific documentation
  • Consultation with hospital ethicist (if available) or independent consultant (second opinion).

• In-depth case conference: medical/moral/ethical discussion.

Parents in the decision-making process

Although parents are usually the best-qualified advocates for their infant, they should not be left to shoulder the burden entirely. Rather, a shared decision should be made.

All 'proxy decision-makers', whether they be parents, physicians or courts of law, must be fully informed and cognizant of the relevant facts. Whatever approach is adopted it is vital that the process is made transparent and that the physician communicates clearly with parents and other members of the health care team.

It is rare for there to be major disagreement between clinical staff caring for the baby and parents, provided that there are careful and repeated discussions between all parties. Tape-recording of conversations has been shown to be a useful way to give the parents time to reflect on what was said. A major dispute between clinicians and family represents a failure in communication.

However, in the unusual situation of conflict when parents prefer no active treatment, the wishes of the parents may be overridden to sustain life. The reverse situation (i.e. parents wishing the continuation of life support and medical staff wishing to withdraw) occasionally arises and must be handled compassionately.

Circumstances in which parents' wishes might be overruled, or when parents are incapable of decision-making

It is not the doctor's role to override the wishes of parents, particularly when their decision is arrived at after careful consideration and reflection. Often religious beliefs have a very strong influence on their decision and it may be helpful to engage religious advisers in the conversation if the family is happy with this.

Where major dispute arises there are three possible courses of action. The first is to ask another neonatologist from a different hospital to give an independent opinion. Discuss this with the family and ask them whether they will agree to this as a way forward. Secondly, in hospitals with clinical ethical committees, the case may be reviewed by them and advice given.

In the UK the courts become involved in the rare cases where there remains a major disagreement about the continuation of care. This usually arises when the parents feel that care should be continued and the clinical staff feel that care is not going to save the baby's life or where survival will involve significant pain or suffering. The court will make a decision on the basis of an independent assessment of the evidence.

Role of the case conference

A suggested approach to deal with issues regarding the withdrawal of life support is the case conference. This involves all relevant staff (medical, nursing, allied health, pastoral care) and parents to work through the complex series of medical, social and ethical issues.

Purpose of conference

A case conference can serve several purposes.
• Ensuring staff are comfortable with the decision.
• Enhancing communication between staff.
• Developing a future care plan:
  further information (investigation)
  time frameworks.
• Providing guidance for counselling parents.
• Mapping out a process for withdrawal of life support.
• Enabling staff to understand the decision-making process.

• Giving an opportunity for all opinions to be expressed.

Communication of withdrawal of life support

The decision to withdraw life support entails several procedures that must be followed:
• The attending physician clearly annotates the medical facts in the chart.
• At times a second neonatologist is consulted and their opinion is documented in the chart.
• Rarely the hospital ethics committee is convened if there is ethical uncertainty.
• The decision-making process is annotated in the chart.
• The decision is communicated to relevant persons, e.g. charge nurse, director of nursing, medical superintendent.
• Cases with unique aspects are documented in detail and archived by the ethics committee.

Care of parents

The care and support of the parents is a necessary part of the decision-making process and its aftermath.
• The parents, preferably together, receive progressive counselling from the neonatologist.
• Ongoing support is provided by nursing staff, social workers and pastoral care staff.
• Parents are informed of the case conference and are counselled afterwards.
• Life and death decisions are made jointly by the neonatologist and the parents – the final decision is parental.
• Offer a bereavement review meeting.

SUMMARY

Key concepts underlying ethical care in the neonatal intensive care units involve:
• respecting parental autonomy
• applying the 'best interest of the patient' philosophy
• minimizing 'harm' to the patient

• establishing sound parent–doctor (professional) relationship
• empowering and informing parents
• respecting parents' values, culture and religious beliefs
• applying a family-centred care approach.

CHAPTER 29
Practical procedures

Key topics

Introduction

Where possible a procedure should be witnessed at least twice and then performed under supervision before doing it independently. Valuable experience in most of the procedures can be gained by practicing on manikins and simulators. Neonatal Life Support and similar courses offer the opportunity to gain practical skills in life saving procedures and those working with newborns should be encouraged to participate and update their skills. One should realize that in ill infants who are not stable, some of these procedures may be potentially harmful, even when performed by experienced staff.

Essential Neonatal Medicine, Fifth Edition. Sunil Sinha, Lawrence Miall, Luke Jardine.
© 2012 John Wiley & Sons, Ltd. Published 2012 by John Wiley & Sons, Ltd.

General guidance

Ensure that all equipment is prepared and that both the operator and assistants are familiar with the procedure. Maintain adequate thermal care during the procedure, as newborn babies are prone to lose heat fast, and ensure that adequate analgesia and anaesthesia have been provided except for emergency situations. Do not persist beyond two failed attempts – seek a colleague's help or take a break and try again.

All procedures should be clearly documented in the notes and any complication arising from the procedure recorded in the critical incident report (CIR) which can be used for audit and practice development.

Adherence to strict aseptic measures is mandatory and operator should be aware of local policies regarding disposal of sharps and needles.

No procedure, unless an emergency, should be carried out without informed consent from the parents.

Mask ventilation

It is important for any nurse, midwife or doctor who is involved in the delivery or care of newborn infants to learn how to use a face mask for emergency assisted ventilation. Traditionally the most commonly used bags on labour wards and in neonatal units were self-inflating bags with pressure-relief safety valves which can be overridden when necessary. However, most units now use a T-piece system (Tom Thumb circuits, Fig. 29.1a) which seems to be more effective in tidal volume delivery, and come with facilities to set up peak pressure and positive end expiratory pressure (PEEP.)

There are several different types of face mask in different sizes to suit premature and full-term infants (Fig. 29.1b). Choose a face mask that fits snugly over the baby's mouth and nose but does not overhang the chin or cover the eyes. Round masks with a cushioned rim are preferable as it is easier to make a tight seal.

Technique

1 Place infant flat with the head in the neutral position, on a firm surface, remove any obstruction

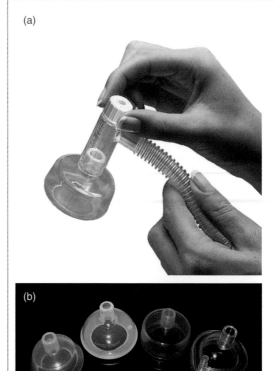

Figure 29.1 (a) T-piece (Fischer Pykell Health Care). (b) Face masks designed for use in face mask ventilation of term and preterm newborns. The masks shown are the Laerdal size 0/1, Armstrong size 1 (Large Infant), Fisher & Pakell 60 mm and Intersurgical size 1 Large Anatomical mask. (Courtesy Dr Fiona Wood.)

(e.g. meconium) with appropriate suction equipment.

2 Place face mask firmly over the nose and mouth with either an air or oxygen flow rate as advised by the manufacturer of the device (e.g. 8 L/min for Neopuff).

3 Hold face mask on firmly (but do not occlude nares) and apply jaw thrust (Fig. 29.2).

4 Inflate at a rate of about 30–40 breaths/min with a T-piece. If using a T-piece circuit with a PEEP value, ensure the PEEP valve is set to an appropriate pressure before use (PEEP 4–6 cm H_2O).

Make sure there is good chest wall movement, good air entry on auscultation of the lungs, and

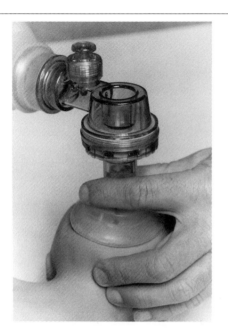

Figure 29.2 Bag-and-mask ventilation. Note fingers lifting the jaw and holding mask securely.

improvement in the infant's colour and heart rate. If chest wall movement is poor, check position of the airway and that the airway is clear. You may need to reposition. Frequently, the application of a jaw thrust or the insertion of an appropriate infant oral pharyngeal airway (Guedel) will improve air entry. Once chest wall movement has been achieved, the lowest pressure to maintain lung inflation should be used. The infant's lungs can be damaged by excessive inflation pressures. If there is no improvement in condition after effective lung inflation for 1–2 min, consider the need for intubation.

Endotracheal intubation

The ability to hand ventilate using a mask/T-piece system or bag-valve-mask is a more vital skill than intubation (Fig. 5.2 and Fig. 29.2). Endotracheal intubation is universally performed using an uncuffed tube (uniform-diameter tube). Use sizes 2.5, 3.0 and 3.5 mm for infants weighing 1.0, 2.0 and 3.0 kg, respectively. Premedication with suitable analgesia and sedation (such as short-acting

opiate), should always be used except for emergency resuscitation. Neuromuscular paralysis can sometime be used as it makes intubation quicker and easier, but if it is already known that intubation in a particular baby is likely to be difficult, one should ensure that a suitably experienced person is present.

Orotracheal intubation

1 Select tube size and insert the introducer almost to the end of the tube and bend it slightly. The introducer makes the tube more rigid but must not protrude out of the end as it can cause airway trauma. Check laryngoscope, suction apparatus, T-piece, and mask. Prepare a means to secure the endotracheal tube once it is in place. This is covered in the next section.
2 Place baby on a firm surface with head in neutral position and ventilate by mask. Give the sedation.
3 Place baby's head in 'sniffing' position by extending the neck. Ensure the face is in the midline. An assistant may press directly on the cricoid cartilage to push the glottis up into view.
4 Pass laryngoscope blade gently along right side of mouth and pull tongue and epiglottis forward by exerting traction parallel to the handle of the laryngoscope (**not** by tilting the blade upwards, and being careful not to damage the gum or palate) (Fig. 29.3).

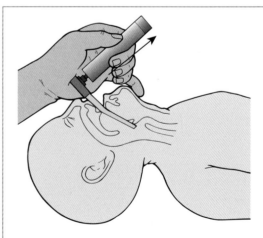

Figure 29.3 Laryngoscopy. The laryngoscope blade displaces the tongue and lifts the epiglottis anteriorly to expose the cords. (Reproduced with permission of Baillière Tindall.)

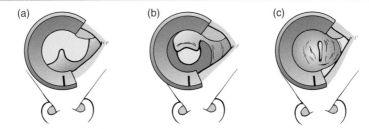

Figure 29.4 The stages of intubation. Visualization of the uvula and oropharynx (a). The epiglottis is seen with the oesophagus beyond it (b). The cords are also seen (c).

Table 29.1 Recommendations for neonatal intubation

Infant's weight (g)	Tube diameter (mm)	Distance (cm)	
		Nasal tube (anterior nares to mid-trachea)	Oral tube (lip to tip)
500–750	2.5	7.5	6.5–6.8
750–1250	2.5	8.5	6.8–7.3
1250–2000	3.0	9.5	7.3–8.0
2000–3000	3.5	10.5	8.0–9.0
3000–4000	3.5	11.0–12.0	9.0–10.0

5 Suction the airway (if required) and pull the laryngoscope blade back until the epiglottis and vocal cords come into view (Fig. 29.4).
6 Pass the endotracheal tube through the vocal cords until the black marking of the tube is below the cords (a slight 'give in' can sometimes be felt as the tube passes into the larynx, **but no force is needed for insertion**). Hold the tube firmly and remove the introducer and apply gentle inflation of the lungs. Table 29.1 gives the approximate distance for tube insertion.
7 Once inserted, tube position can be confirmed clinically by equality of breath sounds (ideally compared under the axillae), no large leak, good symmetrical excursion of chest wall and appropriate physiological response in heart rate, respiratory rate and oxygen saturation.

Disposable end-tidal CO_2 detectors are now available and should be used to confirm that the tube is in the trachea but this can give false results in infants under 1 kg and in low cardiac output states.

Nasotracheal intubation

Nasal intubation is not normally used for emergency intubation but some units prefer this for long-term intubation (and ventilation) as fixation is more stable. Therefore, this is mostly carried out as an elective procedure. The overall preparation and procedure is similar to oral intubation.
1 Select tube and check Magill's forceps. An introducer is not used. Visualize the back of the mouth with a laryngoscope.
2 A lubricated endotracheal tube is gently passed down the right nostril until it just appears behind the soft palate.
3 The tip of the endotracheal tube is picked up by the Magill's forceps and placed gently between the vocal cords. The tube is then advanced down the trachea as the operator guides it with Magill's forceps.

Fixation of the endotracheal tube

Each unit has its own methods for securing an endotracheal tube (Fig. 29.5). It is most important that the tube is fixed securely on to the face to avoid accidental extubation, and also to ensure that the

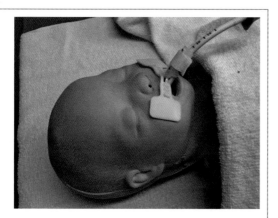

Figure 29.5 Commercial endotracheal tube fixator.

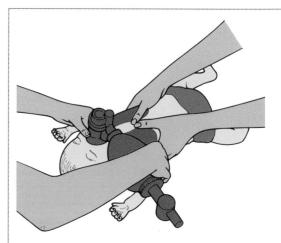

Figure 29.6 External cardiac massage over the lower third of the sternum. Simultaneous ventilation is also necessary as shown.

infant's sensitive skin is not traumatized by the procedure.

Extubation procedure

This should be a planned procedure and performed only after careful assessment of the baby's suitability for extubation. Despite this careful judgement, a baby may not tolerate extubation and require reintubation, and hence there should be a resuscitation trolley at hand. Prophylactic treatment with caffeine, and postextubation switch to nasal continuous positive airway pressure (CPAP) (especially in low birthweight babies) may aid successful extubation and reduce the need for reintubation. Individual units must develop their own protocols.

Cardiopulmonary resuscitation

Cardiopulmonary resuscitation (CPR) is necessary in cases of cardiac arrest or severe bradycardia not responding to airway opening, oxygenation and ventilation.

There are two methods for chest compressions. The most effective method is the two-handed approach but this can be difficult to do if space around the baby is limited, and vascular access is being obtained. To do this:

1 Encircle the hands around the chest, with fingertips around the back and both thumbs at mid to lower third of the sternum (Fig. 29.6).

2 Compress the chest by the thumbs about a third of the chest wall, at a ratio of three compressions to one ventilation breath.

3 Assess the effect by following the NLS guidelines.

The second method is the one-handed technique:

1 Two fingers are placed over mid to lower sternum.

2 The chest is compressed as outlined above.

Drainage of a pneumothorax

If there is a sudden deterioration in an infant with respiratory distress, whether he/she is receiving mechanical ventilation or not, a pneumothorax should be considered and the following carried out.

1 Observe chest movement and auscultate. Is air entry different between the two sides?

2 Transilluminate the chest using a cold fibreoptic light source. A pneumothorax will cause the affected hemithorax to glow. In very tiny babies the whole chest may transilluminate normally because of the thin chest wall, and this requires careful interpretation.

3 If the baby is not *in extremis*, perform an urgent chest radiograph.

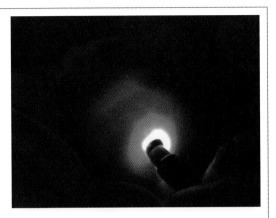

Figure 29.7 Transillumination of a large unilateral pneumothorax.

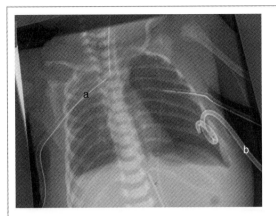

Figure 29.8 Two types of drains used for treating pneumothorax. This child required multiple drains. The top catheters (a), one on each side, are straight catheters whereas the lower one (b) is a pigtail catheter. (Courtsey Dr Shalabh Garg.)

4 If the condition is critical and a pneumothorax is strongly suspected, a therapeutic thoracocentesis is performed by placing a 19G butterfly needle into the second intercostal space in the midclavicular line. It is essential that the other end of the butterfly tube is attached to a three-way stopcock and to a 20 mL syringe. The air can then be aspirated and a clinical improvement should be noted. Alternatively, the end of the butterfly tube can be placed in an underwater container and bubbles seen as the air escapes. Remember that blindly needling the chest may itself produce a pneumothorax.

5 Once the infant's condition is stable, an intercostal catheter is inserted using aseptic precautions.

Placement of a chest drain

There are two positions for drainage insertion:
- anteriorly in the second intercostal space in the midclavicular line (Fig. 29.8a)
- laterally in the fifth or sixth intercostal space in the anterior to mid-axillary line (Fig. 29.8b).

The anterior position appears to be the most successful in draining pneumothoraces, but it is important to avoid trauma to the infant's nipples and unsightly scarring. In most units, the lateral position is the preferred position.

There are two main types of chest drain. The more common are the blunt dissection type.

However, more modern pigtail chest drains are now often used with excellent results. Both techniques are described below.

Chest drain: blunt dissection

1 The skin is cleansed with suitable skin preparations and infiltrated with local anaesthetic (1% lidocaine).

2 A deep incision is made in the site of choice (as above) on the affected side. The intercostal muscle should be breached by the scalpel blade. Blunt dissect through the muscle.

3 A size 10 Fr pleural catheter (size 12 Fr is better for larger infants) is introduced through the chest wall and pleura preferably without the trocar. The catheter is introduced in the direction of the lung apex for a distance of 3–5 cm depending on the size of the infant. For a more laterally sited catheter it is important that the catheter be angled anteriorly, as posteriorly positioned catheters are more likely to obstruct.

4 Once the tip is in the pleural cavity about 2 cm from the chest wall, it is quickly connected to an underwater seal. It is preferable to attach the tube to an underwater seal under low (5–10 cmH$_2$O) continuous suction to prevent obstruction, especially if blood is present in the chest.

5 The catheter is secured with a purse-string suture and strapped to the chest wall with a bridge of Micropore tape or plastic adhesive dressing such as Tegaderm.

A flutter valve is very useful instead of an underwater seal if the pneumothorax occurs during transportation of the infant, ensuring that it does not become wet with blood or moisture.

Chest drain: pigtail catheter

The pigtail chest drain has been used for many years in adult and paediatric practice. It is inserted using a Seldinger technique and so has the advantage that it is less traumatic and often considered easier to insert. The main disadvantage to these drains is that fluid is more likely to occlude the drain.

To insert the drain:

1 Prepare the site of drain insertion with suitable skin preparation and infiltrate the skin with 1% lidocaine for anaesthesia.

2 Insert the provided needle with a 10 mL syringe into the chosen site, aspirating as you insert. Stop inserting when air or fluid is obtained. Now disconnect the syringe but hold the needle in position carefully.

3 Pass the guide wire through the needle into the thoracic cavity. Always hold the guide wire and stop advancing when any resistance is felt.

4 While holding the guide wire, slide the needle out over the guide wire, keeping the guide wire in place.

5 Slide the dilator over the guide wire, to dilate a tract into the chest wall. You may need to make a very small incision where the guide wire is, to assist passage of the dilator into the chest. Once the dilator has created a tract, remove the dilator, keeping the guide wire *in situ*.

6 Pass the chest drain over the guide wire until all the small holes in the drain are within the thoracic cavity. Now remove the guide wire, leaving the drain in place.

7 Connect the chest drain to an underwater seal.

8 Fix the chest drain in place using Steri-strips and Tegaderm. You do not need to suture this type of drain, as it 'curls up' inside the chest like a pig's tail! The chest radiograph in Fig. 29.8 shows this.

Removal of intercostal chest drain

The chest tube is clamped when there has been no bubbling for 24 h, and it is removed after a further 12–24 h if there is no deterioration clinically or reaccumulation of the pneumothorax on chest radiograph. Take care that air is not sucked into the chest after catheter removal. The intercostal catheter is removed slowly and pressure applied to the site. The skin edges can be closed with Steri-strips and an adhesive dressing applied to the site. Purse-string sutures should not be used as they can leave unsightly scars.

Pericardial aspiration

This procedure is indicated for cardiac tamponade due to pneumopericardium or a large pericardial effusion or haemorrhage.

1 Use a 23G needle connected to a three-way stopcock and a 10 mL syringe.

2 Enter under the thorax to the left of the xiphisternum and advance upwards and to the left at 45° to vertical and 45° to the midline while applying gentle suction.

3 The pericardium is entered and air or fluid withdrawn. An echocardiogram should be performed as soon as possible after the procedure.

Umbilical vessel catheterization

Umbilical arterial catheterization

Umbilical arterial catheterization (UAC) is performed for intermittent sampling of arterial blood and continuous direct monitoring of arterial PO_2 and blood pressure especially in a baby who is receiving mechanical ventilation. The following catheter sizes are used:

- 3.5 Fr for infants weighing less than 1500 g
- 5 Fr if greater than 1500 g.

There are two common positions for placement of the tip of the umbilical artery catheter:

- **High**: in the aorta at the level of the diaphragm (T10).
- **Low**: below the level of the renal arteries (L4–L5).

There is no convincing argument in favour of high or low position but the usual practice is to aim

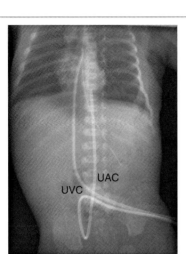

Figure 29.9 Umbilical artery catheter (high position in aorta at or above diaphragm) and umbilical vein catheter based on the infant's shoulder-to-umbilical distance. Following insertion, the UAC always dips down into the internal iliac artery before climbing up in the aorta (the catheter on the right side) as compared to UVC (umbilical venous catheter) which goes up straight into portal vein and inferior venae cava (the catheter on the left). In this case, the tip of the UAC was noted to be higher and hence pulled back. Ideal position of the UAC tip should be at the level of T8–T10. (Courtsey Dr Fiona Wood.)

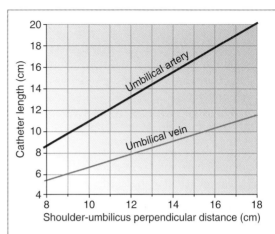

Figure 29.10 Distance in centimeters between the umblicus and the shoulder tip as a guide for the length of umblical catheter to be inserted to reach the level of the diaphragm.

for the tip of the catheter at the level of the diaphragm, or just above it.

An estimate can be made of how far to pass the catheters on the basis of the distance in centimetres between the umbilicus and the shoulder tip. The length to be inserted can then be read directly from Fig. 29.10. Alternatively the formula

$$UAC\,(cm) = (weight \times 3) + 9\;cm$$

can be used.

Technique

1 Measure the shoulder-to-umbilicus distance and estimate the distance to pass the catheter from Fig. 29.10. The calculated distance is for placement in the aorta at T10.

2 Use full surgical scrub technique with gloves, gown and mask. Cleanse cord and abdominal wall with suitable cleaning solution. Attach a three-way stopcock and a syringe of normal saline to the catheter and flush it with heparinized saline solution.

3 Apply a piece of ribbon gauze around the cord before cutting the cord with a scalpel. Pull the cord tie if bleeding occurs from the cord. Cut cord horizontally about 1 cm above the abdominal wall. Identify the three cord vessels and dilate the mouth of one of the arteries with a pair of fine iris forceps or dilator.

4 Cannulate the artery and introduce the catheter the calculated distance. Check position of catheter radiologically after the UAC is secured in place.

5 The catheter is secured *in situ* preferably by placing a zinc oxide tape across the catheter and then suturing it to umbilical stump (NLS manual).

6 The catheter is connected to a pressure transducer for blood pressure monitoring. Circulation to the lower limbs is closely observed. A heparin–saline infusion should then be started to reduce the risk of thrombosis.

7 An abdominal radiograph must be taken to confirm the correct placement and locate the catheter tip. This can only be confirmed by visualization of whole length of the catheter and confirming its anatomy (and hence the necessity to include chest and abdomen in the radiograph) (Fig. 29.10).

If the catheter is sited too low it should not be advanced as it carries the risk of introducing infection; instead, it should be withdrawn to the lower position.

Umbilical venous catheterization

Umbilical venous catheterization (UVC) is useful in any infants for a number of reasons:
- Urgent resuscitation in the labour ward.
- Central venous access for fluid administration.
- Exchange transfusion.
- Difficult venous access, e.g. hydrops fetalis.
- Central venous pressure (CVP) monitoring.
- Performance of balloon septostomy for transposition of the great arteries (TGA).
- Administration of drugs and total parenteral nutrition (TPN).

Technique

Emergency resuscitation
1 Ensure full resuscitation is taking place as per NLS guidelines.
2 Place a cord tie around the base of the cord, ready to pull tight if the cord bleeds after cutting.
3 Flush the UVC with 0.9% sodium chloride solution.
4 Cut the cord with a horizontal incision and identify the larger vessel, the umbilical vein.
5 Quickly insert the UVC into the vein in as aseptic manner as possible in the circumstances and aspirate the syringe while advancing. Fix the UVC in place with tape when blood is aspirated.
6 You can now administer emergency drugs through the UVC without radiography of the line. As this line is not inserted under aseptic conditions it needs replacing on the neonatal intensive care unit (NICU) when the baby is stable.

Elective insertion
1 Preparation as for umbilical artery.
2 Measure the shoulder–umbilical distance and calculate insertion distance using Fig. 19.10.
3 Umbilical vein must be clearly distinguished from two umbilical arteries (see Fig. 29.9). Rarely is it necessary to spend much time on dilatation,

---

Box 29.1 Complications of exchange transfusion

The possible complications can be summarized in several categories:

- **Vascular**: air/clot embolization, thrombosis.
- **Cardiac**: dysrhythmia, volume overload, arrest.
- **Electrolyte**: hyperkalaemia, hypernatraemia, hypocalcaemia, acidosis.
- **Infective**: bacteraemia, hepatitis B, cytomegalovirus (CMV).
- **Other**: hypoglycaemia, necrotizing enterocolitis (NEC).

---

but clot may need to be removed. Advance the catheter to the calculated distance.
4 Check blood aspirates before suturing purse-string as catheter can easily slip out.
5 Radiograph the line position before use.

Exchange transfusion

Exchange transfusion is practised much less frequently these days than formerly. The operator must be fully acquainted with the technique before embarking on it, as this may lead to serious complications (Box 29.1). The only real indication for exchange transfusion is unconjugated hyperbilirubinaemia; the technique has been tried in a number of other conditions but without strong scientific evidence.

The blood should be less than 48 h old, ABO compatible with mother and infant and rhesus negative. If the baby is critically ill, blood may be buffered with trishydroxyaminomethane (THAM) 3.5% to correct the pH. The volume to be exchanged is usually 180 mL/kg for a double-volume exchange.

Techniques

- **Isovolaemic.** Blood is removed from the umbilical artery and given via the umbilical vein.
- **Single catheter.** Preferably umbilical vein, but the artery may be used.
- **Peripheral vessels.** A peripheral artery catheter and venous cannula are used.

1 Donor blood is warmed via a heating coil in a water bath. Generally, 10 mL aliquots are used (i.e. remove 10 mL of infant's blood then replace). The first 10 mL aliquot is sent for serum bilirubin (SBR), haematocrit (Hct), full blood count (FBC), electrolytes, proteins, glucose-6-phosphate dehydrogenase (G6PD), liver enzymes, serology, etc.

2 The heart rate, blood pressure, temperature and respirations should be monitored continuously throughout the exchange transfusion.

3 A careful record is kept of all blood sampled and transfused.

4 At the end of the exchange transfusion, blood is sent to the laboratory for haemoglobin, total and direct bilirubin, electrolytes, calcium, sugar and blood culture.

5 Do not feed the infant for at least 2 h before and at least 4 h after exchange transfusion. Instead give maintenance IV fluids.

Dilutional exchange transfusion for polycythaemia

The indications for an isovolaemic dilutional exchange transfusion are:
• venous haematocrit Hct greater than 75% in an asymptomatic baby
• venous Hct greater than 70% in a symptomatic baby.

In this situation the technique is the same as above but exchange with 0.9% sodium chloride or 4.5% albumin with an aim of reducing haematocrit.

The exchange transfusion should be performed via a blood vessel with a good blood flow (usually an umbilical vein).

The volume to be exchanged can be calculated using the following formula:

$$\text{Volume to be exchanged} = \frac{\text{infant's Hct} - \text{desired Hct} \times \text{kg body weight} \times 90}{\text{donor Hct}}$$

Peripheral arterial catheterization

Cannulation of either the radial or the posterior tibial artery is equally effective as cannulation of the umbilical artery, but for some operators it is technically more difficult, especially in very small babies.

Technique

1 Palpate the vessel and visualize it with a fibreoptic cold transillumination light.

2 Collateral circulation must be assessed by the Allen test. The wrist is held firmly on the radial side and the blood squeezed out of the hand. If the colour returns rapidly to the hand while pressure is maintained on the radial artery, it is safe to cannulate the radial artery.

3 The wrist is cleansed with suitable cleaning solution. The transillumination light can be held under the wrist while a 24G catheter is advanced slowly in the direction of the radial artery at an angle of about 20° to the skin. Once blood is seen in the clear plastic chamber the catheter is advanced a further 0.5 mm, and then, while advancing the catheter slightly, the stylet is withdrawn. The index finger is placed over the radial artery to prevent blood loss. The technique is the same as for vascular venous cannulation.

4 The catheter is attached to an extension tubing, three-way stopcock with Luer lock adaptors, and connected to an infusion pump with heparinized saline set at 1–2 mL/h (1 U heparin per mL of solution). The catheter should be attached to a pressure transducer. The line must be clearly labelled as arterial so that under no circumstances will drugs, blood or any other solutions except normal saline be infused through this line. The catheter must be firmly strapped and taped to an armboard, which is immobilized.

Complications

One of the major complications of peripheral arterial cannulation is ischaemia of the limb, which presents as discoloration and poor perfusion – fingers and toes. This should be recognized straight away and dealt with by immediate removal of the cannula and infusion of saline or low molecular weight dextran to facilitate reperfusion.

Intermittent arterial sampling

This may be performed most safely from the radial or posterior tibial arteries, as a one-off sampling procedure where arterial blood gas assessment is required. The brachial artery should not be used because limb ischaemia may occur. Femoral artery puncture is particularly hazardous as it is done blindly and carries a risk of haemorrhage and infection. If frequent arterial gases are needed, it may be worth inserting an arterial line.

Technique

1 Palpate the vessel.
2 Prepare either a 25G needle with a clear barrel or a 25G short butterfly and attach to a millilitre syringe that has been lightly coated with heparin (1000 U/mL).
3 Cleanse skin with an alcohol/chlorhexidine swab and insert the needle at an angle of 30° to the skin surface (Fig. 29.11). The landmark at the wrist is just proximal to the proximal crease and lateral to the flexor carpi radialis tendon. Transfix the artery and then withdraw the needle slowly until blood spurts into the syringe.
4 Remove 0.3 mL of blood and then withdraw the needle. Apply pressure over the artery for at least 3–4 min.

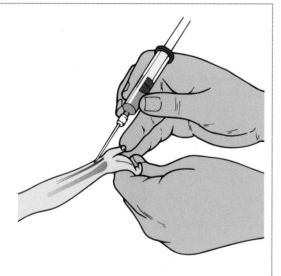

Figure 29.11 Technique for radial artery sampling. The needle transects the artery and is then withdrawn while aspirating the syringe.

Blood sampling

Venepuncture

This is a commonly performed procedure. Try to avoid using large veins that maybe needed for vascular access later. Giving oral sucrose to baby prior to the procedure reduces pain and is recommended.
1 Visualize and palpate the vessel. Apply a tourniquet (usually a tight finger grip) proximal to the vessel. Cleanse the skin with alcohol/chlorhexidine swab.
2 Use a 21 or 23G winged needle and enter the vein until blood exits the end of the needle. Blood will usually drip fully from the needle into a specimen container. Universal precautions including gloves must be used when dealing with blood sampling, and the operator should be conversant with the local procedure for dealing with any inadvertent needlestick injury.

Heel-prick capillary blood sampling

Most laboratory tests can be carried out readily on small quantities of blood. In newborn infants capillary blood obtained from a heel-prick is usually the method of choice. Up to 1 mL of blood can be sampled by this method. It is often used to obtain capillary blood gas samples. Remember analgesia – prior administration of oral sucrose to the baby alleviates pain.
1 Wash hands carefully and put on gloves and clean the heel with a 70% alcohol Mediswab.
2 Hold the leg around the ankle with thumb and fingers (do not hold the leg around the calf or shin as this may cause extensive bruising) (Fig. 29.12).
3 Prick the heel with a disposable lancet or Autolet, on the most medial or lateral portion of the plantar surface (see shaded areas on Fig. 29.13). Heel punctures should be performed on the plantar surface of the heel, but beyond the lines defined by the lateral and medial limits of the calcaneus (Fig. 29.13). The heel-prick should not be deeper than 2 mm, and should not be on the posterior curvature of the heel, nor at previous sites that may be infected.).
4 Collect the blood into a capillary tube held horizontally or catch drops in blood bottles.

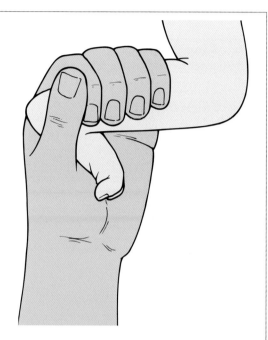

Figure 29.12 Method for holding the heel for blood sampling.

It may be necessary to squeeze the foot beforehand to get a good flow of blood. Warming the foot using a warm wrap may improve the blood supply.

Insertion of a percutaneous long line

This is a useful technique which provides long-lasting central venous access.

A peripherally inserted central line (PICC) pack is used which contains the insertion needle (splits for easy removal), the PICC line and all the other equipment needed for insertion (see Fig. 29.14).

This procedure must be carried out using strict aseptic precautions and the operator should be fully masked and gowned. The veins in the antecubital fossa, long saphenous or superficial temporal veins are the most suitable for cannulation.

1 The area is exposed and thoroughly cleansed with alcohol/chlorhexidine. Before inserting the butterfly, the length of silastic tubing necessary to place the tip in the right atrium is estimated. Pre-flush the longline with saline.

2 The butterfly is inserted into the vein as for venepuncture. When blood is seen to drip out of the needle, the silastic catheter is threaded through the inside of the 19G butterfly until the correct length is reached. The insertion butterfly is then split and removed from the catheter, being careful to not pull out the long line.

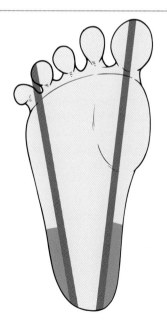

Figure 29.13 Preferred areas of the foot suitable for heel-prick in very small babies.

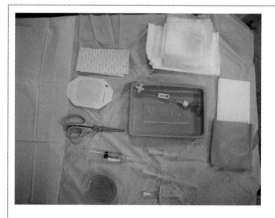

Figure 29.14 Equipment required for insertion of percutaneous intravenous central catheter (PICC). (Courtsey Dr Shalabh Garg.)

3 The whole line should then be gently flushed with heparinized saline.

4 Secure the line firmly with sterile adhesive strips, and cover with a sterile transparent dressing (e.g. OpSite).

5 Before commencing the infusion the position of the catheter tip should be checked to ensure it is in a central vein, by radiography. If the tip is in too far it may be pulled back to a more suitable position. The tip of the line must not lie within the heart as there is a risk of pericardial tamponade.

Complications of long line

The following observations, indicative of possible complications, should be made following insertion of a long line:
- site – blood loss/leakage
- infection
- thrombosis
- reduced perfusion of limbs.

Extravasation injury

Subcutaneous extravasation of fluids and drugs is a common complication in neonatal intensive care units. Minor extravasations do not cause any problem but if the volume of the leaked fluid is large or the fluid is irritant or hypertonic, such as calcium injection or TPN, this can cause significant problems including skin blistering, ischaemia and tissue necrosis. Although not completely unavoidable, the incidence of this complication can be greatly reduced by improved vigilance.

Where significant extravasation has occurred, certain measures should be used to minimize the pain and extent of the damage. One way to reduce further damage is to dilute the effect of irritation caused by the infusate by injecting hyaluronidase into the subcutaneous tissue under the area of damaged skin either by injecting through the cannula itself (if still *in situ*) or, better still, by making 3–4 small openings in the skin overlying the damaged tissue with either a fine scalpel or wide bore needle, and irrigating the tissue through these openings in turn with 20–100 mL of 0.9% normal saline. The saline should run out of these openings like a fountain. The remaining fluid can be mas-

saged out of the openings by gentle manipulation. The damaged skin is then kept reasonably moist with dressings such as paraffin gauze. Document the lesion before and after flushing using photographs, and refer early to plastic surgery if there is extensive tissue damage.

Collection of cerebrospinal fluid

The indications for lumbar puncture (LP) may be diagnostic (e.g. suspected meningitis, metabolic screen, differentiating between communicating and non-communicating hydrocephalus) or therapeutic (progressive ventricular dilatation).

Lumbar puncture

1 A full surgical aseptic technique is necessary with gloves, gown and mask.

2 An experienced nurse needs to hold the baby in the left lateral position with the head, hips and knees well flexed. The back needs to be completely parallel to the edge of the table. Make sure the airway is not obstructed.

3 The skin is cleansed with a suitable cleaning agent. Generally a 22G LP needle with stylet is used.

4 Use lumbar spaces L3–L4 or L4–L5. Use topical anaesthetic (EMLA cream) over the area for 30 min. The lumbar puncture needle is then inserted and directed towards the umbilicus. Once the subarachnoid space is penetrated, the stylet is removed and cerebrospinal fluid (CSF) is allowed to drip into each of three bottles. Sometimes the needle needs to be gently rotated to check for CSF flow. It is easy to push the needle too far into the anterior vertebral venous plexus.

5 Measurement of lumbar CSF pressure may be necessary in infants with poshaemorrhagic ventricular dilatation (see Chapter 22). This can be done by attaching a Luer locking pressure transducer directly to the hub of the needle or by using a manometer tube. Pressure measurements are only valid if the infant is breathing quietly and not crying. The head and trunk must be flat and in the same plane, and the infant not too tightly curled up.

6 CSF should always be sent for cell count, Gram stain and culture and glucose and protein

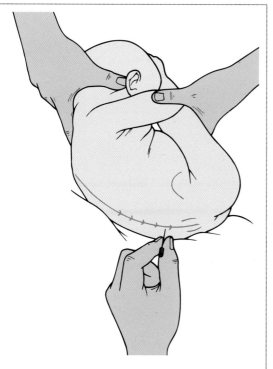

Figure 29.15 Showing position of infant during lumber puncture while taking care to avoid excessive bending.

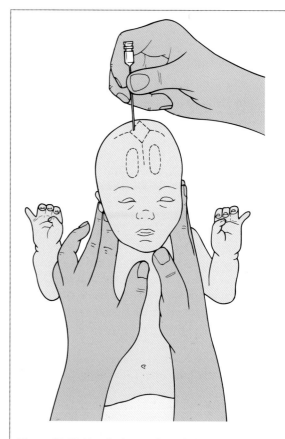

Figure 29.16 Ventricular tap through the anterior fontanelle using a styletted needle.

estimations. Other tests may include viral polymerase chain reaction (PCR) studies, syphilis serology or metabolic studies (lactate, glycine).

Ventricular tap

Rarely, a ventricular tap will be needed to diagnose ventriculitis, and decompress posthaemorrhagic hydrocephalus pending a VP shunt, or to instil antibiotics. Generally, the procedure will be performed by a neurosurgeon or other experienced staff.

1 The baby is placed in a supine position with the nose upwards and the neck and face parallel to the mattress (Fig. 29.15).
2 A full aseptic technique should be used. A long 20G or 22G LP needle with stylet is gently inserted at the lateral angle of the anterior fontanelle and angled towards the medial canthus of the eye on the same side (Fig. 29.16).

3 Once the skin and dura have been pierced, the stylet may be removed and the needle gently advanced until CSF wells up from the needle.
4 CSF from the ventricles should be collected by allowing it to drip into sterile bottles. Never aspirate.

Collection of urine

This may be performed by a 'clean-catch' bag method, suprapubic aspiration or urethral catheter. Suprapubic puncture is best done once the presence of a full bladder has been confirmed with ultrasound. It is a relatively painful procedure and ideally should be discouraged. The most reliable way to get an uncontaminated sample of urine is through ure-thral catheterization.

Bag collection

A clean-catch bag sample of urine may provide useful information. However, an inexpertly collected sample provides confusing or misleading information.

1 Cleanse a wide area of the perineum and penis with sterile saline-soaked swabs using a no-touch technique. In females the vulva will need to be separated, but in males the foreskin must not be retracted although it needs to be cleaned.

2 Wait for the perineum to dry before attaching a sterile urine-collecting bag.

3 Inspect the bag periodically, and as soon as the baby has voided remove the bag and immediately pour the urine into a universal sterile container.

4 Send the sample to the laboratory immediately. If there is any delay in transporting the sample, refrigerate it.

5 If no urine has been obtained after 1 h, the skin should be cleansed again and a fresh collecting bag applied.

A suitable alternative to bag collection in babies and small children is to put a pad inside the nappy and when it is wet, to suck out the urine using a small syringe. This is considered to be as sterile as a bag sample, and widely practised in many centres.

Suprapubic aspiration

The indications for this procedure are an inconclusive culture from a bag specimen, or the presence of vulvovaginitis or balanitis when urinary tract infection is suspected.

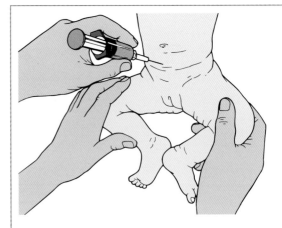

Figure 29.17 Suprapubic aspiration of urine from the bladder. The needle should be aimed slightly superiorly in the midline and 0.5 cm above the pubis.

1 The bladder must be full before commencing the procedure (confirm with ultrasound if possible).

2 A wide area of skin over the lower abdomen is prepared with povidone-iodine solution and alcohol.

3 A 21G needle attached to a 10 mL syringe is used to puncture the skin 1 cm above the pubic symphysis in the midline.

4 The needle is advanced into the bladder, angled slightly upwards to the perpendicular. As the needle is slowly advanced gentle suction is applied. The needle usually only needs to be advanced 1.5–2.0 cm below the skin surface (Fig. 29.17). Ultrasound guidance can be used for insertion of the needle

5 The urine can then be sent to the laboratory.

 Now visit **www.essentialneonatalmed.com** to test yourself on this chapter.

Index

Note: Page numbers in *italics* refer to figures, those in **bold** refer to tables.
